IN VIVO IMMUNOLOGY

Regulatory Processes during Lymphopoiesis and
Immunopoiesis

ADVANCES IN EXPERIMENTAL MEDICINE AND BIOLOGY

Recent Volumes in this Series

A Continuation Order Plan is available for this series. A continuation order will bring delivery of each new volume immediately upon publication. Volumes are billed only upon actual shipment. For further information please contact the publisher.

IN VIVO IMMUNOLOGY

Regulatory Processes during Lymphopoiesis and Immunopoiesis

Edited by

E. Heinen
M. P. Defresne
J. Boniver

and

V. Geenen

University of Liège
Liège, Belgium

PLENUM PRESS • NEW YORK AND LONDON

Library of Congress Cataloging-in-Publication Data

In vivo immunology : regulatory processes during lymphopoiesis and
  immunopoiesis / edited by E. Heinen ... [et al.].
       p.   cm. -- (Advances in experimental medicine and biology ; v.
  355)
     "Proceedings of the 11th International Conference on Lymphoid
  Tissues and Germinal Centers, held July 4-8, 1993,in Liège,
  Belgium"--T.p. verso.
    Includes bibliographical references and index.
    ISBN 0-306-44726-6
    1. Cellular immunity--Congresses. 2. Immune response--Regulation-
  -Congresses.   I. Heinen, E. (Ernst) II. International Conference
  on Lymphatic Tissues and Germinal Centers in Immune Reactions (11th
  : 1993 : Liège, Belgium) III. Series.
    [DNLM: 1. Lymphoid Tissue--immunology--congresses. 2. Immunity,
  Cellular--immunology--congresses.   W1 AD559 v. 355 1994]
  QR185.5.I5   1994
  616.4'1--dc20
  DNLM/DLC
  for Library of Congress   94-37496
                                                               CIP

Proceedings of the 11th International Conference on Lymphoid Tissues and Germinal Centers,
held July 4–8, 1993, in Liège, Belgium

ISBN 0-306-44726-6

©1994 Plenum Press, New York
A Division of Plenum Publishing Corporation
233 Spring Street, New York, N.Y. 10013

Printed in the United States of America

PREFACE

The 11th International Conference on Lymphoid Tissues and Immune Reactions was held in Spa-Liège (Belgium), from 4 to 8 July 1993. The regular devotees refer to these conferences as the "Germinal Centre Conferences or GCC". In the 1960s, the germinal centres were the subject of such considerable study and speculation that a group of dynamic people decided to devote an international conference centered on that topic. This led to the first GCC organized in Bern in 1966.

Following the success of this initial meeting, further sessions have been organized at regular intervals and, over the years, the scope of the GCC has been broadened. Nowadays, the GCC conferences are dedicated to *in vivo* immunology and deal mainly with cellular, functional and molecular aspects of the lymphoid system. The credo of these conferences is *"in vivo veritas,"* implying that the sole investigation of components (like molecules or cell populations) only gives a partial truth. Ultimately, the components have to be explored in their global context in order to see how they interact with other parts and how they are integrated as a whole to ensure the homeostasis of the immune system. In 1966, the GCC lasted 3 days and included 57 contributions "which were discussed at length." The present conference lasted 4 days and accommodated 2 honorary lectures, 80 free papers and 209 poster presentations. Out of those presentations, a selection was performed by the Chairpersons to compose the present volume.

At this meeting, the organizers restricted topics to those related to the structure and the function of the immune system. Positive and negative selection was considered either at the level of T or B cells, but in close relationship with their tissular environments. New data and hypotheses related to non-lymphoid effector and regulatory cells, to the cell traffic, and to the emerging field of neuroendocrine-immune interactions were presented and discussed during separate sessions. Pathologic aspects of the immune defences such as in AIDS and in lymphoproliferative diseases received thoughtful attention. The germinal centres and the MALT were two topics which attracted high interest, numerous presentations, and lively discussions.

Thus, the present conference covered the lympho- and immunopoiesis of B and T cells, the interactions of lymphoid populations with accessory cells, and some dysregulatory aspects of the immune system. It was a convincing manifestation that cellular and tissular approaches of immunology fruitfully interact with molecular immunology. The Germinal Centre Conferences continue to provide a unique forum for progress in all those fields.

The success of this meeting resulted from the joint efforts of many people, notably Paul Nieuwenhuis, as well as the scientific and technical staffs of the laboratories of Pathology, Neuroendocrine-Immunology, and Human Histology of the University of Liège. Maddalena Basiglini and Monique Leroi-Niesten deserve a very special mention for all of the work they have accomplished in the Secretariat of the local Committee.

The Organizing Committee of the 11th International Conference on Lymphoid Tissues and Germinal Centres in Immune Reactions wishes to sincerely acknowledge the generous support from the Mayor and the City of Spa, the National Fund of Scientific Research of Belgium, the French Community of Belgium, and the University of Liège.

Ernst Heinen
Marie-Paule Defresne
Vincent Geenen
Jacques Boniver

CONTENTS

POSITIVE AND NEGATIVE SELECTION

NONLYMPHOID EFFECTOR AND REGULATORY CELLS

CELL TRAFFIC

AIDS AND LYMPHOPROLIFERATIVE DISEASES

GERMINAL CENTRES

B CELL DIFFERENTIATION AND MUCOSAL IMMUNITY

POSITIVE AND NEGATIVE SELECTION

ANALYSIS BY IN SITU HYBRIDIZATION OF CYTOKINE mRNAS EXPRESSION IN THYMIC NURSE CELLS

Johanne Deman, Chantal Humblet, Marie Thérèse Martin, Jacques Boniver and Marie Paule Defresne

Laboratory of Pathological Anatomy
CHU-B35 University of Liège
B4000 Liège Belgium

INTRODUCTION

Several observations showed that thymocytes and thymic epithelial cell lines can produce cytokines (Ceredig et al., 1986; Denning et al., 1988; Eshel et al., 1990; Ransom et al., 1987; Van der Pouw Kraan et al. 1992) and respond to their actions (Defresne et al., 1990; Everson et al., 1990; Hodgkin et al., 1990; Palacios et al., 1987; Plum et al., 1990; Ranges et al., 1988; Suda et al., 1990 a,b; Takashi et al., 1991; Watson et al., 1989). However, most of these data were obtained in vitro, often after stimulation with non physiological agents such as PMA or calcium ionophores. The first demonstration of the presence of cytokines in the thymus in situ was the detection of IL-2 and IL-4 transcripts in suspensions of non stimulated thymocytes isolated from foetuses of CBA mice (Carding et al., 1989). Later on, we demonstrated on frozen sections that mRNAs for IL-1, IL-2, IL-4, IL-6, TNFα and γIFN were present in the thymus during ontogeny following a chronological sequence (Deman. et al., 1992, 1993).

This presence of cytokine mRNAs under physiological conditions support the hypothesis that cytokines really play a role in T cell differentiation. To understand this role,

In Vivo Immunology, Edited by E. Heinen *et al.*
Plenum Press, New York, 1994

it seems necessary to characterize cytokine producing cells and to know whether stromal cells participate to this production. In a first step, we have looked for the presence of cytokine transcripts in TNC: to this purpose we used RNA-RNA in situ hybridization on thymic nurse cells frozen sections.

MATERIALS AND METHODS

Mice

C57BL/Ka mice originating from Stanford University were raised in our animal colony.

Isolation of thymic nurse cells

Thymic nurse cells (TNC) are obtained after enzymatic dissociation of pooled adult thymuses and repeated sedimentations at 1g. After centrifugation, the pellet of TNC was frozen in liquid nitrogen.

Preparation of probes

All the probes used for this study are listed in table 1.

Table 1. Description and origin of probes (*AS: antisense probe; S: sense probe).

Probes	Plasmids	Restriction enzymes	(pb)	References	Origin
IL-1 AS* IL-1 S	PGem4zf(-)	SalI EcoRI	652	Gray et al, 1986	Dr.E.Hooghe-VUB
IL-2 AS IL-2 S	PGem4zf(-)	BamHI ScaI	331	Yokota et al, 1985	Dr.T.Astier-Gin-INSERM-Bordeaux
IL-4 AS IL-4 S	PGem4zf(-)	EcoRI SalI	725	Noma et al, 1986	Dr.T.Astier-Gin-INSERM-Bordeaux
IL-6 AS IL-6 S	PGem4zf(-)	BamHI NarI	1089	Simpson et al, 1988	Dr.E.Hooghe-VUB
γIFN AS γIFN S	PGem4zf(-)	BamHI HindIII	311	Gray et al, 1983	Prof.W.Fiers-Gent
TNFαAS TNFαS	PGem4zf(-)	HindIII BamHI	1644	Fransen et al, 1985	Prof.W.Fiers-Gent

These DNA probes were transferred by cloning into p-GEM. After linearization of the plasmid, RNA can be selectively transcribed from either strand of the cloned DNA using either SP6 or T7 RNA polymerase in order to obtain sense and antisense probe which were labelled with ^{35}S UTP and CTP according to the supplier's recommendations (Boehringer Mannheim, Mannheim, FRG). The specific activity was approximately 1×10^8cpm/mg.

In Situ Hybridization

Cryosections of TNC pellets placed on glass slides coated with 0,1mg/ml of poly-L-lysine were fixed in paraformaldehyde (4% in PBS, containing 20mM vanadyl ribonucleosides complexes (VRC) and 5mM MgCl2) during 15 min. at room T°. After permeabilization with 0,25% Triton X-100 in PBS, 20mM VRC, 5mM MgCl2 during 10 min. at room T° and dehydratation, slides were incubated overnight at 50°C with 50ml of probe mixture prepared as follows: 50ml of 50% formamide, NaCl (0,6M), TrisHCl (10mM), EDTA (1mM), 1% SDS, DDT (10mM), yeast t-RNA (0,25mg/ml), 1X Denhardt's (50X Denhardt's = 1% Ficoll, 1% polyvinylpyrrolidine, 1% BSA), 10% PEG-6000 (Polyethylene glycol-6000) and 1 ml of ^{35}S labeled probe (150.000 cpm/ml).

Controls were slides pretreated with RNAse or treated with the sense probe.

Slides were washed in several solutions: 2X5 min in PBS + 5mM MgCl2; 30 min in 0,5M NaCl, 10mM Tris HCl containing 20mg/ml of RNAse, 37°C; 30 min in 0,5M NaCl, 10mM Tris HCl; 30 min in 50% formamide/2XSSC (1XSSC = 0,3M NaCl/0,03M sodium citrate), 50°C and 30 min in 50% formamide/1XSSC, 0,05% Triton X, 37°C. Dehydratation in 30%, 50%, and 70% ethanol in 300mM ammonium acetate was realized and the slides were finally autoradiographed. We considered as positive cells (cells expressing mRNAs) those cells that had >8 grains per cell.

RESULTS

Presence of cytokine mRNAs in thymic nurse cells (TNC)

The presence of cytokine transcripts in TNC was analysed on cryosections of TNC pellets.

It appears that TNC are never labeled by IL-4 and γIFN probes whereas they possess mRNAs for IL-1, IL-2, IL-6 and TNFα (table 2). The labeling is generally localized on epithelial cells in the case of IL-1, IL-6 and TNFα, whereas mRNAs for IL-2 are exclusively present within engulfed thymocytes.

Table 2. Cytokine transcripts in TNC.

PROBES	PRESENCE OF CYTOKINE TRANSCRIPTS IN THYMIC NURSE CELLS (TNC)	CELL TYPE LABELLED
IL-1	+	epithelial cells
IL-2	+	thymocytes
IL-4	-	-
IL-6	+	epithelial cells
γ-IFN	-	-
TNF-α	+	epithelial cells

DISCUSSION

We previously showed on fetal thymic frozen sections that, under physiological conditions, thymic cells produced cytokine transcripts and that this production varied according to developmental stages (Deman et al., 1992,1993). From our results and those of others (Carding et al., 1989; Dallman et al., 1991; Moore et al., 1993), it was suggested that there exists a dynamic interplay of cytokines that control the T cell differentiation.

To understand their role, it seems necessary to identify the nature of producing cells, and particularly to define whether stromal cells participate to this production. We have chosen to undertake this study with TNC given the important role of these complexes in T-cell differentiation (De Waal Malefijt et al., 1986; Kyewski, 1986; Shortman and Vremec, 1991; Wick and Oberhuber, 1986). Our results show that epithelial TNC possess IL-1, IL-6 and TNFα mRNAs whereas the engulfed thymocytes are able to produce IL-2 transcripts.

The production of IL-1 and IL-6 by thymic epithelial cell lines was previously demonstrated (Denning et al., 1988; Eshel et al., 1990), as well as the presence of IL-1 within thymic epithelial cells in situ (Robert et al., 1991). However, to our knowledge, this work is the first demonstration of the presence of TNFα mRNAs within thymic epithelial cells.

In vitro, TNC lymphocytes produce IL-2 in response to an allostimulus (Vakharia, 1983) and it was demonstrated that they contain precursors of helper-lineage (Andrews et al., 1985) : it is thus not surprising to observe the presence of IL-2 transcripts within this lymphocyte population.

What could be the role of these cytokines within these lymphoepithelial complexes ?

-some of them such as IL-1, IL-6 or TNFα have been shown in vitro to support the proliferation of immature thymocytes (Everson et al., 1990; Hodgkin et al., 1990; Suda et al., 1990 a, b), most often in the presence of a co-stimulus such as mitogen or phorbol esters.

-they also can be implicated in thymocyte maturation: for example, IL-1 induces the maturation of progenitor thymocytes (Takashi et al., 1991)

-it had also been shown that TNFα can modulate the interactions between epithelial cells and immature thymocytes within TNC (Defresne et al., 1990)

-and finally, it can be suggested that they play a role in repertoire selection: IL-1 and IL-2 can inhibit anti-CD3 induced apoptosis in vitro (Mac Conckey et al., 1990; Nieto et al., 1990) whereas TNFα can induce thymocytes apoptosis (Deman et al, in preparation).

Cytokines are therefore likely to play a crucial role within TNC: it will be of considerable importance to analyse the signals inducing their secretion by the epithelial TNC as well as to identify the cells bearing lymphokine receptors to understand their network of interactions within TNC.

We also intend to continue these studies by the identification of cytokines produced by macrophages and interdigitating cell forming T-rosettes.

REFERENCES

Andrews, P., Boyd, R.L., Shortman, K., 1985, The limited immunocompetence of thymocytes within murine thymic nurse cells, Eur.J.Immunol. 15:1043.

Carding, S.R., Jenkinson, E.J., Kingston, R., Hayday, A.C., Bottomly, K., Owen, J.J.T., 1989, Developmental control of lymphokine gene expression in fetal thymocytes during T-cell ontogeny, Proc.Natl.Acad.Sci.USA. 86:3342.

Ceredig, R., 1986, Proliferation in vitro and interleukine production by 14-day fetal and adult CD8$^-$CD4$^-$ thymocytes, J.Immunol. 137:2260.

Dallman, M.J., Montgomery, R.A., Larsen, C.P., Wanders, A., Xells, A.F., 1991, Cytokine gene expression : analysis using northern blotting, polymerase chain reaction and in situ hybridization, Immunological Reviews. 119:164.

Defresne, M.P., Humblet, C., Rongy, A.M., Greimers, R., Boniver, J., 1990, Effect of γIFN and TNFα on lymphoepithelial interactions within thymic nurse cells, Eur.J.Immunol. 20:429.

Deman, J., Delvenne, P., Martin, M.T., Boniver, J., Defresne, M.P., 1992, Analysis by in situ hybrization of cells expressing mRNA for TNFα in the developing thymus of mice, Dev. Immunol. 2:103.

Deman, J.,Humblet,C., Martin, M.T., Boniver, J., Defresne, M.P., 1993, Analysis by in situ hybrization of cells expressing cytokine mRNAs in the murine developing thymus, Int. Immunol. submitted

Denning, S.M., Kurtzberg J., Le P.T., Tuck D.T., Singer K.H., Haynes B.F., 1988, Human thymic epithelial cells directly induce activation of autologous immature thymocytes, Proc. Natl. Acad. Sci. U.S.A. 85: 3125.

De Waal Malefijt, R., Leene, W, Roholl, P.J.M., Wormmeester, J., Hoeben, K.A., 1986, T cell differentiation within thymic nurse cells, Lab. Invest. 55:25.

Eshel, I., Savion N., Shoham J., 1990, Analysis of thymic stromal cell subpopulations grown in vitro on extracellular matrix in defined medium. II. Cytokine activities in murine thymic epithelial and mesenchymal cell culture supernatants, J. Immunol. 144: 1563.

Everson, P., Eldridge, H., Koopman, J., 1990, Synergism of Interleukin-7 with the thymocyte growth factors IL-2, IL-6 and TNFα in the induction of thymocyte proliferation, Cel. Immunol.. 127:470.

Fransen, L., Muller, R., Marmenout, A., Tavernier, J., Van der Heyden, J., Kawaschima, E., Chollet, A., Tizard,R., Van Heuverswyn, H., Van Vliet, A., Ruysschaert, M.R., Fiers, W., 1985, Molecular cloning of mouse tumour necrosis factor cDNA and its eukayotic expression, Nucleic.Acids.Res. 13:4417.

Gray, P.W., Goeddel, D.V., 1983, Cloning and expression of murine immune interferon cDNA, Proc.Natl.Acad.Sci.U.S.A. 80:5842.

Gray, P.W., Glaister, D., Chen, E., Goeddel, D.V., Pennice, D., 1986, Two interleukin 1 genes in the mouse: cloning and expression of the cDNA for murine Interleukin 1β, J. Immunol.. 137:3644.

Hodgkin, P.D., Cupp, J., Zlotnik, A., Howard,M., 1990, IL-2, IL-6 and IFNγ have distinct effects on the IL-4 plus PMA-induced proliferation of thymocyte subpopulations, Cell. Immunol. 126:57.

Kyewski, B.A., 1986, Thymic nurse cells: possible sites of T-cell selection, Immunol. Today. 7:374.

Mac.Conkey, D.J., Hartzell, P., Chow, S.C., Orrenius, S., Jondal, M., 1990, IL-1 inhibits T cell receptor-mediated apoptosis in immature thymocytes, J..Biol..Chemistry. 265:3009.

Moore N.C., Anderson G., Smith C.A., Owen J.J.T., Jenkinson E.J., 1993, Analysis of cytokine gene expression in subpopulations of freshly isolated thymocytes and thymic stromal cells using semiquantitative polymerase chain reaction, Eur. J. Immunol. 23: 922.

Nieto, M.A., Gonzalez, A., Lopez-Rivas, A., Diaz-Espada, F., Gambon, F., 1990, IL-2 protects against anti-CD3-induced cell death in human medullary thymocytes, J..Immunol. 145:1364.

Noma, Y., Sideras, P., Naito, T., Bergstedt-Lindquist, S., Azuma, C., Severinson, E., Tanabe, T., Kinashi, T., Matsuda, F., Yaoita, Y., Honjo, T., 1986, Cloning of a cDNA encoding the murine IgG1 induction factor by a novel strategy using SP6 promoter, Nature. 319:640.

Palacios, R., Sideras, P., Von Boehmer, H., 1987, Recombinant IL-4/BSF-1 promotes growth and differentiation of intrathymic T cell precursors from fetal mice in vitro, Embo.J..6:91.

Plum, J., De Smedt, M., Leclercq, G., Tison.B, 1990, Inhibitory effect of murine recombinant IL-4 on thymocyte development in fetal thymus organ cultures, J. Immunol. 145:1066.

Ranges, G.E., Zlotnik, A., Espevik, T., Dinarello, C.A., Cerami, A., Pallodino, M.A., 1988, Tumor Necrosis Factor-α /cachectin is a growth factor for thymocytes, J..Exp. Med. 167:1472.

Ransom, J., Fisher, M., Mosmann, T., Yokota, T., Deluca, D., Schumacher, J., Zlotnik, A., 1987, Interferon-γ is produced by activated immature mouse thymocytes and nhibits the IL-4-induced proliferation of immature thymocytes, J.Immunol. 139:4102.

Robert, F., Geenen, V., Schoenen, J., Burgeon, E., De Groote, D., Defresne, M.P., Legros, J.J., Franchimont, P., 1991, Colocalization of immunoreactive oxytocin, vasopressin and interleukin-1 in human thymic epithelial neuroendocrine cells, Brain.Behav.Immunol. 5:102.

Shortman, K., Vremec,D., 1991, Different subpopulations of developing thymocytes are associated with adherent (macrophage) or nonadherent (dendritic) thymic rosettes, Dev..Immunol. 1:225.

Simpson, R.J., Moritz, R.L., Van Roost, Van Snick, J., 1988, Characterization of a recombinant murine Interleukin-6: assigment of disulfide bonds, Biochem.Biophys. Res.Commun. 157:364.

Suda, T., Murray, R., Fisher, M., Yokota, T , Zlotnik, A., 1990a, TNF$_\alpha$ and P40 induce day 15 murine fetal thymocyte proliferation in combination with IL-2, J. Immunol. 144:1783.

Suda, T., Murray, R., Guidos, C., Zlotnik, A., 1990b, Growth-promoting activity of IL-1α, IL-6 and TNFα in combination with IL-2, IL-4 or IL-7 on murine thymocytes, J. Immunol. 144:3039.

Takashi, T., Gause, W.C., Wilkinson, M., Mac Leod, C., Steinberg, A.D., 1991, IL-1 induced maturation of progenitor thymocytes, Eur. J. Immunol. 21:1385.

Vakharia D.D., 1983, Demonstration of keratin filaments in thymic nurse cells (TNC) and alloreactivity of TNC-T cell population, Thymus 5: 43.

Van der Pouw-Kraan, T., Van Kooten, C., Rensink, I., Aarden, L., 1992, IL-4 production by human T cells: differential regulation of IL-4 vs. IL-2 production, Eur..J. Immunol. 22:1237.

Watson, J.D., Morrissey, P.J., Namen, A.E., Conlon, P.J., Widmer, M.B., 1989, Effect of IL-7 on the growth of fetal thymocytes in culture, J. Immunol.143:1215.

Wick, G., Oberhuber, G., 1986, Thymic nurse cells: a school for alloreactive and autoreactive cortical thymocytes?, Eur.J.Immunol. 16:855.

Yokota, T., Arai, N., Lee, F., Rennick, D., Mosmann, T., Arai, K.I., 1985, Use of a cDNA expression vector for isolation of mouse interleukin 2 cDNA clones: expression of a T-cell growth-factor activity after transfection of monkey cells, Proc.Natl.Acad.Sci. USA 82:68.

GENETIC EXPRESSION OF THE C-CBL PROTO-ONCOGENE IN HUMAN THYMOCYTES

Sabine Thaon[2], Jean-François Quaranta[2], and Daniel Régnier[1,2]*

[1]Laboratoire de Physiol. Animale, U.L.B., Rhode-SaintGenèse
1640 Brussels, Belgium* and [2]INSERM U.343, Faculté de Médecine
06100 Nice, France

INTRODUCTION

A very new proto-oncogene, called c-*cbl,* has recently been described. This oncogene was discovered as a virally transduced oncogene responsible for inducing pre B cell lymphoma in mice (Holmes et al., 1986; Langdon et al., 1989a).

Chromosomal mapping has shown that, in mice, two c-*cbl* loci exist (Regnier et al.,1989); but in humans, only the CBL-2 locus was found (Savage et al., 1991). The cDNA cloning and sequencing make c-*cbl* a very likely transcriptional factor of the leucine zipper family, even though the encoded protein has not yet been identified (Langdon et al., 1992). Furthermore, v-*cbl* is a 3' truncated form of c-*cbl*.and its sequence is identical to that of its c-*cbl* counterpart. Finally, there is 98 % homology within the v-*cbl* region between mice and human proto-oncogenes (Blake et al.,1991).

The mRNA expression of c-*cbl* was first analyzed in the mouse: It is spontaneously highly expressed mainly in the thymus and in the testis. Moreover, it was found in a range of diverse hemopoietic murine and human cell lines (Langdon et al., 1989b). The mRNA expression was identified as three transcripts of 10.7, 5.6 and 3.5 kb with a relative pattern of expression depending on the cells.

Here we report the spontaneous and potentialized mRNA expression of c-*cbl* in humans through the addition of diverse inductors into the cultures. This study largely focused on the mRNA expression in human thymocytes. The last part of our work, currently under progress, will give an acount of the genetic regulation of c-*cbl* expression.

1* Corresponding author

In Vivo Immunology, Edited by E. Heinen *et al.*
Plenum Press, New York, 1994

RESULTS

Spontaneous and *in-vitro* Potentialized CBL mRNA Expression in Thymocytes

If not specified, all Northern blots were done with total RNA. All experiments were carried out three to four times and the cells were in a resting state before being activated in culture. A v-*cbl* probe was used. Thymus came from five month to six year old children undergoing surgery for a congenital heart-malformation. The 10.7 kb transcript was very well represented and thus was the only one analyzed, while the 5.6 and 3.5 kb transcripts were often weak or absent. The spontaneous expression of c-*cbl* in the human thymus was high as well as in the mouse (Data not shown) and after 3 hours in culture, the expression readily fell down (Table1, Basal).

For each experiment, we either hybridized with an IL-2 probe or we checked the viability of the cells through an Elisa assay for the secretion of IL-2. TPA +PHA, wich is quite mitogenic for T cells, always gave a strong signal, as expected.(Data not shown). Northern blots were hybridized with a house-keeping gene (GAPDH) which made it possible to establish the relative hybridization intensity of CBL mRNA for each condition through scanning densitometry.

Table 1, which gives a synoptic view of several compiled experiments, shows that 12-O-tetradecanoylphorbol-13-acetate (TPA) had a strong effect 3 hours after the addition of this inductor into the culture upon CBL mRNA expression. Conversly, the signal was repeatedly very weak after one hour of culture. The phyto-haemaglutinine (PHA) highly increased CBL expression only after an overnight culture. A pair of soluble anti-CD2 monoclonal antibodies never gave a high expression of the oncogene. Interestingly, it appeared that TPA+PHA together clearly reduced the CBL expression obtained with one or the other inductor.

Table 1. Synoptic view of c-*cbl* total RNA expression of *in-vitro* activated human thymocytes (Relative hybridization intensity measured through scanning densitometry).

	TIME AFTER STIMULATION (HOURS)			
STIMULATORS	1/2	1	3	18
BASAL (+3 H)	+/-	+/-	+/-	-
PHA	+/-	++/-	++	++++
TPA	+/-	-	+++++	+/-
TPA+PHA	+/-	+	+++	++
Anti-CD2	NT	+/-	+	++

In order to analyze a more physiological mitogenic cell signal, we used anti-CD3 antibodies immobilized to plastic with or without Interleukine-1β (IL-1β) , as *in vitro*-activators. We then extracted polyA⁺mRNA and made the Northern as usual. Results are shown on table 2.

This experiment shows that anti-CD3 gave a strong signal (10.7 and 5.6 kb) as soon as half an hour after the cell contact with the anti-CD3 antibodies; it decreased more or less rapidly afterwards. In the presence of IL-1β, the signal given through the CD3 complex drasticallly decreased and this effect was confirmed by other experiments done with total mRNA. Moreover, anti-CD3+TPA completely abolished the expression of c-*cbl* obtained with antibodies alone. This latter effect was also observed with a Jurkat cell line (Data not shown).

Table 2. c-*cbl* polyA⁺RNA expression in human thymocytes cultured with anti-CD3 monoclonal antibodies immobilized to plastic.

	TIME AFTER STIMULATION (HOURS)		
STIMULATORS	1/2	1	3
BASAL (+3H)	+/-	NT	-
Anti-CD3	++++	+++	++/-
Anti-CD3+IL-1	++/-	+	+/-
Anti-CD3+TPA	-	NT	-

Spontaneous and *in-vitro* Potentialized CBL mRNA Expression in Peripheric Blood Cells (PBL)

A series of experiments done with human PBL, monocytes, and purified T cells (Data not presented) repeatedly showed that the CBL expression of these cells was very weak compared with the CBL expression in the thymus (in the same experimental conditions). Moreover, the spontaneous CBL expression of these mature blood cells was totally absent. It thus confirms that the expression of c-*cbl* is quite specific of cells in the process of maturation/differentiation.

Effects of Cycloheximide and Actinomycine upon CBL mRNA Expression of *in-vitro* Thymocytes

In order to analyze the mechanisms of CBL activation led by anti-CD3 as well as TPA in human thymocytes, we performed experiments using Cycloheximide (CHX) which blocks the Neo-synthesis of protein and/or Actinomycine (ACT) wich blocks the transcription.

Preliminary data (not presented here) showed that the CD3-complex signal stabilizes CBL mRNA through a post-transcriptional process, wich is often the case for early activated genes, as c-*cbl* stimulated by anti-CD3 antibodies. The effects of TPA are mainly to raise the CBL mRNA degradation mechanisms and to increase the level of transcription. In view of the drop of the signal after one hour and of the peak after three hours of culture in the presence of TPA, we can assume that these mechanisms are sequential. On the other hand, the paradoxical effect of TPA upon the CD3 response could be explained by TPA early RNase activity. Run on assays are in progress to confirm these experiments.

DISCUSSION

We can put forward that c-*cbl* is an early activated gene via the CD3 complex. As such, it is likely to play a role in the Go-G1 phase transition or in the G1 phase of the cell cycle. Futhermore, it has been proved that a number of TPA-treated cell lines are able to differentiate in culture (Auwerx et al., 1988; Makover et al., 1991) and that TPA-treated HL-60 cells accumulate in the G1 phase of the cell cycle (Rovera et al., 1980). TPA is thus likely to place thymocytes in a very early phase of the cell cycle (after 3 hours of culture) when c-*cbl* is strongly expressed.

A co-mitogenic signal, like IL-1β or the TPA, wich are known to display progression factor effects when used as cofactors, decreases or abrogates the initial activation. Thus, c-*cbl* expression probably has to be repressed for the cells to continue through the cell cycle.

Cell-maturation/differentiation or thymocyte-apoptosis -- which are respectively considered as a delayed cell cycle (Kirschner et al., 1985; Lohka et al., 1988) or an occurence in an abnormal cell cycle (Colombel et al., 1992)-- can be closely linked to the c-*cbl* activation. Therefore, this oncogene may be involved in one of the alternative pathways wich seem to occur during an early phase of the cell cycle.

It is noteworthy that c-*cbl* expression has features similar to that of Apoptosis: It is an active process which could be triggered by the CD3 complex, knocked out in the presence of some co-mitogenic factors as IL-1; it could possibly take place in an early phase of the cell cycle and it is also specific of some tissues such as the thymus. In this regard, it may play a role in the selection of the T-cell repertoire.

REFERENCES

Auwerx, J.H., Deeb, S., Brunzell, J.D., Peng, R. and Chait A., 1988, Transcriptional activation of the lipoprotein lipase E genes accompanies differentiation in some human macrophage-like cell lines, *Biochemistry* 27:2651.

Blake, T.J., Shapiro, M., Morse III, H.C. and Langdon W.Y., 1991, The sequences of the human and mouse c-cbl proton-oncogenes show v-*cbl* was generated by a large truncation encompassing a proline-rich domain and a leucine zipper-like motif, *Oncogene.* 6:653.

Colombel, M., Olsson, C.A., Ng P-Y and Buttyan, R., 1992, Hormone-regulated apoptosis results from re-entry of differentiated prostate cells into a defective cell cycle, *Cancer Res.* 52:4313.

Holmes, K.L., Langdon, W.Y., Fredrickson, T.N., Coffman, R.L., Hoffman, P.M., Hartley, J.W. and Morse III, H.C., 1986, Analysis of neoplasms induced by Cas-Br-M tumor extracts, *J. Immunol.* 137:679.

Langdon, W.Y., Hartley, J.W., Klinken, S.P., Ruscetti, S.K. and Morse III, H.C., 1989a, V-*cbl*, an oncogene from a dual recombinant murine retrovirus that induces early B-lineage lymphomas, *Proc. Natl. Acad. Sci. USA* 86:1168.

Langdon, W.Y., Heath, K.G. and Blake, T.J., 1992, The localization of the products of the c-*cbl* and v-*cbl* oncogenes during mitosis and transformation, *Current topics in Microbiol. and Immunol.* 182:467.

Langdon W.Y., Hyland, C.D., Grumont, R.J. and Morse III, H.C., 1989b, The c-*cbl* proton-oncogene is preferentially expressed in thymus and testis tissue and encodes a nuclear protein, *J. Virol.* 63:5420.

Lohka, M.J., Hayes, M.K. and Maller J.L., 1988, Purification of maturation-promoting factor, an intracellular regulator of early mitotic events, *Proc. Natl. Acad. Sci. USA* 85:3009.

Makover, D., Cuddy, M., Yum, S., Bradley, K., Alpers, J., Sukhatme, V. and Reed, J. C., 1991, Phorbol ester-mediated inhibition of growth and regulation of proto-oncogene expression in the human T cell leukemia line Jurkat, *Oncogene,* 6:455.

Regnier, D., Kozak, C.A., Kingsley, D.M., Jenkins, N.A., Copeland, N.G., Langdon, W.Y. and Morse III, H.C., 1989, Identification of two murine loci homologous to the v-*cbl* oncogene, *J. Virol.* 63:3678.

Rovera, G., Olashaw, N. and Meo, P., 1980, Terminal differentiation in human promyelocytic leukaemic cells in the absence of DNA synthesis, *Nature.* 284:69.

Savage, P.D., Shapiro, M., Langdon, W.Y., Geurts van Kessel, A.D., Seuanez, H.N., Akao, Y., Croce, C., Morse III, H.C. and Kersey, J.H., 1991, Relationship of the human protooncogene CBL2 on 11q23 to the t(4;11), t(11;22), and t(11;14) breakpoints, *Cytogenet Cell Genet.* 56:112.

Warner, A., 1985, The role of gap junctions in amphibian development, 1985, *J. Embryol. Exp. Morphol., Suppl.* 81:365.

PRODUCTION AND SELECTION OF B LYMPHOCYTES IN BONE MARROW:

LYMPHOSTROMAL INTERACTIONS AND APOPTOSIS IN NORMAL, MUTANT

AND TRANSGENIC MICE

Dennis G. Osmond

Department of Anatomy and Cell Biology
McGill University
Montreal, Canada H3A 2B2

INTRODUCTION

The primary genesis of B lymphocytes in mouse bone marrow shares many features in common with the development of T lymphocytes in the thymus. Both processes involve a proliferative expansion of phenotypically differentiating precursor cells, an ordered rearrangement of gene loci for antigen-recognition receptors and a rigorous selection of suitably competent cells. In particular, intimate interactions between lymphocyte precursors and local stromal cells play key roles in regulating both cell proliferation and cell selection. To conclude the section of this Volume on positive and negative selection in primary lymphoid tissues, which deals mainly with intrathymic lymphopoiesis, the present article will review briefly our recent work on B lymphopoiesis in the bone marrow. The work deals with the microenvironmental organisation and dynamics of B cell genesis under normal conditions in vivo.

PRODUCTION AND LOSS OF PRECURSOR B CELLS IN BONE MARROW

We have previously defined a developmental sequence of six phenotypically distinct populations of precursor B cells in mouse bone marrow based on immunofluorescence labeling of intranuclear terminal deoxynucleotidyl transferase (TdT), surface B220 glycoprotein and μ heavy (H) chains of IgM.[1,2] Cells prior to the expression of μ chains, termed pro-B cells, pass through three stages: early pro-B (TdT$^+$B220$^-\mu^-$), intermediate pro-B (TdT$^+$B220$^+\mu^-$) and late pro-B (TdT$^-$B220$^+\mu^-$). The latter give rise to classical pre-B cells distinguished by intracytoplasmic μ chains (cμ), subdivided into large dividing cells and small post mitotic forms that finally mature into B lymphocytes expressing surface IgM (sIgM). Rearrangements of H chain gene loci occur during the pro-B stage, followed by light (L) chain gene rearrangements in pre-B cells. The pro-B cells in this model correspond largely with populations designated in other systems either as A,B,C, based on the expression of S7,HSA,BP1 and B220,[3] or as pre-B I, based on cloned cell lines responding to IL-7 and stromal cell contact.[4]

In Vivo Immunology, Edited by E. Heinen et al.
Plenum Press, New York, 1994

Two opposing processes are apparent in B cell genesis. We have quantitated the population dynamics of cells at each differentiation stage by measuring the number of cells normally flowing through cell cycle per unit time, using mitotic arrest techniques in vivo. Pro-B and large pre-B cells undergo a series of divisions, estimated to total 5-6, resulting in a progressive clonal expansion at successive stages. This is apparently associated, however, with a large-scale (>70%) cell loss at the pre-B cell stage. In addition, the data do not preclude the possibility of loss at earlier stages, notably among late pro-B cells, some of which could represent cells with nonproductive rearrangements of Ig H chain gene loci. Similarly high degrees of cell loss occur in rat bone marrow,[5] sheep Peyer's patch[6] and chicken bursa of Fabricius.[6] Thus, the final output of B cells from the bone marrow represents a balance between cell proliferation and cell loss.

Factors Promoting Proliferation of Precursor B Cells

Local stromal cell factors are of paramount importance in controlling the proliferation of pro-B and pre-B cells in mouse bone marrow. IL-7 remains the prime factor, greatly augmented in effect by coincident exposure to either the ligand for the tyrosine receptor kinase, c-kit, or insulin-like growth factor 1 (IGF-1)[7,8,9] IL-7 is also effective when administered systemically. When either infused or introduced as a functional transgene linked to an MHC class II promoter, the sustained high expression of IL-7 produces proliferative expansion of pro-B cells as well as pre-B cells, suggesting that these cells all constitute receptive target cells (H. Valenzona, S. Dhanoa, R. Plyam, R. Ceredig and D.G. Osmond, unpublished).

Stromal cells appear to respond to systemic cytokines. Various foreign agents can stimulate pro-B and pre-B cell proliferation, mediated by the products of activated macrophages in the spleen.[10] Pathological conditions associated with intense macrophage activity, eg. murine malaria and peritoneal oil-granuloma, produce prolonged pro-B cell stimulation.[11] IL-1 is a candidate mediator, being stimulatory when infused at low dose rates (L. Fauteaux and D.G. Osmond, unpublished).

Intrinsic signals may promote increased precursor B cell proliferation, notably as a result of oncogene dysregulation, an important factor in initiating B cell lineage neoplasias. Eµ-myc transgenic mice, in which c-myc is constitutively expressed in the B cell lineage, show prolonged polyclonal expansion of proliferating pro-B and pre-B cell pools, before eventually developing monoclonal malignant B lymphomas.[12,13]

Significantly, however, many of the foregoing stimuli, in addition to promoting proliferation, are associated with disproportionately high degrees of cell loss.

Factors Promoting Loss of Precursor B Cells at Various Stages

Functional Ig gene expression appears to be needed for the survival of precursor B cells in vivo. In scid mice, unable to rearrange successfully the Ig H chain gene loci, precursor cells feed into the B cell lineage and pass through the TdT-expressing pro-B cell stages quite normally but part way through the late pro-B cell stage virtually every cell is deleted.[14] The introduction of a functional L chain transgene into scid mice produces no effect on this deletion, but a µ chain transgene allows further development into cµ⁺ cells before complete deletion again occurs, while double µ and λ transgenes permit a complete development to sIgM⁺ B lymphocytes, though in subnormal numbers (D.G. Osmond, R.A. Phillips, R. Plyam and S. Rico-Vargas, unpublished).[15] In each case, the particular precursor cells present in the bone marrow continue to proliferate and to flow through mitosis in normal numbers. Defects in Ig gene expression thus result not in a static developmental "block" or "arrest" but in a dynamic stream of cell development leading to deletion. Precursor B cells in vivo may thus be deleted at various points in differentiation depending upon the degree of successful Ig gene rearrangement and expression. Proliferative stimuli do not permit the cells to escape deletion. Scid mice stimulated either by the introduction of the Eμ-myc transgene or by IL-7 still completely delete all late pro-B cells (N. Kim and D.G. Osmond, unpublished).

Pre-neoplastic states are associated with enhanced precursor B cell loss, mainly at the late pro-B stage in pristane oil-treated and malaria-infected mice, and at the pre-B stage in Eμ-myc transgenic mice.[11,13] Speculatively, these conditions may all predispose to genomic instability and illegitimate Ig gene recombinations.

Mice treated repeatedly with anti-IgM antibodies from birth fail to develop B cells, all precursor cells being lost at the pre-B cell stage when they would normally begin to express sIgM, apparently a model of central clonal deletion of B cells.[16]

The normal large-scale loss of precursor B cells may thus represent a negative selection of cells with autoreactive specificities, defective Ig gene rearrangements or illegitimate recombinations causing oncogene dysregulation. The selection mechanisms, however, are not necessarily identical in each case.

LYMPHOSTROMAL INTERACTIONS REGULATING PRECURSOR B CELL PROLIFERATION

We have shown that B220$^+$ precursor B cells develop in intimate association with stromal reticular cells in mouse bone marrow and can thus be directly exposed to stromal cell regulatory factors in vivo.[17] There is much interest in the nature of cell adhesion and other molecules at the lymphostromal interface which mediate regulatory signals for cell proliferation, localization and migration by cell-cell or cell-matrix interactions.

The binding of radiolabeled mAB M/K-2[18] administered iv and detected by electron microscope radioautography has revealed VCAM-1, a member of the Ig superfamily, heavily and uniformly expressed along the processes of stromal reticular cells in normal mouse bone marrow.[19] Individual processes are associated with precursor cells of various lineages (lymphoid, erythroid and granulocytic) which all express the ligand for VCAM-1, the integrin VLA-4 (α_4B_1). VCAM-1 and VLA-4 thus appear to constitute a common cell adhesion mechanism for multiple hemopoietic cell lineages.

In contrast, a 110 kD protein detected by mAb KMI-6 is heavily expressed by stromal reticular cell processes only around cells of immature lymphoid morphology, apparently restricted to the actual area of lymphostromal contact.[20] The highly restricted expression of this protein in the form recognized by mAb KMI-6 suggests that the stromal reticular cells may be polarized, vectorially directing products into interacting areas of surface membrane to produce lineage-specific niches. These observations may begin to explain how individual reticular cells in bone marrow may simultaneously regulate more than one interacting lineage and how the stimulation of one lineage may produce concomitant depression of another by competition for stromal adhesion sites.

Kit ligand is expressed by stromal cells in bone marrow, while c-kit is expressed on early precursor B cells. We find that an anti-c-kit blocking antibody, mAb ACK-2, binds to approximately one half of TdT$^+$ cells and one quarter of B220$^+$ cells, all of which are proliferating actively (D.G. Osmond, S-I. Nishikawa, B. Weiskopf and S. Rico-Vargas, unpublished), in accord with in vitro indications that c-kit plays an important role in early B lymphopoiesis.[21,22] However, we find that in vivo treatment with mAb ACK-2, which virtually eliminates erythropoiesis and granulopoiesis, actually increases the proliferative output of pro-B and pre-B cells. One speculation to account for this finding is that alternative signalling pathways, notably IGF-1[9], may augment IL-7 responses in the absence of c-kit, while B lymphopoiesis enjoys advantageous access to stromal reticular cells in the absence of competing lineages.

Early precursor B cells are often surrounded by an unusually thick layer of electron dense extracellular matrix.[23] While the matrix in bone marrow has been shown to include fibronectin, laminin and collagen type IV, the particular composition of the matrix involved in lymphostromal interactions remains undefined.

LYMPHOSTROMAL INTERACTIONS INVOLVED IN PRECURSOR B CELL SELECTION

B220$^+$ precursor B cells in normal mouse bone marrow are frequently observed to be enfolded within complex processes of resident macrophages which contain numerous inclusion bodies.[16,24] The B220$^+$ cells themselves sometimes show irregular nuclear profiles and peripheral chromatin condensation suggesting the early stages of programmed cell death (apoptosis). Mice expressing the bcl-2 transgene in the B cell lineage show markedly increased numbers of B lymphocytes within the bone marrow, though whether these result from either a central or peripheral block in apoptosis remains to be determined (D.G. Osmond, A. Harris, A. Straser and H. Valenzona, unpublished).

Macrophage-lymphocyte interactions are enhanced in conditions of increased precursor B cell loss. Both macrophages and the apparent ingestion of large B220$^+$ cells are unusually prominent in scid mice, suggesting this to be the mechanism for deleting aberrant late pro-B cells.[14] The latter are not evidently apoptotic, however, in ultrastructural appearance. B lineage cells from scid mice can remain viable and proliferate in vitro if given IL-7 and supportive stromal cells.[25] The findings suggest that B lineage cells whose Ig gene loci either remain in germline configuration or are aberrantly rearranged are not necessarily programmed intrinsically for premature death, but they are nevertheless normally recognized and subjected to rapid negative selection by macrophages within the in vivo microenvironmental architecture. The fate of precursor B cells in Ig transgenic-scid mice is currently under investigation.

Extreme degrees of apoptosis among B220$^+$ cells together with massive ingestion by macrophages are a prominent feature in the bone marrow of Eμ-myc transgenic mice[13] (K. Jacobsen, C.L.Sidman and D.G. Osmond, unpublished). Constitutive overexpression of c-myc in the B cell lineage thus appears to initiate both a premature programmed death and macrophage-mediated deletion of many pre-B cells. Excessive macrophage activity and much apparent apoptosis also characterize the bone marrow of anti-IgM treated mice. Similar studies of other models of central clonal B cell deletion are underway.

CONCLUSION

Precursor B cells in mouse bone marrow undergo proliferative expansion in association with stromal reticular cells, whose regulatory influence appears to be mediated by both general and lineage-specific adhesion molecules and growth factors, partially influenced by systemic cytokines and to some extent in competition with other hemopoietic lineages. The expression of regulatory molecules and their control at these lymphostromal interfaces remains incompletely understood.

Many precursor B cells are rapidly ingested by resident macrophages, associated with the concurrent initiation of apoptotic cell death, at least in some circumstances. The rapidity of this process accounts for the apparent discrepancy between the magnitude of cell loss and the paucity of dying cells detectable at a given time. The nature of the molecules recognized by the macrophages on cells to be deleted has yet to be determined. The negative selection process represents, however, an important screening mechanism which is normally able to prevent the dissemination of potentially aberrant, functionless, dysregulated or certain autoreactive B cells.

Surviving B lymphocyte clones enter segments of the bone marrow sinusoids from which they are released into the systemic blood circulation. Whether this final step involves a positive selection of Ig specificities and the nature of the ligands that could determine such a selection are, as yet, unknown.

Acknowledgments

This work was supported by grants from the Medical Research Council of Canada and the National Cancer Institute of Canada.

REFERENCES

1.   D.G. Osmond, B cell development in the bone marrow, *Semin. Immunol.* 3:173 (1990).
2.   Y-H. Park and D.G. Osmond, Dynamics of B lymphocyte precursor cells in mouse bone marrow: proliferation of cells containing terminal deoxynucleotidyl transferase, *Eur. J. Immunol.* 19:2139 (1989).
3.   R.R. Hardy, C.E. Carmack, S.A. Shinton, J.D.Kemp and K. Hayakawa, Resolution and characterization of pro-B and pre-pro-B cell stages in normal mouse bone marrow, *J. Exp. Med.* 173:1213 (1991).
4.   A. Rolink and F. Melchers, Molecular and cellular origins of B lymphocyte diversity, *Cell* 66:1081 (1991).
5.   G.J. Deenen, I.V. Balen, D. Opstelten, In rat B lymphocyte genesis sixty percent is lost from the bone marrow at the transition of nondividing pre-B cell to sIgM$^+$ B lymphocyte, the stage of Ig light chain gene expression, *Eur. J. Immunol.* 20:557 (1990).
6.   B. Motyka and J.D. Reynolds, Apoptosis is associated with the extensive B cell death in the sheep ileal Peyer's patch and the chicken bursa of Fabricius: a possible role in B cell selection. *Eur. J. Immunol.* 21:1951 (1991).
7.   A.E. Namen, S. Lupton, K. Hjerrilk, J. Wagnall, D.Y. Mochizuki, A. Schmierer, B. Mosley, C. March, J. Urdal, S. Gillis, D. Cosman, J. Good-Urdal, S. Gillis, D. Cosman and R.G. Goodwin, Stimulation of B-cell progenitors by clonal murine interleukin-7, *Nature* 333:571 (1988).
8.   L.G. Billips, D. Petitte, K. Dorshkind, R. Narayanan, C-P. Chur and K.S. Landreth, Differential roles of stromal cells, Interleukin-7, and *kit*-ligand in the regulation of B lymphopoiesis, *Blood* 79:1185 (1992).
9.   K.S. Landreth, N. Ramaswamy and K. Dorshkind, Insulin-like growth factor-I regulates pro-B-cell differentiation, *Blood* 80:1207 (1992).
10. Y.H. Park and D.G. Osmond, Regulation of early B cell proliferation in mouse bone marrow: Stimulation by exogenous agents mediated by macrophages in the spleen, *Cell. Immunol.* 134:111 (1991).
11. D.G. Osmond, S. Priddle and S.R. Rico-Vargas, Proliferation of B cell precursors in bone marrow of pristane-conditioned and malaria-infected mice: Implications for B cell oncogenesis, *in*: "Current Topics in Microbiology and Immunology", M. Potter and F. Melchers, eds., Springer Verlag, Heidelberg.

12. A.W. Harris, C.A. Pinkert, M. Crawford, W.Y. Langdon, R.L. Brinster and J.M. Adams, The Eμ-myc transgenic mouse. A model for high-incidence spontaneous lymphoma and leukemia of early B cells, *J. Exp.Med.* 165:353 (1988).

13. C.L. Sidman, D.J. Shaffer, K. Jacobsen, S. Rico-Vargas and D.G. Osmond, Cell populations during tumorigenesis in Eμ-myc transgenic mice, *Leukemia* (in press).

14. D.G. Osmond, N. Kim, R. Manoukian, R.A. Phillips, S.A. Rico-Vargas and K. Jacobsen, Dynamics and localization of early B-lymphocyte precursor cells (Pro-B cells) in the bone marrow of scid mice, *Blood* 79:1695 (1992).

15. M. Reichman-Fried, R.R. Hardy and M.J. Bosma, Development of B-lineage cells in the bone marrow of *scid/scid* mice following the introduction of functionally rearranged immunoglobulin transgenes, *Proc. Natl. Acad. Sci. USA* 87:2730 (1990).

16. G. Fulop, J. Gordon and D.G. Osmond, Regulation of lymphocyte production in the bone marrow. I. Turnover of small lymphocytes in mice depleted of B lymphocytes by treatment with anti-IgM antibodies, *J. Immunol.* 130:644 (1983).

17. K. Jacobsen and D.G. Osmond, Microenvironmental organisation and stromal cell associations of B lymphocyte precursor cells in mouse bone marrow, *Eur. J. Immunol.* 20:2395 (1990).

18. K. Miyake, J. Medina, K. Ishihara, M. Kimoto, R. Auerbach and P.W. Kincade, A VCAM-like adhesion molecule on murine bone marrow stromal cells mediates binding of lymphocyte precursors in culture, *J. Cell Biol.* 114:557 (1991).

19. D.G. Osmond, K. Miyake, P.W. Kincade, J. Kravitz and K. Jacobsen, Interactions between stromal reticular cells and lymphoid precursor cells in mouse bone marrow: in vivo expression of KM16, V-CAM-1 and VLA-4 determinants, *Anat. Rec.* 232(4):68A (1992).

20. K. Jacobsen, K. Miyake, P.W.Kincade and D.G. Osmond, Highly restricted expression of a stromal cell determinant in mouse bone marrow in vivo, *J. Exp. Med.* 176:927 (1992).

21. M. Ogawa, Y.Matsuzaki, S. Nishikawa, S-I. Hayashi, T. Kunisada, S. Sudo, T. Kina, H.Nakauchi and S-I. Nishikawa, Expression and function of *c-kit* in hemopoietic progenitor cells, *J. Exp.Med.* 174:63 (1991).

22. A. Rolnik, M. Streb, S.I. Nishikawa and F. Melchers, The c-kit encoded tyrosine kinase regulates the proliferation of early pre-B cells, *Eur. J. Immunol.* 21:2609 (1991).

23. K. Jacobsen, J. Tepper and D.G. Osmond, Early B lymphocyte precursor cells in mouse bone marrow: substeal localization of B220+ cells during post-irradiation regeneration, *Exp. Hematol.* 18:304 (1989).

24. K. Jacobsen and D.G. Osmond, Cell deletion in B cell genesis and the role of bone marrow macrophages, *in:* "Lymphatic Tissues and In Vivo Immune Responses", S. Ezine, S. Berrih-Aknin and B. Imhof, eds., Marcel Dekker, New York.

25. P.W. Kincade, Experimental models for understanding B lymphocyte formation, *Adv. Immunol.* 41:181 (1987).

THYMIC NEUROENDOCRINE SELF PEPTIDES AND T CELL SELECTION

Vincent Geenen[1], Henri Martens[1], Eric Vandersmissen[1], Ouafae Kecha[1], Abdellah Benhida[1], Nadine Cormann-Goffin[1], Pierre J. Lefèbvre[2], and Paul Franchimont[1]

Institute of Pathology CHU-B23, [1]Department of Endocrinology, Immuno-Endocrinology Unit, [2]Laboratory of Experimental Diabetology University of Liège, B-4000 Liège (Sart-Tilman), Belgium

INTRODUCTION

Our previous studies have shown that the thymic epithelial cells (TEC) of different animal species were the site for synthesis of polypeptide precursors belonging to the neurohypophysial (NHP), tachykinin (TK), and insulin neuroendocrine families[1,2,3,4,5]. However, at least in basal conditions, cultured human TEC do not secrete NHP-related peptides, neurokinin A (NKA) nor insulin-like growth factor 2 (IGF2); the existence of a classical secretory pathway in the thymic epithelium may thus be questioned. We also failed to detect immunoreactive (ir) thymic NHP-related peptides in classical secretory granules and a very elegant recent study has demonstrated that ir oxytocin (OT), the dominant thymic NHP-related peptide, was located diffusely in the cytosol and in clear vacuoles of murine TEC[6]. The term *cryptocrine* has been introduced in the word-list of Endocrinology to describe this particular type of cell-to-cell signaling in specialized microenvironments constituted by large "nursing" epithelial cells (like TEC/TNC in the thymus, or Sertoli cells in the testis) enclosing cell populations that migrate and differentiate at their very close contact (respectively, T cells and spermatids)[7]. In the general evolution of cell-to-cell communication, the cryptocrine type of signaling is located at a rather primitive step, between intercellular adhesion and paracrine exchanges of soluble signals. Moreover, in the thymus, the cryptocrine stage is closely associated with the presentation of the self molecular structure to the developing T cell system. Therefore, the thymus appears as one crucial meeting point for the two major systems of intercellular communication: therein, the endocrine system may influence the early steps of the immune response, whereas the immune system is educated in self neuroendocrine principles[8]. We would like to present here our experimental arguments that permit to transpose at the level of the thymic repertoire of neuroendocrine-related peptides the dual physiological role of this primary lymphoid organ in T cell positive and negative selection.

THYMIC CRYPTOCRINE SIGNALING AND T CELL POSITIVE SELECTION

We and other authors have reported the expression of NHP peptide receptors in the rat thymus, by rat thymocytes[9], by a murine cytotoxic T cell line (CTL-L2), as well as by a murine pre-T cell line (RL12-NP)[10,11]. These receptors were functional since the binding of NHP peptides to CTL-L2 or RL12-NP cells was followed by a phosphoinositide breakdown and a mobilization of inositol phosphates within those cells. Through the use of various NHP pharmacological agonists and antagonists, it was shown that immature T cells were expressing a NHP V1-subtype receptor, whereas NHP OT-type receptors were detected on mature cytotoxic T cells. This observation strongly suggests that a shift in the molecular type of the NHP receptor system expressed by T cells occurs in parallel with their stage of differentiation. Finally, the addition of different NHP peptides to the cultures of human or murine freshly isolated thymocytes induced a significant increase of their incorporation of [^{3}H]TdR incorporation, provided the cells are cultured in serum-free media devoid of mercaptoethanol (which could reduce the disulfide bridge of NHP-related peptides and inhibit their bioactivity)[11].

Within the thymus, physico-chemical conditions are encountered to render functional *in vivo* the cell-to-cell signaling through NHP-related signals and receptors. Indeed, while the precise biochemical nature of the thymic NHP-related signal, as well as the genetic mechanisms leading to its specific expression within TEC are still under current investigation in our Department, their intrathymic concentrations are in agreement with the high affinity (0.1 nM) Kd of NHP peptide receptors expressed by pre-T cells. These conditions cannot be applied to the much lower blood concentrations of the neurohormones vasopressin (VP) and OT (in the picomolar range). Therefore, on the basis of these observations, it can be concluded that a functional interaction is engaged within the thymus between a NHP-related signal synthesized within TEC and specific NHP peptide receptors expressed by pre-T cells. Given the cellular activation that follows the binding of NHP signals to their cognate T cell receptors, this type of signaling might be involved as an accessory pathway during the process of T cell differentiation.

This model of cryptocrine signaling also applies to other neuroendocrine-related peptides synthesized in TEC. With regard to the TK-related dominant thymic peptide, NKA (but not substance P) was previously shown to exert an interleukin 1-like bioactivity and to increase the mitotic index of murine thymocytes[12]. Although this point has not been definitively demonstrated, it is most plausible that thymic NKA exerts this action through specific TK receptors expressed by target thymocytes. In the case of thymic IGF2, specific type 1 and 2 IGF receptors have been shown to be expressed in the thymus, on human PHA-activated T lymphocytes, and on anti-CD3-activated human T lymphocytes[13,14]. These findings also strongly support that thymic IGF2 (originating from TEC) and its cognate receptors (expressed by thymocytes) might intervene as an additional accessory pathway in T cell differentiation.

At this stage, it is more and more apparent that T cells encounter during their differentiation within the thymus various neuroendocrine-related signals synthesized by TEC. A functional signalling may occur since the specific receptors for these signals are expressed by T cells at different levels of maturation. Therefore, the various signaling events generated by all those molecular interactions in the thymic environment are physiologically relevant as distinct accessory pathways leading to the final T cell positive selection.

THYMIC NEUROENDOCRINE SELF PEPTIDES AND T CELL NEGATIVE SELECTION

Besides its role in the growth of immature T lymphocytes and in the development of the whole T cell repertoire, the thymus is the site for the induction of central immunological self-tolerance by negative selection of autoreactive T cells[15,16,17]. This action was longly thought to be mediated by thymic interdigitating cells, but there is more and more evidence that TEC are also strongly implicated in the tolerogenic action of the thymus[18,19]. Since neuroendocrine-related peptides are mainly synthesized within TEC (including TNC), it was therefore of interest to investigate their putative involvement in central T cell tolerance.

Through various polyclonal and monoclonal antibodies directed to different epitopes of the NHP peptide family, immunocytochemical (ICC) analyses have shown that the dominant NHP epitope identified in TEC from different species is located, at least partially, within the six amino acid cyclic part of the OT molecule[20,21]. The sequence **CYIXNC** (single letter amino acid code) characterizes all members of the OT lineage, as well as one putative ancestral precursor vasotocin (VT) of the NHP family. In the thymus, this epitope is associated with a neurophysin-like protein domain which is present in the structure of all identified NHP polypeptide precursors. This NHP self epitope also possesses a hydrophobic residue Tyr (Y) in a position which has been found to be important for the anchorage of antigenic sequences in the groove of MHC class I molecules[22]. A second epitope representative of the NHP family is also present in the central highly conserved part of the neurophysin domain. Our most recent studies have evidenced an association between thymic ir neurophysin and immunoaffinity-purified human thymic MHC class I molecules[23], and this preliminary result argues for the presentation of NHP epitopes by thymic MHC-derived proteins to the developing T cells. Given the importance of OT-related peptides in the control of reproductive functions (parturition, lactation, maternal behaviour and paracrine regulation of gonadal functions), it seems logical that their intrathymic expression would result in a stronger tolerance by the immune system. Since the water metabolism-regulating neurohormone VP differs from OT by one single amino acid in the NHP dominant epitope, it might be less tolerated by the immune system. Interestingly, some cases of idiopathic diabetes insipidus were shown to result from an autoimmune aggression against hypothalamic VP-producing neurons[24]. Therefore, further investigation of neuroendocrine-related self peptides should help our understanding of the central immune tolerance to various neuroendocrine functions.

In this perspective, we have recently provided solid evidence that IGF2 was the dominant thymic peptide of the insulin superfamily[4]. After alignment of the peptide sequences from different members of the insulin family (Table 1) and following the criteria established for the presentation by MHC class I[22], one can predict that the IGF2-derived sequence **CGGELVDTL** is a T cell epitope. This sequence is highly conserved throughout the family and may thus be considered as a self peptide for the B domain of the insulin family. Therefore, through thymic IGF2, the molecular self identity of the pancretic islet ß cell (synthesis and endocrine secretion of insulin) is indeed represented in face of the developing T cell system. This is of high physiological significance with regard to its central immune tolerance and we postulate that the above sequence might be one important tolerogenic factor for the pancreatic islet ß cell, at least during fetal development. The breakdown of immune tolerance to endocrine ß cells is more and more implicated as the major etiopathogenic event in the emergence of type I diabetes or insulin-dependent diabetes (IDDM). This breakdown is thought to induce an autoimmune cascade leading to the final disappearance of insulin-secreting ß cells, although the primary autoantigen remains to be further deciphered[25]. Interestingly, using another completely different experimental approach, some authors have identified the sequence of residues 7-15 (CGSHLVEAL) of the bovine insulin B chain as a target *autoantigen* for H-2K[b]-restricted cytotoxic T cells[26]. Those authors have also suggested that antigenic determinants of insulin B chain were dominant over peptide sequences derived from insulin A chain. That sequence is highly homogous to the human IGF2-derived *self antigen* since 5/9 amino acids are identical (55% homology). It is not identical however, and the biochemical difference between an insulin autoantigen and an insulin self antigen could result in dramatically opposed immune responses. From these observations, the classical implication of *"altered self"* in autoimmunity is progressively reappearing and this point could be fundamental in the establishment of an effective and safe procedure for the prevention of IDDM in humans.

Table 1. The insulin peptide superfamily (single letter code).

	B domain	*A domain*
IGF2		
Human	RPSETL**CGGEL**V**DTL**QFVCGDRGFYF	GIVEECCFRSCDLALLETYCA
Cow		
Rat	S	
Mouse	G G	S
IGF1		
Human	GPETL**CGAEL**V**D**ALQFVCGDRGFYFNKPT	GIVDECCFRSCDLRRLEMYCA
Cow		
Rat	P	
Mouse	P	
Insulin		
Lymnæa	PHRRGV**CG**SA**LA**D**L**VDFACSSSNQPAMV	NIVCECCMKPCTLSELRQYCP
Bombyx	QAVHTT**CGRH**L**AR**TL**ADLCWEAGVD	GIVDECCLRPCSVAVLLSYC
Hagfish	RTTGHL**CGKD**L**VNAL**TIACGVRGFFYDPTLM	GIVEQCCHKRCSIYNLQNYCN
Guinea pig	FVSRHL**CGSN**L**VETL**TSVCQDDGFFYIPKD	GIVDQCCTGTCTRHQLQSYCN
Rat	FVNQHL**CGSHL**VEA**L**YLVCGERGFFYTPLT	GIVDQCCTSICSLYQLENYCN
Human	FVNQHL**CGSHL**VEA**L**YLVCGERGFFYTPLT	GIVEQCCTSICSLYQLENYCN
Relaxin		
Porcine	NDFIKA**CGRE**L**V**RLWVEICGVWS	TLSEKCCEVGCIRKDIARLC

CONCLUSION

By focusing our research interest towards the impact of thymic neuroendocrine-related peptides upon the process of T cell differentiation, the model of neurosecretion has shifted to the novel model of cryptocrine cell-to-cell signalling. At the molecular level, the classical neuropeptide concept was replaced by those of neuroendocrine self peptides and of the molecular self identity of neuroendocrine families. As discussed in this chapter, thymic neuroendocrine self peptides might exert a dual role in T cell differentiation depending on the type of intercellular dialogue in which they are engaged between TEC and pre-T lymphocytes (cryptocrine signalling or presentation by MHC-derived proteins coexpressed by TEC).

ACKNOWLEDGMENTS

These studies are supported by the Special Research Fund of University of Liège Medical School, by grants FRSM n° 3.4562.90 and Télévie-FRSM n° 7.4611.91, and by the European Science Foundation.

REFERENCES

1. V. Geenen, J.J. Legros, P. Franchimont, M. Baudrihaye, M.P. Defresne, and J. Boniver. The neuroendocrine thymus: Coexistence of oxytocin and neurophysin in the human thymus, *Science* 232: 508 (1986).
2. V. Geenen, F. Robert, H. Martens, A. Benhida, G. Degiovanni, M.P. Defresne, J. Boniver, J.J. Legros, J. Martial, and P. Franchimont, At the Cutting Edge. Biosynthesis and paracrine/cryptocrine actions of "self" neurohypophysial-related peptides in the thymus, *Mol. Cell. Endocrinol.* 76: C27 (1991).
3. V. Geenen, N. Cormann-Goffin, H. Martens, A. Benhida, F. Robert, J.J. Legros, J. Martial, and P. Franchimont, Thymic neurohypophysial-related peptides and T cell selection, *Regul. Peptides* 45: 273 (1993).
4. A. Ericsson, V. Geenen, F. Robert, J.J. Legros, Y. Vrindts-Gevaert, P. Franchimont, S. Brené, and H. Persson, Expression of preprotachykinin-A and neuropeptide-Y messenger RNA in the thymus, *Molec. Endocrinol.* 4: 1211 (1990).
5. V. Geenen, I. Achour, F. Robert, E. Vandersmissen, J.C. Sodoyez, M.P. Defresne, J. Boniver, P.J. Lefèbvre, and P. Franchimont, Evidence that insulin-like growth factor (IGF2) is the dominant thymic peptide of the insulin superfamily, *Thymus* 21: 115 (1993).
6. M. Wiemann and G. Ehret, Subcellular localization of immunoreactive oxytocin within thymic epithelial cells of the male mouse, *Cell Tissue Res.*, in press.
7. J.W. Funder, At the Cutting Edge. Paracrine, cryptocrine, acrocrine, *Mol. Cell. Endocrinol.* 70: C21 (1990).
8. V. Geenen, F. Robert, H. Martens, D. De Groote, and P. Franchimont, The thymic education of developing T cells in self neuroendocrine principles, *J. Endocrinol. Invest.* 15: 621 (1992).
9. J. Elands, A. Resink, and E.R. de Kloet, Neurohypophysial hormone receptors in the rat thymus, *Endocrinology* 126: 2703 (1990).

10. V. Geenen, F. Robert, M. Fatemi, M.P. Defresne, J. Boniver, J.J. Legros, and P. Franchimont, Vasopressin and oxytocin: thymic signals and receptors in T cell ontogeny, *in*: "Recent Progress in Posterior Pituitary Hormones," S. Yoshida and L. Share, eds., Elsevier, New York (1988).

11. H. Martens, F. Robert, J.J. Legros, V. Geenen, and P. Franchimont, Expression of functional neurohypophysial peptide receptors by immature and cytotoxic T cell lines, *Prog. NeuroEndocrinImmunol.* 5: 31 (1992).

12. O. Söder and P. Hellström, The tachykinins neurokinin A and physalaemin stimulate murine thymocyte proliferation. *Int. Arch. Appl. Immunol.* 90: 91 (1989).

13. R.W. Kozak, J.F. Haskell, L.A. Greenstein, M.M. Rechsler, T.A Waldmann, and S.P. Nissley, Type I and II insulin-like growth factor receptors on human phytohemagglutinin-activated T lymphocytes. *Cell. Immunol.* 109: 318 (1987).

14. E.W. Johnson, L.A. Jones, and R.W. Kozak, Expression and function of insulin-like growth factor receptors on anti-CD3-activated human T lymphocytes, *J. Immunol.* 148: 63 (1992).

15. G.J.V. Nossal, Immunologic tolerance: Collaboration between antigen and lymphokines, *Science* 245: 147 (1989).

16. M. Blackman, J. Kappler, and P. Marrack, The role of the T cell receptor in positive and negative selection of developing T cells, *Science* 248: 1335 (1990).

17. H. von Boehmer and P. Kisielow, Self-nonself discrimination by T cells, *Science* 248: 1369 (1990).

18. J.C. Salaün, A. Bandeira, I. Khazaai, F. Calman, M. Coltey, A. Coutinho, and N.M. Le Douarin, Thymic epithelium tolerizes for histocompatibility antigens, *Science* 247: 1471 (1990).

19. S.R. Webb and J. Sprent, Tolerogenecity of thymic epithelium, *Eur. J. Immunol.* 20: 2525 (1990).

20. F. Robert, V. Geenen, J. Schoenen, E. Burgeon, D. De Groote, M.P. Defresne, J.J. Legros, and P. Franchimont, Colocalization of immunoreactive oxytocin, vasopressin and interleukin 1 in human thymic epithelial neuroendocrine cells, *Brain Behav. and Immun.* 5: 102 (1991).

21. F. Robert, H. Martens, N. Cormann-Goffin, A. Benhida, J. Schoenen, and V. Geenen, The recognition of hypothalamo-neurohypophysial functions by developing T cells, *Dev. Immunol.* 2: 131 (1992).

22. K. Falk, O. Rôtzschke, S. Stevanovic, G. Jung, and H.G. Rammensee, Allele-specific motif revealed by sequencing of self-peptide eluted from MHC molecules, *Nature* 351: 290 (1991).

23. V. Geenen, E. Vandersmissen, H. Martens, G. Degiovanni, and P. Franchimont, Evidence for the association between human thymic MHC class I molecules and a dominant neurohypophysial peptide, *J. Immunol.* 150: 39A (1993).

24. W.A. Scherbaum and G.F. Bottazzo, Autoantibodies to vasopressin cells in idiopathic diabetes insipidus: Evidence for an autoimmune variant, *Lancet* I: 897 (1983).

25. L. Castano and G.S. Eisenbarth, Type I diabetes: A chronic autoimmune disease of human, mouse, and rat, *Annu. Rev. Immunol.* 8: 647 (1990).

26. J.M. Sheil, S.E. Shepherd, G.F. Klimo, and Y. Paterson, Identification of an autologous insulin B chain peptide as a target antigen for H-2K^b-restricted cytotoxic T lymphocytes, *J. Exp. Med.* 175: 545 (1992).

HUMAN FETAL LIVER CELLS DIFFERENTIATE INTO THYMOCYTES IN CHIMERIC MOUSE FETAL THYMUS ORGAN CULTURE

Magda De Smedt, Georges Leclercq, Bart Vandekerckhove, and Jean Plum

Department of Clinical Chemistry, Microbiology, and immunology
University of Ghent, University Hospital
Blok A, De Pintelaan 185
B-9000 Ghent, Belgium

INTRODUCTION

The production of hematopoietic cells in blood-forming organs requires interaction between progenitor cells and stromal elements. The ability of these early cells to differentiate along multiple lineages can be experimentally reproduced *in vitro*. This is the case for myelopoiesis and B lymphocyte production where convenient *in vitro* stem cell assays in both murine and human models (1, 2) are available.

In contrast, the maintenance of the three-dimensional structure of the thymic epithelium appears to be a prerequisite for driving the full differentiation of stem cell into mature T lymphocytes. In the mouse, experimental T cell differentiation can be achieved quantitatively by transfer of precursor cell candidates into irradiated hosts, either systematically (3) or by direct intrathymic injection (4,5). Another possibility is to introduce precursor cell candidates into thymic rudiments using a hanging drop method and to monitor the differentiation in fetal thymic organ cultures (FTOC) (6).

These interesting assay systems can not be applied to human. Péault et al. (7) explored the possibility of the SCID-hu mouse, a chimera obtained by transplantation of human hematolymphoid tissue into congenitally immunodeficient host, to provide an in vivo culture system for dissecting the human T cell differentiation process (8). They have described (7) a system in which microinjection of CD34⁺ fetal precursor cells into HLA-mismatched fetal human thymus fragments, partially depleted of hematopoietic cells by low temperature culture, allowed to develop upon engraftment into immunodeficient SCID mice.

Merkenshlager et al. (9, 10) have shown recently that introduction of unseparated fetal human thymocytes into fetal murine thymic rudiments by the hanging drop method allowed differentiation of human T cells in the murine microenvironment.

In Vivo Immunology, Edited by E. Heinen *et al.*
Plenum Press, New York, 1994

Here, we show that total fetal liver cells and CD3, CD4, CD8 immunomagnetic depleted liver cells, when transferred by hanging drop into thymic rudiments of SCID mice of day 14-15 of gestation are capable to fully differentiate into human CD4$^+$CD8$^+$ and CD4$^+$ and CD8$^+$ single positive cells. These experiments indicate that stromal interactions between epithelial cells and hematopoietic precursors are either non species-specific or can be compensated by dendritic human cell interaction for complete T cell differentiation in the thymus. Furthermore, this system provides an easy tool to study critical factors in human T cell differentiation process.

MATERIALS AND METHODS

The methods have been detailed elsewhere (Hematopoietic Stem Cell Manual, Eds. E. Wunder & S. Serke, AlphaMed Press, Dayton, Ohio, USA, in press october 1993). Briefly, precursor cells were from human fetal liver of 20-22 week old fetuses. Fetal liver cells were isolated by lymphoprep gradient (Nyegaard, Oslo, Norway) centrifugation. The cell population was frozen and kept in liquid N_2 until use. These cells were thawed and washed once before transfer. A single fetal day 14 SCID thymic lobe was placed into each well of a Terasaki microwell plate (60x10 μl, Nunc, Roskilde, Denmark) containing 25 μl of IMDM complete medium with 100,000 fetal liver cells. The plate was then inverted and cultured for 48 h in a humidified petri dish. The lobes were removed after this period and set up as organ cultures for different length of time. At various times, a cell suspension was made of each thymic lobe separately, total cell count was done, cells were labeled with CD45 human versus CD45 murine, and with human CD4, CD8 and CD3 in three color fluorescence (Becton Dickinson Immunocytometry systems, Mountain View, CA, USA). Flow cytometric analysis was carried out on a FACScan (Becton Dickinson) using low-angle light scatter and forward scatter to gate out dead cells. In some experiments, fetal liver cells were depleted for CD3, CD4, CD8 positive cells with immunomagnetic depletion (Dynabeads, Dynal, Oslo, Norway).

RESULTS AND DISCUSSION

Because unseparated human fetal thymocytes can repopulate and differentiate in murine thymic rudiments when transferred by hanging drop and cultured in FTOC (9,10), we looked if precursor cells at an earlier stage of differentiation had the same capacities. We found that the mouse SCID thymocytes stained with anti-mouse CD45, remained at a low absolute number throughout the whole length of observation of the organ culture, whereas the human cells stained with anti-human CD45 increased progressively in function of time of the culture, with a maximal cell number of 120,000 to 150,000/lobe achieved after 4 weeks of culture. Anti-human CD45 does not stain SCID mouse thymocytes aspecifically (data not shown). As approximately 2,000 cells enter the thymus lobe, at least a 50-70-fold increase in human cells was seen.

When human differentiation markers were studied, the appearence of different subsets were noted. After one week of culture CD4^{low+}CD3$^-$ cells were the first cell to appear in FTOC. After two weeks of culture CD4$^+$CD8$^+$ cells and CD3$^+$ cells (fig. 1)

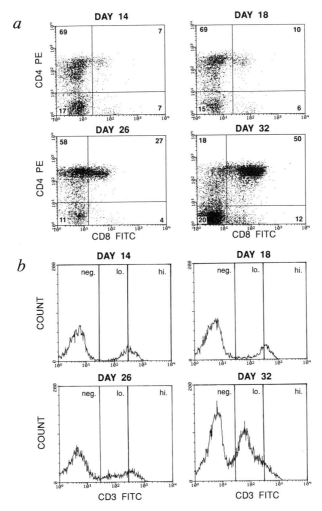

Fig. 1. Kinetic analysis of CD4, CD8 and CD3 expression on human cells in chimeric fetal thymus organ culture.
Human fetal liver cells were transferred to fetal murine SCID thymic lobes. At the indicated days of culture, cells were labeled with anti-human CD8 FITC and anti-human CD4 PE, or with anti-human CD3. Dot plots are shown for CD4-CD8 expression, histograms for CD3 expression.

were detectable . Almost all cells were CD1$^+$ (data not shown). After 4 weeks of culture single CD4$^+$ and CD8$^+$ thymocytes appear with high CD3 expression (fig. 1). These phenotypes indicate that full T cell maturation of human lymphocytes in a murine thymus' microenvironment can be obtained starting from precursor cells present in fetal liver. Another finding was that when total fetal liver cells were transferred into fetal SCID thymus CD4$^+$ γ/δ T cells were found. It is possible that this population represents a thymus independent subset of γ/δ T cells. It has been shown that in human fetal liver approximately 20% of γ/δ T cells had a CD4$^+$CD8$^-$ phenotype that is infrequent among γ/δ T cells in the thymus and the blood (11). As both α/β and γ/δ T cells can be cultured from human fetal liver (11), it was necessary to address whether the growth of CD3$^+$ cells in the FTOC was not due to the expansion of these extrathymic populations in the murine thymus rather than due to the differentiation of stem cells. This was shown by transfer of fetal liver precursor cells, after depletion of CD4$^+$, CD8$^+$, CD3$^+$ by immunomagnetic depletion, in the murine thymus. In these experiments, the γ/δ CD4$^+$ T cells were absent. These results indicate that in the latter study a complete differentiation was obtained, starting from human precursor cells, in SCID thymus instead of an unphysiological transfer and expansion of extrathymic T cells already present in fetal liver. Taken together these results indicate that starting from fetal liver cells, human precursor cells can differentiate and proliferate in the different T cell subsets in mouse thymus microenvironment.

Our study helps to resolve to delineate in function of time the different stages of T cell differentiation. It is clear that is difficult to address the different stages of differentiation with the use of different clinical samples from abortions, because of the difficulty to time precisely the fetal age, and due to the individual differences, including genetic background of each specimen. Although our system has also its limitations, it offers the possibility to study in function of time the different differentiation steps with the same source of stem cells transferred in a genetically and fetal age identical thymic microenvironment. It is clear that the first human population to emerge is the CD4^{dim+} population. In the mouse, it has been reported that low-CD4 cells represent a very early phase in the T cell development in the thymus. This population is at a phase between the bone-marrow derived stem cell colonizing the thymus and the CD4$^-$CD8$^-$ precursors engaged in T cell rearrangement (12). We did not address whether this CD4^{dim+} cell population differentiates in CD4$^-$CD8$^-$ population or into CD4$^+$ CD8$^+$ population. Our findings are in agreement with those of Alvarez-Vallina et al., who have shown that in human thymus the CD1$^+$CD4$^+$CD8$^-$CD3$^-$ subset contained the highest proportion of cycling cells and concluded that they may represent an early transitional stage between CD4$^-$CD8$^-$ and CD4$^+$CD8$^+$ thymocytes (13).

Our studies provide us with a tool to investigate the effect of cytokines, microbial agents, including HIV, on the differentiation of human T cells in the thymus. It also offers the opportunity to evaluate the hematopoietic stem cell for its T cell differentiation capacity.

ACKNOWLEDGMENTS

We thank Christian De Boever for artwork. This work was supported by grants from VLAB, FGWO and OOA.

REFERENCES

1. Whitlock, C., K. Denis, D. Robertson, and O. Witte. 1985. *In vitro* analysis of murine B-cell development. *Annu. Rev. Immunol.* 3:213.
2. Keller, G. 1992. Hematopoietic stem cells *Curr. Opinion in Immunol.* 4:133.

3. Ezine, S., I. Weissman, and R. Rouse. 1984. Bone marrow cells give rise to distinct clones within the thymus *Nature (Lond.)* 309:629.

4. Goldschneider, I., K.L. Komschlies, and D.L. Greiner. 1986. Studies of thymocytopoiesis in rats and mice. I. Kinetics of appearance of thymocytes using a direct intrathymic adoptive transfer assay for thymocyte precursors. *J. Exp. Med.* 163:1.

5. Guidos, C.J., I.L. Weissman, and B.J. Adkins. 1989. Developmental potential of CD4⁻CD8⁻ thymocytes. Peripheral progeny include mature CD4⁻CD8⁻ T cells bearing *a β* T cell receptor. *J. Immunol.* 142:3773.

6. Williams, G.W., R. Kingston, M.J. Owen and Jenkinson. 1986. A single micromanipulated stem cell gives rise to multiple T-cell receptor gene rearrangements in the thymus *in vitro*. *Nature* 324:6092.

7. Péault, B., I.L. Weissman, C. Baum, J. M. McCune and A. Tsukamoto. 1991. Lymphoid reconstitution of the human fetal thymus in SCID mice with CD34⁺ precursor cells. *J. Exp. Med.* 174:1283.

8. McCune, J.M., R. Nakimawa, R. Kaneshima, L.D., Schultz, M. Lieberman, and I.L. Weismann. 1988. The SCID-hu mouse:murine model for the analysis of human hematolymphoid differentiation and function. *Science (Wash. DC).* 241:1632.

9. Fisher, A.G., L. Larsson, L.K. Goff, D.E. Herstall, L. Happerfield and M. Merckenschlager. 1990. Human thymocyte development in mouse organ cultures. *Int. Immunol.* 2:571.

10. Merckenschlager, M. and A.G. Fisher. 1992. Human postnatal thymocytes generate phenotypically immature CD3(dim), CD5(dim), CD1a(bright) progeny in organ culture. *J. Immunol.* 148:1012.

11. Wucherpfenning, B.K., Y.J. Liao, M. Prendergast, J. Prendergast, D.A. Hafler, and J.L. Strominger. 1993. Human fetal liver γ/δ T cells predominantly use unusual rearrangements of the T cell receptor δ and γ loci expressed on both CD4⁺CD8⁻ and CD4⁻CD8⁻ γ/δ T cells. *J. Exp. Med.* 177:425.

12. Wu, L., R. Scollay, M. Egerton, M. Pearse, G.J. Sprangrude and K. Shortman. 1991. CD4 expressed on earliest T-lineage precursor cells in the adult murine thymus. *Nature* 349:71.

13. Alvarez-Vallina, L., A. Gonzalez, F. Gambon, M. Kreisler, and F. Diaz-Espada. 1993. Delimitation of the proliferative stages in the human thymus indicates that cell expansion occurs before the expression of CD3 (T cell receptor). *J. Immunol.* 150:8.

TOWARDS IDENTIFICATION OF MEMORY B CELLS IN HUMAN TONSILS

Thierry Defrance and Chantal Lagresle

Unité d'Immunologie et Stratégie Vaccinale
Institut Pasteur de Lyon, Avenue Tony Garnier
69365, Lyon Cedex 07, France

INTRODUCTION

Unravelling the mechanisms underlying the generation of B cell memory is an important issue for improvement of the actual modes of vaccination and for the design of new vaccines. However, to this date, our knowledge of the phenotype and properties of memory B cells in humans is still rudimentary, possibly because of the difficulty to assess memory on a functional basis in the human system. It is now widely agreed that memory B cells are generated through a process of positive selection occurring within the germinal centers of secondary follicles. Based on the generally accepted notion that memory B cells express classes of antibodies other than IgM and IgD on their surface, we made the assumption that memory B cells should be searched for in the B cell population lacking expression of surface IgD. Thus, we examined the distribution of several surface markers on purified IgD⁻ B cells isolated from tonsils and found that expression of CD10, CD38 and CD44 distinguished two major B cell subsets among the IgD⁻ B cell compartment. We subsequently separated the two B cell types and performed further phenotypical analysis and functional studies which showed that one of these IgD⁻ B cell populations displays most of the features commonly ascribed to memory B cells. In the present paper we review the experimental data which support this hypothesis and propose a putative scheme of the memory B cell differentiation pathway.

In Vivo Immunology, Edited by E. Heinen *et al.*
Plenum Press, New York, 1994

33

PHENOTYPICAL HETEROGENEITY OF THE IgD⁻ B CELL COMPARTMENT IN TONSILS

The antibodies tested for their reactivity on purified IgD⁻ B cells included monoclonals directed against: germinal center-related antigens (CD38, CD77), follicular mantle-associated molecules (CD39, CD24), a homing receptor (L-selectin/LECAM-1), the CD44/Hermes/Pgp-1 antigen, different Ig heavy chain isotypes (M, G and A), the cell-cycle related antigen Ki67 and the product of the proto-oncogene bcl-2, implicated in cell survival.

The dual parameter fluorescence analysis of purified IgD⁻ B cells performed by combining anti-CD38 and anti-CD44 mAbs revealed that the expression of these two molecules on IgD⁻ B cells was mutually exclusive and delineated two major non-overlapping B cell subsets displaying the following phenotype : IgD⁻/CD38⁺/CD10⁺/CD44⁻ (CD38⁺ B cells) and IgD⁻/CD38⁻/CD10⁻/CD44⁺ (CD38⁻ B cells). Based on this experimental finding, isolation of CD38⁺ and CD38⁻ B cells was subsequently achieved by negative selection using anti-CD44 and anti-CD38 monoclonals, respectively. The purity of both isolated B cell populations was routinely superior to 90%. The phenotypical characteristics of CD38⁺ and CD38⁻ B cells are summarized in Table 1. The positive staining of CD38⁺ B cells obtained with anti-CD10, CD38 and CD77 monoclonals which react with germinal centers (GC) on tonsil tissue sections[1], strongly suggested that this B cell subset was constituted of GC B cells. This hypothesis was further substantiated by the finding that CD38⁺ B cells were highly enriched for cycling cells (Ki67⁺) and vulnerable to apoptotic cell death, as suggested by the virtual lack of Bcl-2 expression in that population. It is likely that a further level of heterogeneity exists in the cellular composition of this B cell subset, as reflected by the fact that CD77 was distributed on only 40% of CD38⁺ B cells. The possibility that CD77 could discriminate centroblasts and centrocytes among the CD38⁺ B cell population is presently being investigated.

In contrast, several lines of evidence argued against a germinal center localization of CD38⁻ B cells : i) they expressed CD44, CD39, CD24 and Bcl-2 which are virtually undetectable in GC, ii) they lacked the typical aforementioned GC B cell markers, iii) they were mainly constituted of non-dividing cells (Ki67⁻). Moreover, the CD44 and L-selectin/LECAM-1 molecules which have been described to be involved in cell homing and recirculation, were both expressed on CD38⁻ B cells, thus suggesting that these cells had acquired migratory competence. The predominant expression of secondary heavy chain isotypes on the surface of CD38⁻ B cells indicated that most of these cells had undergone isotype switching.

Table 1. Phenotypical characteristics of CD38$^+$ and CD38$^-$ B cells

	CD38$^+$ B cells		CD38$^-$ B cells	
CD10	+^{1}		-	
CD24	-		(+)	(70 %)
CD38	+		-	
CD39	-		(+)	(70 %)
CD44	-		+	
CD77	(+)^2	(40 %)	-	
LECAM-1	-		(+)	(30 %)
IgM	(+)	(13 %)	(+)	(26 %)
IgG	(+)	(46 %)	(+)	(44 %)
IgA	(+)	(11 %)	(+)	(23 %)
Ki67	(+)	(70 %)	(+)	(11 %)
Bcl-2	-		(+)	(92 %)

^{1} + the antigen is distributed on the entire population

^{2} (+) the antigen is not distributed on the entire population ; the average proportion of positive cells is indicated in brackets

FUNCTIONAL RESPONSES OF CD38$^+$ AND CD38$^-$ B CELLS

Proliferation and differentiation of isolated CD38$^+$ and CD38$^-$ B cells was examined in three distinct *in vitro* activation systems: ligation of sIgs (immobilized anti-Ig antibodies), ligation of CD40 (soluble anti-CD40 mAb), simultaneous crosslinking of sIgs and CD40. CD38$^+$ B cells were virtually unresponsive to most growth-stimulatory signals applied, but modestly proliferated in response to the IL-4 + anti-CD40 antibody combination. The relatively low proliferative capacity of CD38$^+$ B cells *in vitro* is somewhat contradictory with their high proliferation rate *in vivo*. The absence, in the experimental models described above, of an essential component of the GC microenvironment responsible for their sustained proliferation *in vivo*, could be a possible explanation for this observation. T cells stand as a plausible candidate for that missing component since we have recently observed that contact-mediated signals provided by activated T cells were able to greatly enhance the proliferative response of CD38$^+$ B cells *in vitro*. The differential efficiency of activated T cells and anti-CD40 antibodies to stimulate CD38$^+$ B cells for DNA synthesis raises the possibility that a signalling pathway other than the CD40/CD40 ligand interaction could be instrumental in supporting growth of centroblasts during GC formation.

In striking contrast, CD38⁻ B cells proliferated vigorously and produced large amounts of antibodies in response to cytokines (IL-2, IL-4, IL-10), whatever the activation stimulus applied. IgG constituted by far the predominant Ig isotype secreted by CD38⁻ B cells (92% of the overall Ig production, on average) following *in vitro* stimulation. This finding was consistent with their surface Ig phenotype and demonstrated that CD38⁻ B cells are representative of a mature population enriched for post-switch IgG-committed precursors. Finally, the production of specific IgG antibodies against recall antigens such as measles virus or tetanus toxoid, which can be considered as good indicators of an anamnestic response, was found to be confined to the CD38⁻ B cell subset.

THE PHENOTYPIC AND FUNCTIONAL FEATURES OF CD38⁻ B CELLS ARE CONSISTENT WITH THE DEFINITION OF MEMORY B CELLS

From the large litterature devoted to this field emerge a few characteristic features defining memory B cells (for a review[2,3]) : a) they are long-lived/non-dividing cells, b) they express classes of antibodies other than IgD on their surface, c) they express mutated antibody molecules with high affinity antigen-binding capacities, d) they are migratory competent, e) they express L-selectin/LECAM-1, high levels of CD44 and low levels of the molecule recognized by the mAb J11D (in the mouse). Although we have not addressed the question whether CD38⁻ B cells have undergone somatic mutations, our results indicate that this B cell subset fulfil most of the criteria described above. So far, the exact localization of CD38⁻ B cells on tissue sections has been impaired by the fact that the markers which identify this population are also distributed on follicular-mantle B cells (CD24, CD39, CD44) or on other cell lineages (CD44). However, it is interesting to note that there is a striking similarity between the phenotype of the CD38⁻ B cell population described herein and that of B cells of the marginal zone of the spleen (IgD low/CD39⁺/CD44⁺) reported by others[4]. This would fit with the well-documented notion that memory B cells accumulate in the marginal zones during T-cell-dependent antibody responses in the mouse[5]. Figure 1 depicts the possible steps of the B cell maturation process leading to the generation of memory B cells. Direct evidence that CD38⁻ B cells derive from CD38⁺ B cells was provided by our finding that the latter population gradually lost expression of CD38 and CD10 while acquiring CD44 upon culturing with activated T cells or anti-CD40 antibodies and IL-4.

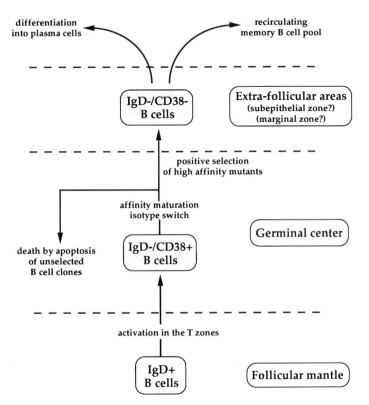

Figure 1. Hypothetical pathway of differentiation of memory B cells

High affinity B cell clones which have been positively selected in the GC have the potential to further differentiate into plasma cells or to integrate the memory B cell pool. If one assumes that CD38⁻ B cells are representative of the whole population of selected high affinity mutants then it is possible that this B cell subset includes both the precursors of plasma cells and those of memory B cells. In line with this hypothesis, the heterogeneous distribution of L-selectin/LECAM-1, CD24 and CD39 on CD38⁻ B cells is evocative of the existence of different maturational stages within this B cell compartment.

REFERENCES

1. D.L. Hardie, G.D. Johnson, M. Khan and I.C.M. MacLennan, Quantitative analysis of molecules which distinguish functional compartments within germinal centers, *Eur. J. Immunol.* 23: 997 (1993).

2. E.S. Vitetta, M.T. Berton, C. Burger, M. Kepron, W.T. Lee and X-M Yin, Memory B and T cells, *Annu. Rev. Immunol.* 9: 193 (1991).

3. D. Gray, Immunological memory, *Annu. Rev. Immunol.* 11: 49 (1993).

4. I.C.M. MacLennan, Y-J Liu, S. Oldfield, J. Zhang and P.J.L. Lane, The evolution of B-cell clones, *Curr. Top. Microbiol. Immunol.* 159: 37 (1990).

5. Y-J. Liu, S. Oldfield, and I.C.M. MacLennan, Memory B cells in T cell-dependent antibody responses colonize the splenic marginal zones, *Eur. J. Immunol.* 18: 355 (1988).

PROLONGED IL-4 TREATMENT DECREASES THE TNP-SPECIFIC MEMORY FORMATION FOR IgG1

René van Ommen and Huub F.J. Savelkoul

Department of Immunology
Erasmus University
Rotterdam
The Netherlands

INTRODUCTION

IL-4 is a pleiotropic lymphokine, produced mainly by activated T-cells, which has a number of activities on B cells[1]. It is obligatory for IgE synthesis, and has an enhancing effect on the IgG_1 production[2]. Whereas it is impossible to detect IgE in nematode infected mice which are made IL-4 deficient by gene targetting, IgG_1 can be detected, but the level is only one-sixth that of control mice[3]. The aim of this study was to investigate the effect of prolonged IL-4 treatment on the total and antigen-specific serum IgG_1 levels. Furthermore, we investigated the effect of such treatment on the memory formation for IgG_1. To that end, BALB/c mice were treated for a period of three months with IL-4 after primary TNP-RIgG immunization. We used a method for cytokine administration that allowed persistent IL-4 levels for a prolonged period of time[4].

MATERIALS AND METHODS

Mice: Female BALB/c mice were bred and maintained at the Department of Immunology of the Erasmus University. All mice were at an age of 12-16 weeks at the start of the experiments. They were held in light-cycled rooms and had access to acidified water and pelleted food ad libitum.

IL-4 treatment: Mice were implanted i.p. with 2×10^6 CV-1/IL-4 cells (kind gift of Dr. N. Arai, DNAX Research Institute, Palo Alto, CA, USA) encapsulated in alinate every two weeks as described earlier[4,5].

Immunization: Rabbit IgG (RIgG) (Sigma Chemical Co., St. Louis, MO, USA) was trinitrophenylated to a level of 25 TNP residues per 10^5 Da of RIgG (as determined spectrophotometrically) by using trinitrobenzenesulphonic acid (Eastman Kodak, Rochester, NY, USA). Mice were injected with 0.2 ml PBS containing either 10 or 100 μg TNP-RIgG adsorbed on 2 mg alum i.p.

In Vivo Immunology, Edited by E. Heinen *et al.*
Plenum Press, New York, 1994

Isotype specific ELISA: Total and TNP-specific IgG_1 levels were measured by isotype-specific ELISA as described previously[5], both with a detection limit of 0.2 ng/ml.

ELISA-spot assay: Nitrocellulose bottomed 96-wells Multiscreen HA plates (Millipore Co., Bedford, MA, USA) were coated with GAM/IgG_1, 1 μg/ml (Southern Biotechnology, Birmingham, AL, USA), and blocked with PBS containing 1% BSA. The plates were then incubated with spleen cell samples for four hours in a humidified and vibration free 5% CO_2 incubator. Plates were washed once with 0.05% Tween 20 in distilled water and twice with PBS containing 0.1% BSA and 0.05% Tween 20. Subsequently, the plates were treated as in a normal ELISA. Development was done by using AEC substrate which was prepared by dissolving 25 mg of 3-amino-9-ethyl carbazole (AEC) (Sigma, St. Louis, MO, USA) in 2 ml dimethylformamide, followed by addition of 95 ml of 0.05 M acetate buffer, pH 5.0 and 40 μl of 30% H_2O_2. The substrate solution was filtered (0.2 μm). Developed plates were dried and the red spots were enumarated under low magnification 10x using a dissecting microscope (Stemi SV 6, Zeiss, Oberkochen, FRG) equipped with a coaxial reflected light source.

Preparation of B cells: Splenic B cells were prepared from control and IL-4 treated mice. T cells were cytotoxically eliminated by treatment of the spleen cells with anti-Thy-1.2 (clone F7D5; Serotec, Oxford, U.K.) and low-tox guinea pig complement (Cederlane, Hornby, Ontario, Canada) in a two-step procedure at 0^0 and 37^0 C, respectively.

T-B cell culture: CDC35, an $I-A^d$ restricted rabbit-Ig specific Th2 clone[6], a kind gift of Dr. D.C. Parker, was maintained by 2-weekly stimulation with irradiated BALB/c spleen cells (30 Gy) and 50 μg/ml rabbit IgG (RIgG) (Sigma) in complete RPMI 1640 medium supplemented with 10% heat inactivated FCS, 2 mM glutamin, 0.1 M pyruvate, 100 IU/ml penicillin, 50 μg/ml streptomycin, 50 μM 2-mercapto-ethanol and 20 IU/ml IL-2. Cells were washed prior to culture with B cells and viability was assessed by trypan blue exclusion. Routinely, viability was >98%. T-cell depleted spleen cells at 2.5×10^5 cells /ml were cultured in 8 replicate wells of flat-bottom microtiter plates together with 5×10^4 cells/ml of irradiated CDC35 cells (30 Gy) in 0.2 ml of complete RPMI 1640 medium at 5% CO_2 and 37^0 C^5. The following antigens were used for stimulation: 30 ng/ml TNP-RIgG, 10 ng/ml TNP-KLH + 10 ng/ml RIgG, 10 ng/ml RIgG, 10 ng/ml RAM/IgE, or 10 ng/ml RAM/IgG_1. After 5 days of culture, cells were harvested for ELISA-spot assay and supernatants for ELISA.

RESULTS

Prolonged IL-4 Treatment Increases Total Serum IgG_1 Levels

Previous studies have demonstrated the involvement of IL-4 in IgG_1 responses *in vivo* and *in vitro*[2]. In order to study the effect of continuous IL-4 treatment during primary immunization on the booster IgG_1 response, mice were immunized with 100 μg TNP-RIgG. Subsequently, mice were treated with recombinant IL-4 by injecting alginate encapsulated CV-1/IL-4 cells every two weeks. This treatment was carried out for three months. During this period the serum level for total IgG_1 increased to a plateau level of 14.5 mg/ml, whereas in control treated mice the level of total serum IgG_1 stayed at 2.1 mg/ml (Figure 1).

To determine if mice with elevated total serum IgG_1 levels were at a plateau for this isotype or still could respond on a secondary immunization, mice were boosted with 10 μg TNP-RIgG. In both groups it was possible to evoke a secondary response with normal kinetics. The total serum IgG_1 level is increased 1.7 mg/ml in the control treated group and 2.6 mg/ml in the IL-4 treated group, between day 4 and 7(Figure 1).

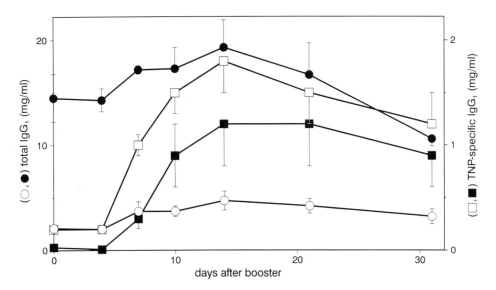

Figure 1. Effect of IL-4 on total and TNP-specific IgG_1 serum levels. Mice were immunized with 100 μg TNP-RIgG adsorbed on alum followed by a control treatment (open symbols) or an IL-4 treatment (closed symbols) every two weeks. Serum levels of total and TNP-specific IgG_1 were determined by ELISA and are expressed as arithmetic mean $\pm$ SEM (n=5).

In IL-4 treated mice the memory TNP-specific IgG_1 response was 29% of the response seen in control treated mice on day 7 (Figure 1). These data suggest that the TNP-specific IgG_1 memory formation is decreased by prolonged IL-4 treatment. Booster immunization did not result in an increase of serum IgG_{2a} levels in control and IL-4 treated mice (data not shown). This indicates that IL-4 treatment does not disturb the isotype regulation during a secondary immune response.

Continuous IL-4 Treatment Increases the Number of IgG_1 and/or IgE Positive-B Cells

A cognate T-B cell culture system previously described[6] was used to determine whether prolonged IL-4 treatment had resulted in an increase of secondary B cells expressing IgG_1 and/or IgE. In this system T cell depleted splenocytes (T cells $<< 2\%$) were stimulated with antigen and CDC35 cells, a Th2 cell-line specific for Rabbit IgG. RAM/IgE and RAM/IgG_1 were used to selectively stimulate ϵ^+ and γ_1^+ B cells. TNP-RIgG was used to stimulate antigen-specific B cells, whereas TNP-KLH and RIgG served as controls.

After five days of culture the number of IgG_1-secreting cells was determined in an ELISA-spotassay. Stimulation with RAM/IgG_1 in the presence of exogenous IL-4 (100 U/ml) revealed an 4.5 fold increase in the number of IgG_1 spot-forming cells (SFC) when compared to control treated mice (Figure 2). A similar increase was seen when no exogenous IL-4 was added during the culture period, although the numbers of IgG_1-SFC in absence of exogenous IL-4 during the culture were lower than when IL-4 was present. These two observations indicate that IL-4 can act as a proliferation factor in this *in vitro* culture system.

The increase of γ_1^+ positive B cells was reflected in the IgG_1 production level. The production of IgG_1 after 5 days of culture of T depleted spleen cells from IL-4 treated mice stimulated with RAM/IgG_1 in the presence of exogenous IL-4 was 4.5 fold higher than when cells from control mice were stimulated. In the absence of IL-4 during the culture period an 13.6 fold increase was observed. No increase in the number of IgG_1-SFC was seen after 5 days of culture with Th2 cells and RAM/IgE when comparing cells from control and IL-4 treated mice (Figure 2), whereas in the same culture more IgG_1 was produced by spleen cells from IL-4 treated mice (Figure 2).

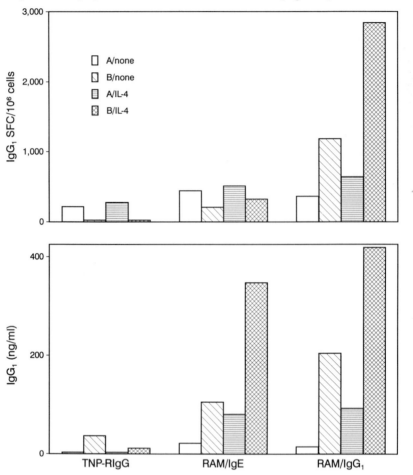

Figure 2. IL-4 treatment increases the number of IgG_1 secondary B cells in the spleen. Thy-1 depleted spleen cells from control treated mice (A) and IL-4 treated mice (B) were cultured with irradiated (30 Gy) CDC35 cells in the presence of either 30 ng/ml TNP-RIgG, 10ng/ml RAM/IgE or 10 ng/ml RAM/IgG$_1$. The number of IgG_1 spot forming cells (SFC) per 10^6 cells and the cumulative IgG_1 production were determined on day 5 by ELISA-spot assay and ELISA, respectively.

A possible explanation for this phenomenon is that during the five days of culture ϵ^+ B cells that were probably also $\gamma_1{}^+$, switch completely to ϵ^+ B cells that are no longer capable of producing IgG_1. This might be the reason that they were not detected in the ELISA-spotassay for IgG_1. IL-4 treatment of mice reduced the number of TNP-specific IgG_1 secreting cells. No IgG_1 secreting cells were found after five days culture of T cell depleted splenocytes of IL-4 treated mice when TNP-RIgG is used as the antigen, whereas in the same situation IgG_1 producing cells were found when cells were used from control treated mice (Figure 2). Prolonged IL-4 treatment also reduced the production of antigen-specific IgG_1 when stimulation took place with RAM/IgG$_1$ (data not shown).

DISCUSSION

The main finding from this study is that prolonged IL-4 treatment after primary immunization with a T cell dependent antigen led to a strong increase in polyclonal but not in antigen-specific IgG_1. The observed effects of IL-4 were specific for IgG_1 as it was shown that the serum IgG_{2a} levels were not influenced by IL-4 treatment. The IgG_1 memory formation specific for TNP decreased as a result of prolonged IL-4 treatment, resulting in a decreased TNP-specific IgG_1 response after booster. On the contrary, the pool of secondary B cells already switched to IgG_1 increased. The use of a culture system in which B cells were stimulated polyclonally in an isotype-specific fashion, independent of their antigenic specificity, allowed this conclusion.

Part of these B cells turned out to be also IgE positive, in that they could be stimulated in a T-B cell culture system by RAM/IgE to produce IgG_1. Such cells have been described by Snapper et al.[7] and are the intermediate cell type in the process of sequential isotype switching from IgM via IgG_1 to IgE[8,9]. Other mechanisms which allow the existence of $\gamma_1 \epsilon$ double positive cells are the alternative splicing of long nuclear RNA and trans-splicing[10]. In both mechanisms switching occurs without DNA recombination.

An explanation for the markedly increased polyclonal IgG_1 production in IL-4 treated mice could be enhanced differentiation of pre-activated B cells as described for IL-6[11] or prolonged survival of pre-activated B cells allowing enhanced clonal out-growth[12]. Another explanation could be the release of the Fc receptor-mediated inhibition of B cell activation by IL-4[13]. This may lead to activation of B cells which can subsequently switch to IgG_1 causing high levels of IgG_1. This high level of polyclonal IgG_1 could possibly inhibit the TNP-specific IgG_1 levels by overruling this antigen-specific response.

Altogether these results indicate that caution has to be taken when IL-4 administration is considered to increase the production of IgG_1 specific for a particular antigen.

Acknowledgments

We thank, Prof.Dr. R. Benner for critically reading the manuscript. This work was supported by the Netherlands Foundation of Medical Research.

REFERENCES

1. Mosmann, T.R., and A. Zlotnik, Springer-Verlag Berlin Heidelberg. A.Habenicht (Ed.); p129 (1990).
2. Finkelman, F. D., J. Holmes, I.M. Katona, J.F. Uraban, M.P. Beckman, L.S. Park, K.A. Schooley, R.L. Coffman, T.R. Mosmann, and W.E. Paul, *Annu. Rev. Immunol.* 8:303 (1990).
3. Kuhn, R., K. Rajewsky, and W. Muller, *Science* 254:707 (1991).
4. Savelkoul, H.F.J., B.W.P. Seymour, L. Sullivan, and R.L. Coffman, *J. Immunol.* 146:1801 (1991).
5. Van Ommen, R., A.E.C.M. Vredendaal, and H.F.J. Savelkoul, Submitted for publication.
6. Tony, H.P., and D.C. Parker, *J. Exp. Med.* 161:223 (1985).
7. Snapper, C.M., F.D. Finkelman, D. Stefany, D.H. Conrad, and W.E. Paul. *J. Immunol.* 141:489 (1988).
8. Yoshida, K., M. Matsuoka, S. Usuda, A. Mori, K. Ishizaka, and H. Sakano. *Proc. Natl. Acad. Sci. USA.* 87:7829 (1990).
9. Mandler, R., F.D. Finkelman, A.D. Levine, and C.M. Snapper. *J. Immunol.* 150:407 (1993).
10. Harriman, W., H. Volk, N. Defranoux, and M. Wabl. *Annu. Rev. Immunol.* 11:361 (1993).
11. Croft, M., and S.L. Swain, *J. Immunol.* 146:4055 (1991).
12. Hodgkin, P.D., N.F. Go, J.E. Cupp, and M. Howard, *Cell. Immunol.* 134:14 (1991).
13. Sinclair, N.R.StC., and A. Panoskaltsis, 1988. *Curr. Opin. in Immunol.* 1:228 (1988).

SELECTION OF ANTI-ARSONATE IDIOTYPE (CRIA) IN A/J MICE BY THE IMMUNE NETWORK

Maryse Brait, Marion Ryelandt, Jamila Ismaili, Robert Miller*, Georgette Vansantem, Roy Riblet* and Jacques Urbain

Laboratoire de Physiologie Animale, Université Libre de Bruxelles, 67, rue des Chevaux, 1640 Rhode St Genese, Belgium
* Medical Biology Institute, La Jolla, Ca 92037, USA

INTRODUCTION

A/J mice immunized against arsonate (ARS) coupled to hemocyanin (KLH) synthesize a cross reactive idiotype named CRIA (Kuettner et al., 1972). This idiotype is encoded by a single combination of genes called the canonical combination which is constituted of one VH gene (VHIdCR11), one D segment (DFL16.1), one JH segment (JH2), one VK gene (VKIdCR) and one JK segment (JK1).

The extensive studies of Gefter group (Manser et al., 1987 and references therein) have shown that during the primary response, several genetical combinations are used, i.e. the VHIdCR11 is associated with different D, JH segments and Kappa light chains. But as the response proceeds, the canonical combination emerges and dominates the secondary immune response. This germ line combination is the target of a somatic hypermutation mechanism which gives rise to a set of variants. The antigen selects the higher affinity variants, leading to affinity maturation of the anti-arsonate response.

Our laboratory has prepared a set of monoclonal anti-idiotypic antibodies which allows an extensive idiotypic study of the anti-arsonate response (Leo et al., 1985). Together with the group of Capra, we have defined several idiotopes on CRIA positive antibodies (Jeske et al., 1986; Hasemann and Capra, 1991). One of which named 2D3 is located in the second hypervariable region of the germline VHIdCR11; three other idiotopes (E3, E4, H8) are mainly assigned to the D-JH part of the CRIA molecules. We can easily follow the emergence of the canonical combination in term of E3, E4, H8 and 2D3 positive antibodies.

It is widely assumed that the dominance of recurrent CRIA idiotype is due to a Darwinian clonal selection of the canonical combination. This genetic combination is able to sustain the ability to generate useful somatic variants of higher affinity for the antigen (Manser et al., 1984).

Using these anti-idiotypic antibodies, our group has published some data which do not fit with the classical interpretation of the recurrence of the CRIA idiotype (Willems et al., 1990). Namely when naive irradiated A/J mice are reconstituted with syngeneic naive bone marrow or spleen cells (around 2x107 cells) and are subsequently immunized with arsonate-KLH, the anti-arsonate response exhibits a normal level of anti-arsonate antibodies if we compare with the non irradiated A/J mice but there is a dramatic repertoire shift. The CRIA idiotype does not dominate the anti-arsonate response (2D3+/-, E3-, E4-). Moreover there is a lack of affinity maturation although an increase in anti-arsonate antibody levels occurs between the primary and secondary responses and class switching is nearly normal in irradiated recipients. Naive irradiated A/J mice with limbs partially shielded in order to allow self reconstitution give rise to anti-arsonate response with the same characteristics. This phenomenon is observed in 75-80% of irradiated recipients and persists as long as two months after irradiation.

At first sight these observations are highly paradoxical since the absence of CRIA per se cannot explain the lack of affinity maturation. Other CRIA negative but anti-arsonate binding B cells can undergo somatic mutations and exhibit affinity maturation. This is the law imposed by the clonal selection. Several groups have shown that after idiotypic suppression of the CRIA, immunization with arsonate-KLH leads to a very efficient anti-arsonate response, devoided of CRIA but displaying a similar or even higher affinity for the antigen (Gaya et al., 1988).

Our observations suggest that in some way the immunological memory is impaired in irradiated recipients reconstituted with naive lymphoide cells. Some hallmarks of immunological memory are expressed, anti-arsonate antibody titers increase between primary and secondary responses and a nearly normal class switching is observed but other hallmarks, affinity maturation and idiotype expression are lost.

To explain these data, we have analyzed several non exclusive working hypotheses.

RESULTS

Could these results be due to irradiation effects? The killing of cells by irradiation could lead to the release of self antigens which could anergize the CRIA B cell clones or irradiation could induce retrovirus expression including superantigens which could alter the T cell repertoire. To assess these problems, we repopulated non irradiated Scid mice with naive spleen cells from C.AL-20 mice (the C.AL-20 strain bears the IgH locus from AL/N and is therefore a CRIA expressor). The anti-arsonate response of such reconstituted Scid mice displays the same phenomenon, namely the absence of the CRIA idiotype.

On the other hand, transfer of Ars-KLH primed spleen cells into naive irradiated recipients does give rise to CRIA idiotype expression and affinity maturation. This clearly suggests that the irradiated environment is not "hostile" to idiotype expression.

Could these results be explained just by statistical factors? Is the loss of idiotype dominance due to a too low frequency of CRIA precursor cells in the inoculum? Although this hypothesis may a part of the explanation it cannot explain the lack of affinity maturation in the anti-arsonate response. We tried to increase the number of naive donor cells up to 108. Increasing numbers of normal spleen cells do not improve the dominance of CRIA idiotype and do not restore affinity maturation.

Could these results be due to the absence of one particular subpopulation of T or B lymphocytes? In our previous work and in unpublished data, we have been unable to restore idiotype expression and affinity maturation by supplying naive irradiated and partially shielded A/J mice with naive peritoneal cells or T cells primed against KLH (Willems et al., 1990). Since our observations suggest clearly that the immunological memory is impaired, we considered the possibility that the missing subpopulation could belong to the J11D low B cell subset. The work of Klinman's group has shown that memory B cells and primary B cells belong to two distinct lineages (J11D low and J11D high B cells) (Linton et al., 1989). A large part of splenic B lymphocytes bind the J11D monoclonal antibody (this antibody reacts with the heat stable antigen). Traitment of naive spleen cells with anti-Thy-1 supernatant and J11D supernatant plus complement leads to recover 10 to 15 % of immunoglobulin positive cells with low binding of J11D monoclonal antibody.

To assess the potential role of J11D low spleen cells, we transferred highly enriched naive J11D low B lymphocytes into KLH primed irradiated A/J mice. Several experimental designs were explored. The figure depicts one of them.

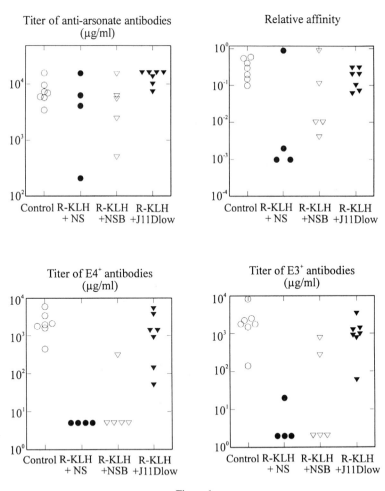

Figure 1.

KLH carried primed irradiated A/J mice were transferred either with 1.5x107 naive spleen cells (R-KLH+NS) or with 1.5x107 naive spleen cells depleted in Thy-1+ cells (R-KLH+NSB) or with 5x107 naive spleen cells depleted in Thy-1+ and J11D high cells (R-KLH+J11Dlow). The secondary anti-arsonate responses of these experimental groups were compared to the response of normal A/J mice immunized with Ars-KLH (control). Only mice engrafted with J11D low B cells express the recurrent CRIA idiotype in the same manner as control mice. Other groups are largely devoid of CRIA expression. Although there is great variability in the other groups among relative affinity determinations, only control mice and J11D low reconstituted mice display strong affinity maturation. Fifty percent of carrier primed A/J mice transferred with 2x106 J11D low exhibit idiotype expression (data not shown).

DISCUSSION AND CONCLUSIONS

These data suggest strongly that the J11D low B cell subset plays a major role in the recurrent CRIA idiotype expression and in affinity maturation of the anti-arsonate response. Nevertheless it is intriguing that an inoculum of 108 spleen cells (which includes approximately 1.5x107 J11D low B cells) did not lead to idiotype expression and affinity maturation. Perhaps the environment of irradiated recipients favors the proliferation and the engraftment of the J11D high cells at the expense of the J11D low cells. From our results and that of others (Linton et al., 1989), J11D high B cells will be unable to give rise to adaptative responses i.e. affinity maturation either there is no mutation or somatic mutations occur but there is no selection. Experiments are underway to distinguish between these possibilities.

Our data lead us to a major paradox. The J11D low B cell subset has a special repertoire, already selected before antigen arrival. We have transferred naive J11D low B cells. Moreover Ryelandt et al. (1993) have shown that the presence of arsonate in the perinatal period does not induce tolerance to arsonate but provokes selectively the loss of the CRIA expression during subsequent arsonate immunization. It seems therefore that the J11D low subset with its special repertoire including the CRIA idiotype is present very early during the development of the immune system. How can we explain the selection of this special repertoire in a period where only self antigens are present? Since the anti-arsonate response is not an autoimmune response only immunological self can select the CRIA idiotype i.e. auto anti-idiotypic antibodies. The repertoire of the J11D low B cells could be built by idiotypic network and the presence of arsonate in immature system prevents these idiotypic selections. Some recurrent idiotypes could be in fact anti-antiself antibodies. This is formalized by Urbain et al., (1989) in the Broken Mirror Hypothesis.

Our data suggest that the Darwinian game, proposed by Gefter, operates on a subset of B lymphocytes which is preselected before antigen arrival.

Acknowledgments

We are indebted to Dr. Klinman, N., and Dr. Linton, P.J., for their numerous suggestions and for providing us the reagents needed in this study. This work presents research results of the Belgian programme on Interuniversity Poles of attraction initiated by the Belgian State, Prime Minister's Office, Science Policy Programming. The Scientific responsability is assumed by its authors.

REFERENCES

Kuttner, M.G., Wang, A., and Nisonoff, A., 1972, Quantitative investigations of idiotypic antibodies, J. Exp. Med. 135:579.

Manser, T., Wysocki, M., Margolies, N., and Gefter, M.L., 1987, Evolution of antibody variable structure during the immune response, Immunol. Rev. 96:141.

Leo, O., Slaoui, M., Marvel, J., et al., 1985, Idiotypic analysis of polyclonal and monoclonal anti-p-azophenylarsonate antibodies of BALB/c mice expressing the major cross-reactive idiotype of the A/J strain, J. Immunol. 134:1734.

Jeske, D., Milner, E.C.B., Leo, O., Moser, M., Marvel, J., Urbain, J., and Capra, J.D., 1986, Molecular mapping of idiotopes of anti-arsonate antibodies, J. Immunol. 136:2568.

Hasemann, C., and Capra, J.D., 1991, Mutational analysis of the crossreactive idiotype of the A strain, J. Immunol. 147:3170.

Manser, T., Huang, S.Y., and Gefter, M.L., 1984, Influence of clonal selection on the expression of immunoglobulin variable region gene, Science 226:1283.

Willems, F., Vansantem, G., De Wit, D., Slaoui, M., and Urbain, J.,1990, Loss of a major idiotype (CRIA) after repopulation of irradiated mice, J. Immunol. 144:1396.

Gaya, A., Alsinet, E., Freixas, M., and Vives, J., 1988, Change in idiotypic predominance in the anti-arsonate response by priming with anti-idiotypic antibodies, Scand. J. Immunol. 28:331.

Linton, P.J., Decker, D., and Klinman, N., 1989, Primary antibody forming cells and secondary B cells are generated from separate precursor cell subpopulations, Cell 59:1049.

Ryelandt, M., De Wit, D., Baz, A., et al., 1993, The perinatal presence of antigen (p-azophenylarsonate) leads to the loss of the recurrent idiotype (CRIA) in A/J mice, submitted.

Urbain, J., Andris, F., Brait, M., et al., 1989, Self-nonself discrimination in the immune system: a broken idiotypic mirror. in the Molecular Basis of the Immune Response. Ed. Bona, C., Ann. N.Y. Acad. of Sci. 546:43.

NONLYMPHOID EFFECTOR AND REGULATORY CELLS

THE LIFE HISTORY AND FUNCTIONAL ROLES OF ACCESSORY CELLS

Sigbjørn Fossum

Immunobiological laboratory
Institute of Basic Medical Sciences
University of Oslo, N-0317 Oslo

1. Accessory cells - ambiguities of the term

Implicit in the designation "accessory cells" is a depiction of the immune system with lymphocytes throning as the ruling class and other leukocytes humbly serving accessory roles. This depiction is fallacious, and for more than one reason. It does not take into account that non-lymphoid cells (NLC) may act independently of lymphocytes, in non-adaptive responses; it obscures the interdependence and interactions of the various members of the immune system; and it envisages our defence system as enrolling only bone marrow derived cells. Immune organs also contain locally derived or autochtonous cells (1), that influence and regulate leukocyte behaviour, selection, proliferation, maturation, migration and immune reactivity. If we take into account also these non-leukocytes, enlist all the cell categories of the immune system, and simply classify them according to origin and migratory behaviour, we get the following scheme:

Table 1 - cell types of immune organs.

Nomads and progeny	Immigrants	Natives
B cells	NK cells	Endothelial cells
B blasts	Dendritic leukocytes	(blood and lymph)
germinocytes	Macrophages	Pericytes
plasma cells	Granulocytes	Fibroblasts/reticulum cells
T cells	Mast cells	Follicular dendritic cells (?)
T blasts	Follicular dendritic	Reticuloepithelial cells
	cells (?)	M cells

The "accessory cell" concept originated with in vitro analyses of B and T cell responses, with the realization that another cell type, which was not a T or B cell had to be present in the mixtures to elicit full-blown responses, in other words the accessory function was first described for the afferent or induction phase of adaptive responses. Today the concept is more complicated. First, the term is context dependent: the same cell types may support lymphocytes in adaptive responses and exercise their functions in non-adaptive responses independent of lymphocytes. Second, even within the domain of adaptive responses the use of the word varies; whereas some authors use "accessory cell" synonymously with "antigen presenting cell", others use it to denote any cell that interact with lymphocytes in their development or that collaborate with lymphocytes in the different phases of adaptive immune responses, as summarized in the following table.

Table 2 - roles of non-lymphoid cells in adaptive immune responses

afferent limb	central limb	efferent limb
Antigen transport	Lymphocyte education	Secretion of
Antigen processing	and selection	inflammatory mediators
Antigen presentation	Antibody affinity maturation	Secretion of
	TH1 vs TH2 responses	antimicrobial agents
	Downregulation of immune	Phagocytosis
	responses	Cell mediated
	Lymphocyte migration	cytotoxicity

2. The life history of dendritic leukocytes (DL) as compared with follicular dendritic cells (FDC) and macrophages (Mφ)

The many cell types that can be labeled accessory, at least in the broadest sense of the term, necessitates selecting the cells to describe. To many immunologists DL represent the archetypal accessory cell; they function primarily in the induction phase of the immune response and seem to be the only cell type capable of stimulating naive T cells (2,3). FDC are central actors in B cell memory formation and antibody affinity maturation, whereas the role of macrophages in stimulating immune responses is still controversial. Here I shall briefly outline what is known about the life history of DL, and where relevant make comparisons with Mφ and FDC.

Origins. DL originate from the bone marrow, as do Mφ. Some workers refer to DL as dendritic macophages, but their relationship to the mononuclear phagocytes system is unclear. Mφ and DL do indeed have several features in common, including phenotypic markers (4). Cell lineage, however, is not a question of markers or functions, but of ontogenetic relationships. Although Mφ and DL appear to have a common bone marrow progenitor (5,6), so do Mφ and neutrophils. If the further differentiation pathway from this progenitor within the bone marrow is separate for Mφ and DL, so that they leave as distinct cell types which do not interconvert in the periphery, there is no more reason to include DL in the mononuclear phagocyte system than to include neturophils. The identity of this progenitor cell is not yet established, but it has recently been shown to be responsive to GM-CSF (6). FDC are sometimes included among DL, partly because of the similarities in names. Until recently the balance of evidence has favoured a local origin of FDC (7) from particular subsets of reticulum cells or reticular fibroblasts (8), but new studies with bone-marrow chimeraes points to a bone marrow origin and possibly a relation to DL (Kapasi et al., this volume).

Migratory routes. DL precursors, probably with monocyte-like features, continuously leave the bone marrow. Despite a massive output to account for the rapid turnover of the peripheral populations, the blood-borne precursors, whatever their identity, can make up only a limited fraction of blood leukocytes, which means that their transit time in blood is short. DL are present in almost all tissues, the most notable exceptions being the brain and the cornea (9). They exhibit somewhat different phenotypes within the various tissues, in particular do Langerhans cells differ from other DL as found e.g. in the gut lamina propria. Microenvironment dependent phenotypic heterogeneity is also a characteristic of Mφ (10,11). The variability probably arises from dissimilar local stimuli, but the possibility remains that it reflects heterogeneous precursors homing to different sites.

At least some DL (4) as well as some Mφ (12) leave the tissues via afferent lymphatics to enter the draining lymph nodes. The fractions proceeding from the peripheral tissues are not known; at least for Mφ it is likely that the majority die in the periphery (12), whereas we can only make guesses about DL. The majority of NLC within the peripheral lymph are DL, indicating that more DL than Mφ proceed from the periphery to the lymph nodes, although this is suggestive and by no means conclusive.

The influx of NLC into lymph nodes is substantial, with flow rates in the sheep of $3x10^5$, $4x10^5$ and $9x10^5$ cells/h in the periperal lymph from limbs, testis and liver, respectively (13). Within the marginal sinus they adhere to and penetrate the lymphendothelium facing the underlying cortex (14) and then proceed to the paracortex where they transform into IDC (15). It should be emphasized that reinjected lymph DL did not enter the thymus, which seems to negate theories that DL sample antigen in the periphery and then proceed to the thymus where they induce tolerance in developing thymocytes. Neither were they found in the lymph node follicles (15), which is of relevance to the claims that FDC may develop from lymph-borne NLC. If FDC do develop from bone-marrow derived precursors, it is unclear how they reach the follicles, but the rate of immigration is likely to be exceedingly low as in mouse bone marrow chimeraes FDC were of donor phenotype even a year after transplantation (7).

There are much fewer NLC in central lymph than in peripheral lymph and no evidence that they leave with the blood, signifying that most are retained and die in the lymph nodes. After having entered the lymph nodes, IDC survive for 1 -2 weeks (4). DL do not enter lymph nodes directly from the blood, i.v. injected intestinal DL go primarily to the liver and the spleen (15). From the liver at least some proceed to the draining celiac lymph nodes, whereas in the spleen they go to the PALS. I.v. injected DL isolated from the spleen also return to the spleen, where they leave the blood stream at the marginal zone to enter the PALS after a curious detour via the red pulp (16).

Transit times, kinetics and fates. It is unclear whether or to what extent peripheral division occurs among DL, but a small fraction of Langerhans cells do divide within the epidermis (rev in 4). After a single i.v. shot of ^{3}H-thymidine labeled DL can be detected in the rat intestinal lymph in less than 24 h. If we disregard the possibility of peripheral division, this gives a minimal transit time of much less than 24 h, as the cells must first finish the last division in the bone marrow, mature sufficiently to leave with blood, and enter the lamina propria before they negotiate their passage to the lymph. With continuous i.v. infusions of ^{3}H-thymidine one can obtain estimates for average transit times from the fractions of unlabeled cells. In the rat, about half the intestinal lymph DL were still unlabeled by day 4, a fraction that had decreased to 7 % by day 10. A semilogarithmic plot gave a straight line, indicating that intestinal DL enter the lymph by random and that they, despite phenotypic variability, make up a single population (unpublished). Following antigenic challenge the influx of DL via lymphatics to the draining lymph nodes is increased (17), but the regulating factors are unknown.

There are up to now few published measurements for the turnover rates of DL within various organs. Bone marrow chimeric studies showed a turnover rate between up to 4 weeks in the rat heart and kidney (9) and up to 7 weeks in the skin (18). These estimates are clearly longer than those of the transit times through the rat gut lamina propria of 4 days. The discrepancies may reflect tissue differences; or that only young DL proceed to the lymph, whereas older DL remain stuck and die in situ; or that the DL that enter peripheral lymph represent a special subpopulation; or, alternatively, that the irradiation and transplantation procedures involved in the chimaeric studies give erroneous results, e.g. the transplanted cells may need time to settle and colonize the bone marrow before export can proceed. Within the lymph nodes the DL remain for up to 2 weeks before dying (unpublished). In the rat spleen and thymus estimates of turnover rates are 2-4 weeks (19).

Mφ also have a rapid turnover, measured in weeks rather than months (12). They do divide in the periphery, but only to a limited extent (12). In contrast, for reasons argued above, if FDC are bone marrow derived they must have a slow turnover. Curiously, they are frequently bi- or even trinucleated (20), indicating occurence of peripheral DNA synthesis and nuclear division without cell division. The ultimate fates of DL, Mφ and FDC are not known. DL probably die within the lymph nodes and spleen, but although the rate of death is high, considering the massive influx and rapid turnover, there are surprisingly few signs of dying DL. It is not known whether death is stochastic or deterministic, i.e. whether they die from senility at a certain age.

3. Functions

That DL are the prime antigen presenting cells for naive T cells is by now well established (2,3). DL have also been shown to transport antigen from the periphery to the draining lymph nodes (21,22), but whether this is valid only for selected antigens or is a general rule is yet unknown. The formidable migratory stream of cells proceeding from the bone marrow via peripheral tissues to the draining lymph nodes is certainly suggestive for an antigen transporting role, with the lymph node paracortex as the crossing point between two different streams of migratory cells, the immigrating DL, vectorially transporting and presenting antigen, and the nomadic T cells. The DL also undergo phenotypic changes along these routes (fig 1, table 3), which has been interpreted as evidence that they may endocytose and process antigen at an early stage and then later upregulate MHC II antigen and transform to predominantly presenting cells (rev in (23)). However, knowledge about the life history of DL is still too patchy to allow final conclusions, and the disturbing fact remains that DL within the T areas of lymph nodes and spleen are voracious phagocytes of allogeneic lymphocytes (4). The evidence for the role of thymic DL in negative selection or tolerance induction is still circumstantial; the idea of DL sampling self antigens in the periphery and presenting to the developing thymocytes seems not to be compatible with migration studies described above.

The functional role of FDC seems to be mainly restricted to antigen presentation to B cells, in particular to germinocytes, of importance for induction of B cell memory formation, antibody affinity formation and possible class switch (23). The roles of macrophages are extensive, particularly in the central and efferent limbs of the immune response, whereas they seem inept in stimulating naive T cells. Here I would only like to point to the the yet largely unexplored roles of these cell types in the morphogenetic development of lympoid tissues. It is thus conceivable that e.g. DL contribute to the development of T areas in the lymphoid tissues. These areas, like the lymph node paracortex and the PALS, organize and are filled with DL in the absence of T cells (14). In the athymic nude rats even the specialized high endothelial venules of the paracortex are present (although with walls flatter than normal) and able to bind and transmit injected T cells. The microenvironmental factors responsible for stimulating the vessels to become HEV and for attracting and retaining T cells are not known, but DL may be important organizatory elements in this development.

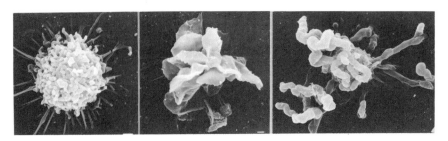

Fig. 1. Scanning micrographs of DL as found in the rat intestinal lymph. Bars 1μm.

Table 3. Functional characteristics of DL along their migratory routes from bone marrow to lymph nodes

Bone marrow ⇒	Blood ⇒	Peripheral tissues ⇒	Lymph ⇒	Lymph nodes
- division - maturation - diversification?	- distribution	- endocytosis - phenotypic and - functional changes - diversification? - division? - antigen presentation? - death?	- antigen transport - antigen presentation	- phenotypic changes - phagocytosis - microenvironmental influences? - death

References

1. Hoefsmit, E.C. 1975. Mononuclear phagocytes, reticulum cells and dendritic cells in lymphoid tissues. In Mononuclear phagocytes in immunity, infection and pathology. R. van Furth, editor. Blackwell Scientific Publications, Oxford. 129-146.

2. Austyn, J.M. 1987. Lymphoid dendritic cells. *Immunology* 62:161.

3. Steinman, R.M. 1991. The dendritic cell system and its role in immunogenicity. *Ann. Rev. Immunol.* 9:271.

4. Fossum, S. 1989. The life history of dendritic leukocytes (DL). In Current topics in pathology. O. H. Iversen, editor. Springer-Verlag, Berlin Heidelberg. 101-124.

5. Klinkert, W.E.F. 1984. Rat bone marrow precursors develop into dendritic accessory cells under the influence of a conditional medium. *Immunobiol* 168:414.

6. Inaba, K., M. Inaba, M. Deguchi, K. Hagi, R. Yasumizu, S. Ikehara, and R. M. Steinman. 1993. Granulocytes, macrophages and dendritic cells arise from a common major histocompatibility complex class II-negative progenitor in the mouse bone marrow. *Proc Natl Acad Sci USA* 90:3038.

7. van Furth, R. 1989. Origin and turnover of monocytes and macrophages. In Cell kinetics of the inflammatory reaction. O. H. Iversen, editor. Springer Verlag, Berlin. 125-150.

8. Dijkstra, C.D., E. W. A. Kamperdijk, and E. A. Døpp. 1984. The ontogenetic development of the follicular dendritic cell. An ultrastructural study by means of intravenously injected horseradish peroxidase (HRP)-anti-HRP complexes as marker. *Cell Tissue Res.* 236:203.

9. Hart, D.N.J. and J. W. Fabre. 1981. Demonstration and characterization of Ia-positive dendritic cells in the interstitial connective tissues of rat heart and other tissues, but not brain. *J Exp Med* 153:347.

10. Dijkstra, D.C., E. A. Döpp, P. m. Joling, and G. Kraal. 1985. The heterogeneity of mononuclear phagocytes in lymphoid organs: distinct macrophage subpopulations in rat recognized by monoclonal antibodies ED1, ED2 and ED3. *Adv Exp Med Biol* 186:409.

11. Damoiseaux, J.G.M.C., E. A. Döpp, J. J. Neefjes, R. H. J. Beelen, and C. D. Dijkstra. 1989. Heterogeneity of macrophages in the rat evidenced by variability in determinants: two new anti-rat macrophage antibodies against a heterodimer of 160 and 95 kD (CD11/CD18). *Journal of Leukocyte Biol.* 46:556.

12. Kaplan, G., A. Nusrat, M. D. Witmer, I. Nath, and Z. A. Cohn. 1987. Distribution and turnover of Langerhans cells during delayed immune responses in human skin. *J. Exp. Med.* 165:763.

13. Smith, J.B., G. H. McIntosh, and B. Morris. 1970. The traffic of cells through tissues: a study of peripheral lymph in sheep. *J. Anat.* 107:87.

14. Fossum, S. 1980. The architecture of rat lymph nodes. II. Lymph node compartments. *Scand. J. Immunol.* 12:411.

15. Fossum, S. 1988. Lymph-borne dendritic leukocytes do not recirculate, but enter the lymph node paracortex to become interdigitating cells. *Scand. J. Immunol.* 27:97.

16. Kupiec-Weglinski, J.W., J. M. Austyn, and P. J. Morris. 1988. Migration patterns of dendritic cells in the mouse. Traffic from the blood, and T cell-dependent and -independent entry to lymphoid tissues. *J Exp Med* 167:632.

17. Kamperdijk, E.W.A., E. M. Raaymakers, J. H. S. de Leeuw, and E. C. M. Hoefsmit. 1982. Lymph node macrophages and reticulum cells in the immune response. The secondary   response to paratyphoid vaccine. *Cell Tissue Res.* 227:277.

18. Chen, H.-D., C. Ma, J. -T. Yuan, Y. -K. Wang, and W. K. Silvers. 1986. Occurence of donor Langerhans cells in mouse and rat chimeraes and their replacement in skin grafts. *J Invest Dermatol* 86:630.

19. Highnam, S.D.M. 1983. Chapter 6: Dendritic cell chimaeras. Ph.D. thesis. University of Oxford, Oxford.

20. Silberberg-Sinakin, I., G. J. Thorbecke, R. L. Baer, S. A. Rosenthal, and V. Berezowsky. 1976. Antigen-bearing Langerhans cells in skin, dermal lymphatics and in lymph nodes. *Cell. Immunol.* 25:137.

21. Macatonia, S.E., S. C. Knight, A. J. Edwards, S. Griffiths, and P. Fryer. 1987. Localization of antigen on lymph node dendritic cells after exposure to the contact sensitizer fluorescein isothiocyanate. Functional and morphological studies. *J. Exp. Med.* 166:1654.

22. Austyn, J.M. 1992. Antigen uptake and presentation by dendritic leukocytes. *Seminars in Immunology.* 4: 227.

23. Liu, Y-J., Johnson, G.D., Gordon, J. and MacLennan,I.C.M. 1992. Germinal centres in T-cell-dependent antibody responses. *Immunol Today.* 13: 17.

THE ROLE OF MACROPHAGES IN REGENERATION OF SPLENIC TISSUE AFTER AUTOLOGOUS TRANSPLANTATION IN RAT

Ellis Barbé, Ed A. Döpp, Jan G.M.C. Damoiseaux, Timo K. van den Berg and Christien D. Dijkstra

Dept. of Cell Biology, Division Histology, Medical Faculty, Vrije Universiteit, Amsterdam

INTRODUCTION

Lymphoid tissues are strictly organized in separated compartments populated by different immune-competent cells. Between these compartments differences exist in the composition of stromal components (Van den Berg et al. 1989). In general, stromal components in lymphoid tissue can be devided into cellular- and extra- cellular components.

There are two major groups of stromal cells. The first group consist of cells which derive from local mesenchymal progenitor cells (Heuserman et al. 1982). An important cell in this group is the reticulum cell, which is characterized by its special relationship to fibers. Cells of the mononuclear phagocyte system constitute the second group of stromal cells. In contrast to the first group these cells are of bone marrow origin (Van Furth 1982). It is a heterogenous population of cells with many different functions in the aspecific defence and the specific immune respons. A relative underestimated function of these cells is their contribution to the microenvironment of lymphoid tissue. A particular population of MΦ, appears to be directly involved in proliferation and differentiation of immune-competent cells (Damoiseaux 1991). However, the exact role of stromal cells and extra cellular components in the formation of compartments is still unknown.

In this paper, the role of MΦ in the development of the splenic microenvironment is being investigated. Therefore, the effect of MΦ elimination on the regenerative capacity of autologous splenic implants is studied. For the characterization of different stromal cell types, a panel of ED monoclonal antibodies (Mabs) is used, recognizing different MΦ subpopulations (Dijkstra et al. 1985) and reticular components (Van den Berg et al. 1989). MΦ were depleted from the spleen by i.v. injection of dichloromethylene-diphosphonate (clodronate, Cl_2MDP)(Van Rooijen & Claassen 1988). We found that depletion of spleen MΦ before transplantation affects the regeneration of the splenic implant to a great extend.

In Vivo Immunology, Edited by E. Heinen *et al.*
Plenum Press, New York, 1994

MATERIALS AND METHODS

Animals

Young adult Wistar rats were obtained from HDS/CPD, Zeist, The Netherlands, and kept under routine laboratory conditions.

Autologous transplantation technique

Splenectomy was performed in 26 rats (Tavassoli et al. 1973). The spleens were cut into 6 pieces of 0.5 cm thickness and placed in the subcutaneous tissue of the abdomen of the same animal. Implants were removed: 7, 14, 21 and 28 days after transplantation. immunohistochemistry was performed on cryostat sections of the implants. Mabs that were used are summarized in table 1.

Macrophage elimination technique

Spleen MΦ were eliminated by i.v. injection of 2 ml liposomes containing Cl$_2$MDP (Van Rooijen & Claassen 1988)

Experimental design

Group A: a control group of 6 rats received no treatment before transplantation.
Group B: 6 rats received a single i.v. injection of liposomes containing Cl2MDP, 5 days before transplantation.
Group C: 6 rats received an i.v. injection of liposomes containing Cl2MDP, 5 days before transplantation. Thereafter they received injections 3, 10 17 and 24 days after transplantation to prevent the influx of MΦ in the implant.

Table 1. Summary of the applied Moabs.

Mab	Specificity in the spleen	References
ED1	Monocytes, MΦ, dendritic cells	Dijkstra et al. 1985
ED3	Recognizes sialoadhesin on marginal zone MΦ and marginal metallophilic MΦ in the spleen.	Dijkstra et al. 1985, Damoiseaux et al. 1991, Van den Berg et al. 1992a
ED14	Recognizes a stromal component found in all compartments of the spleen, probably associated with reticular fibers and extra cellular matrix.	Van den Berg et al. 1989
HIS14	Recognizes kappa chain on B cells	Kroese et al. 1987
OX34	Recognizes CD2 on T cells and splenic MΦ	He 1988

RESULTS

Group A

After almost complete necrosis, the control implants regenerated within 28 days into tissue with a structure almost indistinghuisable from normal spleen as has been described before (Tavassoli et al. 1973, Dijkstra & Langevoort 1982) .

In the first 7 days, a rim of viable cells containing ED1 positive MΦ, that surrounded the necrotic centre of the implant, was observed. After 14 until 21 days, the viable rim increased in size, compared to the necrotic centre. In the viable rim newly formed reticular fibers were observed as was shown by the ED14 Mab. On day 14, a new white pulp started to be formed; reticular fibers that accompanied new central arterioles in the viable rim, were observed. At the same time, separated accumulations of lymphoid cells were seen around these arterioles. A fine meshwork of fibers within the centres of the periarteriolar lymphocyte sheaths (PALS) was developed after 21 days. A subpopulation of ED3 MΦ started to surround the lymphocyte accumulations like the marginal metallophillic MΦ (fig. 1a). On day 28, splenic tissue with a clear red pulp as well as white pulp was seen. Separated B- and T cell compartments could be observed in the new white pulp. There was no necrotic centre observed at this time (fig. 1b).

Group B and C

The implants of rats which were treated with a single i.v. injection of Cl₂MDP before transplantation, showed a decreased tendency to regenerate. The regeneration of the reticulum was strongly disturbed (fig. 2a). Only thick and diffuse reticular components were observed, whereas the delicate meshwork, which is present in control implants, was completely absent. In addition, only a few accumulations of lymphocytes were found, B- and T cell areas herein could not be distinghuised. A small number of swollen MΦ could be observed in the small viable rim surrounding the still large necrotic centre (fig. 2b).

The implants of rats that received multiple i.v. injections of Cl₂MDP before and after transplantation to prevent the influx of MΦ in the implants, showed an even more impaired tendency to regenerate. No newly formed reticular components were seen (fig. 2c). After 28 days, only a few lymphocytes and MΦ with swollen appearance, were found in the very small rim of viable cells that surrounded the necrotic implant (fig. 2d).

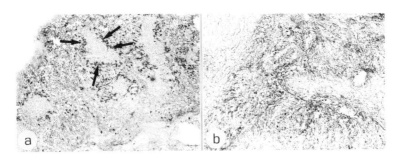

Figure 1. Regeneration of control implants (100x).
a. 21 days after autologous transplantation, ED3 staining: a rim of ED3 positive MΦ (↑) starts to surround the lymphocyte accumulations. *b.* 28 days after transplantation, ED14 staining: the necrotic centre is completely replaced by newly formed reticulum.

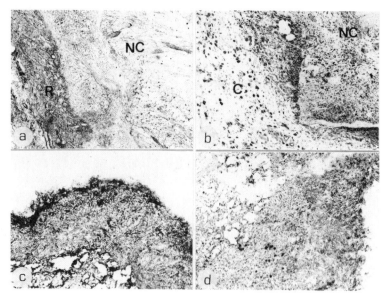

Figure 2. Regeneration of splenic implants after Cl₂MDP liposome treatment (100x).
a. Implants of rats with single treatment, 28 days after transplantation, ED14 staining: a thick diffuse reticular meshwork (R) is formed in the rim of viable cells, notice the still large necrotic centre (NC). *b.* Implants of rats with single treatment, 28 days after transplantation, ED1 staining: under the capsule (C) only a small rim of viable cells is found, surrounding the necrotic centre (NC). *c.* Implants of rats with multiple treatment, ED14 staining: a remnant of reticulum is left, there is no newly formed reticulum. *d.* Implants of rats with multiple treatment, 28 days after transplantation, ED1 staining: there are no signs of regeneration.

DISCUSSION

In this study the role of MΦ in the development of the splenic microenvironment was investigated by studying the effect of MΦ depletion on the regeneration of splenic implants.

After almost complete necrosis, new splenic tissue was formed in the control implants. Like in ontogenic development (Van Rees et al. 1988) and in MΦ depletion studies on in situ spleen (Van Rooijen et al. 1990), the appearance of the different MΦ subpopulations in the implants occurred in the same order. The compartment-specific localization of MΦ subpopulations, as well as the restoration of the reticular meshwork, ocurred simultaneously with the strict localization of lymphocyte subpopulations in their compartments (PALS, follicles, marginal zones). As it seems, the formation of a new spleen environment depends on the interactions between stromal cells and immunecompetent cells. Mutual differences in the construction of stromal components between the compartments, as was described before (Van den Berg et al. 1989), were also observed during regeneration. Probably, lymphocyte subsets maintain their own specific association with different stromal components so compartments can be formed.

With the use of the MΦ depletion technique, we brought to light new evidence for these speculations. Elimination of MΦ before transplantation resulted in profoundly disturbed regenerative capacity of the implants. Especially the development of new reticulum was strongly affected. Without MΦ no splenic compartments were formed at all. A possible explanation is, that without MΦ phagocytosis of the necrotic remnants does not occur. The remnant necrotic centre, which contains toxic enzymes originating from death cells, may not form a suitable environment for regeneration. Furthermore, in the comparable process of wound repair, MΦ play a role in the formation of granulation tissue (Leibovich & Ross 1975). Studies demonstrate that herein MΦ are involved in neovascularization, which is highly important in the development of organs and wound repair. If there is no neovascularization in the implants the influx of new viable cells, like lymphocytes and monocytes is inhibited. Besides stimulation of neovascularization, it is known that MΦ have a direct effect on the proliferation of fibroblasts by production of growth factors (Leibovich & Ross 1975). This might explain the disturbance of reticulum regeneration in the implants. There is evidence that different reticular components contribute to lymphocyte localization and migration (Van den Berg et al. 1992). Therefore, the lack of reticulum in the implants might be responsible for the absence of splenic compartments.

In summary, we showed that MΦ which play a key-role in the development of splenic tissue. Without the presence of MΦ, no reticulum and no separated compartments populated by different immunecompetent cells, are formed.

REFERENCES

Damoiseaux, J.G.C.M., 1991," Macrophage Heterogeneity in the Rat, " Febodruk, Enschede.

Dijkstra, C.D., Döpp, E.A., Joling, P., and Kraal, G., 1985, The heterogeneity of mononuclear phagocytes in lymphoid organs: distinct macrophage subpopulations in the rat recognized by monoclonal antibodies ED1, ED2, ED3, *Immunol.* 54: 589.

Dijkstra, C.D., and Langevoort, H.L., 1982, Regeneration of splenic tissue after autologous subcutaneous implantation: development of non-lymphoid cells in the white pulp of rat spleen, *Cell Tissue Res.* 222: 97.

He, Q., 1988, A role of transmembrane signaling for the cytoplasmic domains of the CD2 T lymphocyte surface antigen. *Cell* 54: 979.

Heuserman, U., Schroeder, L., Zurborn, K.H., and Stutte, H.J., 1982, Structure and function of stroma of lymphoid tissue, *in*: "Lymphoidproliferative Diseases of the Skin," M. Goos, and E. Christopher, eds., Springer-Verslag, Heidelberg

Kroese, F.G.M., Wubbema, A.S., Opstelten, D., Deenen, G.J., Schwander, E.H., De Leij, L., Vos, H., Volberta, J., and Nieuwenhuis, P., 1987, B lymphocyte differentiation in the rat: production and characterization of monoclonal antibodies to B lineage associated antigens, *Eur J. Immunol.* 17; 921.

Leibovich, S.J., and Ross, R., 1975, The role of macrophages in wound repair, *Am. J. Path.* 84: 71.

Tavassoli, M., Ratzan, R.J., and Croby W.H., 1973, Studies on regeneration of heterotopic splenic autotransplants, *Blood* 41: 701.

Van den Berg, T.K., Döpp, E.A., Brevé, J.J.P., Kraal, G., and Dijkstra, C.D., 1989, The heterogeneity of the reticulum of rat peripheral lymphoid organs identified by monoclonal antibodies, *Eur. J. Immunol.* 19: 1747.

Van den Berg, T.K., Brevé, J.J.P., Damoiseaux, J.G.M.C., Döpp, E.A., Kelm, S., Crocker, P., Dijkstra, C.D., and Kraal, G., 1992 a, Sialoadhesin on macrophages: its identification as a lymphocyte adhesion molecule, *J.Exp. Med.* 176: 647.

Van den Berg, T.K., 1992 b, "The Microenvironment in Lymphoid Tissues,"Febodruk, Enschede.

Van Furth, R., 1982, Current vieuw on the mononuclear phagocyte system, *Immunobiol.* 161: 178.

Van Rees, E.P., Dijkstra, C.D., and Sminia, T., 1990, Ontogeny of the rat immune system: an immunohistochemical approach. *Dev. Comp. Immunol.* 14: 9.

Van Rooijen, N., and Claassen, E., 1988, In vivo elimination of macrophages in spleen and liver, using liposome-encapsulated drugs, *in*: " Liposomes as drug carriers, " G. Gregoriadis, ed., Wiley, London.

Van Rooijen, N., Kors, N., Van der Ende, M., and Dijkstra, C.D. , 1990, Depletion and repopulation in spleen, liver of rat after intraveneous treatment with liposome-encapsulated dichloromethylene diphosphonate. *Cell Tissue Res.* 260: 215.

IN VIVO ANTIGEN PRESENTATION CAPACITY
OF DENDRITIC CELLS FROM ORAL MUCOSA
AND SKIN DRAINING LYMPH NODES

Erna van Wilsem, Ingrid van Hoogstraten[1],
John Brevé, Yaved Zaman, and Georg Kraal

Department of Cell Biology, [1]Department of Pathology
Vrije Universiteit, Amsterdam, The Netherlands

INTRODUCTION

Epidermal Langerhans cells (LC) have been implicated as pivotal antigen processing cells in the induction and expression of contact sensitivity. Following epicutaneous exposure with a variety of sensitizing antigens, LC are induced to migrate from the epidermis, via the efferent lymphatics, to regional lymph nodes. Using fluoresceinated antigen, it has been possible to identify the cells within the population of interdigitating dendritic cells (DC) which are extremely potent antigen presenting cells [1,2]. No B-cells, T-cells or macrophages were bearing detectable levels of antigen [3].

In addition to the epidermis, Langerhans cells can also be identified in the epithelium of the oral mucosa [4]. Interestingly, application of antigen at this site predominantly leads to a T-cell mediated "oral" tolerance after sensitization [5].

In spite of the similarities in distribution of antigen presenting cells in the two types of epithelia, it is obvious that antigen deposition leads to opposite immunological responses. Therefore, using a transfer system with isolated dendritic cells, we wished to determine wether differences would exist in antigen presentation capacity in vivo between DC from lymph nodes which drain oral mucosa or skin sites.

MATERIALS AND METHODS

Identification of antigen bearing cells

BALB/c mice were skin painted with 2% Rhodamin B isothiocyanate (Sigma, St. Louis) on the shaved abdomen, fore- and hindlimbs and the dorsal skin of both ears in a total volume of $50\mu l$ DMSO (Merck, Darmstadt)/aceton/dibytylphthalate (Sigma) 1:4.5:4.5.

In Vivo Immunology, Edited by E. Heinen *et al.*
Plenum Press, New York, 1994

Induction of immune tolerance

At day 0, BALB/c mice were given a sublingual dose of 50 μg oxazolone (Sigma, St. Louis) or picrylchloride (PCl, gift of dr J.Garssen,RIVM) in 50μl ointment (unguentum hypromellosi) under light anesthesia. After 1 hour the ointment was removed with a small spatula followed by rinsing with warm (37°C) water. Ten days later 3% oxazolone or 5% PCL in aceton/ethanol (1:3) was applied at the shaved abdomen and fore -and hindlegs (150 μl). The mice were challenged 4 days later, with 0.8% oxazolone or 0.8% PCl in aceton/olive oil (1:4), 10 μl on both ears. The ear thickness was measured 24 hours later and compared with the response of animals that only received a challenge (negative control).

For contact sensitivity the same procedure was followed without pretreatment with a sublingual dose.

Dendritic cell isolation and transfer

Dendritic cells were isolated by the method as described by Knight et al.[6] with modifications according to Vremec et al.[7].

Briefly, draining lymph nodes were pooled, chopped into small fragments, then agitated in a collagenase IV (Sigma 40 U/mg, 0.5 mg/ml)/DNAse I (Boehringer, Mannheim, Germany)(0.02 mg/ml) solution (RPMI/hepes/2% FCS) by rapidly pipetting up and down a wide-bore Pasteur pipette. The pieces were incubated for 30' at 37°C, whereafter 0.1 M EDTA solution was added (10%). The pieces were resuspended and incubated for another 5 minutecs.

The resulting cell suspension that was obtained after enzyme treatment was spun down through 2 ml FCS/EDTA (1ml 0,1M EDTA + 10 ml FCS, incubated for 30'). The pellet was resuspended in HBSS/FCS/EDTA (HBSS + hepes, O.2 mg/ml EDTA, 10% FCS/EDTA) and pipetted through a wire mesh. Living cells were counted by trypan blue exclusion, and 5.10^6 cells/ml were layered onto 2 ml Nycodenz (Nycomed Pharma, Oslo Norway) (14.5 gr/ 100 ml HBSS/FCS/EDTA) and centrifuged for 20 minutes at 600 g.

Cells in the interface were collected, washed once, resuspended in RPMI and 30μl of 3.33 cells/ml were subcutaneously injected into the four foothpads.

RESULTS AND DISCUSSION

The skin epithelium, as well the epitelium of the oral mucosa contains a network of Langerhans cells with similar morphology and distribution [9].

Application of the fluorescent antigen Rhodamin B was used to investigate their confirmity in antigen processing and transportation. Both oral epithelial LC and skin epithelial LC were able to transport the antigen to their draining lymph nodes where antigen bearing, red fluorescent, cells with dendritic morphology could easily be detected by the use of a fluorescent microscope. These cells were not expressing B-, or T-markers but were MHC class II positive.

Despite these similarities in processing and transport, the effect of antigen application on oral mucosa or skin on the final immune response is completely opposite. Pretreatment of mice with oxazolone via the oral mucosa leads to a T-cell mediated tolerance after sensitization, while mice that did not receive this treatment react with a contact sensitivity response after topical application of oxazolone.

Because in both routes of antigen application Langerhans cells and dendritic cells are involved, the question arise wether these cells are responsible for the induction of sensitizing- or tolerogenic signals. Therefore we wished to compare the in vivo antigen presentation capacity of dendritic cells from lymph nodes draining the oral mucosa and skin sites using a transfer system. Both the possibility to transfer immune tolerance with oral mucosa draining DC as well as the potency of these antigen bearing cells to induce contact sensitivity were tested.

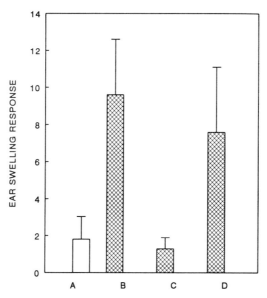

Figure 1. Induction of immune tolerance via the oral mucosa, represented by ear swelling responses. The results are expressed as the mean value of 5 mice. The mice represented by bar A have only received a challenge with oxazolone (oxa) (negative control). Bar B represents the positive control, mice that have been sensitized by application of oxa on the skin followed by a challenge with oxa. The mice of bar C and D have received an oral pretreatment with respectivily 0.5 mg and 0.25 mg oxa, followed by a sensitizing treatment.

To investigate if the signal for immune tolerance was correlated to Langerhans cells arriving from the oral mucosa, we transferred dendritic cells, isolated from lymph nodes draining the oral mucosa 24 hours after antigen application. These cells were subcutaneously injected into four footpads of naive mice and after 10 days followed by 2a sensitizing protocol.

As demonstrated in figure 2a, the ear swelling response of mice injected with DC from LN draining oxazolone painted mucosa was in the same order as the positive control (normally sensitized mice) while the response of orally pretreated mice was suppressed. This indicates that the induction of immune tolerance via the oral mucosa is not totally provided by mucosa derived LC/DC but that other factors are involved. The antigen loading of the cells could play a role but also the microenvironment in which Langerhans cells arrive, e.g. local cytokine profiles could be of more importance [10].

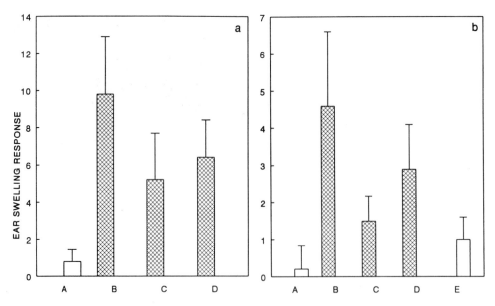

Figure 2a. Transfer of immune tolerance represented by ear swelling responses. The results are expressed as the mean value of 5 mice. The mice represented by bar A have only received a challenge with oxazolone (oxa) and are therefore the negative control. Bar B represents the positive control, mice that have been sensitized by application of oxa on the skin followed by a challenge with oxa. The mice of bar D were injected with DC (100,000/mouse) isolated from LN draining oxazolone painted mucosa. The ear swelling response of these mice should be compared with the response of bar C representing mice that received the "normal" oral tolerizing treatment.

Figure 2b. The potency of DC isolated from LN draining oxazolone painted mucosa to induce contact sensitivity. The results are expressed as the mean ear swelling response of 7 mice. Bar A represents the negative control, mice that only received a challenge with oxazolone (oxa). The mice of bar B and bar C were, respectively, injected with DC (100,000/mouse) isolated from LN draining oxa painted skin and mucosa. The mice of bar D received a 1:1 mixture of the cells of bar B and C. Bar E represents a specificity control of mice injected with DC (100,000/mouse) isolated from LN draining picrylchloride painted skin, followed by oxa challenge.

The previous results could indicate that independent of their origin from oral mucosa or skin Langerhans cells are antigen-presenting cells in *sensu stricto* and that the outcome of the immune response - tolerance versus hypersensitivity - depends solely on the local environment of the draining lymph node.

Therefore DC isolated from mucosa- and skin draining lymph nodes were isolated 24 hours after oxazolone application and transferred to naive mice like in the previous experiment. Four days later the mice were challenged and the ear swelling response was measured one day later.

As illustrated in figure 2b, transfer of DC isolated from skin draining lymph nodes resulted in a positive ear swelling response compared to the negative control [6] and the antigen specific control (picrylchloride painted skin) while injection of DC isolated from mucosa DLN resulted in a lower ear swelling response.

When a mixture (1:1) of mucosa- and skin draining DC was transferred, the ear swelling response was an intermediate between the mucosa- and skin response alone. Therefore we concluded that DC isolated from mucosa draining lymph nodes are not suppressive but less responsive.

We like to conclude the dendritic cells isolated from lymph nodes draining the oral mucosa and skin have the same antigen presentation capacity in vivo but the final height of the respons is not the same. This can be explained by the differences in antigen concentration between the sublingual dose and the peripheral dose which may result in different antigen loading of the dendritic cells.

REFERENCES

1. A.Kinnaird, S.W.Peters, J.R.Foster, I.Kimber, Dendritic cell accumulation in draining lymph nodes during the induction phase of contcat allergy in mice. *Int.Arch.Allergy appl.Immunol.* 89:202(1989)

2. S.E.Macatonia, S.C.Knight, A.J.Edwards, S.Griffiths, P.Fryer, Localization of antigen on lymph node dendritic cells after exposure to the contact sensitizer fluorescein isothiocyanate. Functional and morphological studies.*J.Exp.Med.* 166:1654(1987)

3.E.J.G.van Wilsem, J.Brevé, M.Kleijmeer, G.Kraal, Antigen bearing cells in skin draining lymph nodes. Phenotype and kinetics of migration.*Submitted*

4. I.Silberberg, R.L.Baer, S.A.Rosenthal, G.J.Thorbecke, V.Berezowsky, Langerhans cells at sites of passively induced allergic contact sensitivity. *Cell.Immunol.*18:435(1975)

5. I.M.W.van Hoogstraten, D.Boden, B.M.E.von Blomberg, G.Kraal, R.J.Scheper Persistent immune tolerance to nickel and chromium by oral administration prior to cutaneous sensitization. *J.Invest.Dermatol.*

6. S.C.Knight, J.Krejci, M.Malkivsky, V.Colissi, A.Gautam, G.L.Asherson, The role of dendritic cells in the initiation of immune responses to contact sensitizers. I In vivo exposure to antigen. *Cell.Immunol.* 94:427(1985)

7. D.Vremec, M.Zorbas, R.Scollay, D.J.Saunders, C.F.Ardavin, L.Wu, K.Shortman, The surface phenotype of dendritic cells purified from mouse thymus and spleen:investigation of the CD8 expression by subpopulation of dendritic cells. *J.Exp.Med.* 176:00(1992)

8.A.Bhattacharya, M.E.Dorf, T.A.Springer, A shared alloantigenic derminant on Ia antigens encoded by the I-A and I-E subregion: evidence for the I region gene duplication. *J.Immunol.* 127:2488(1981)Figure 1a illustrates the dose dependency of this tolerogenic response while figure 1b demonstrates this phenomenon is not antigen dependent

9. B.R.J.Rittman, M.W.Hill, G.A.Rittman,I.C.Mackenzie, Age-associated changes in Langerhans cells of murine oral epithelium and epidermis. *Archs.oral Biol.*32:885(1987)

10. R.A.Daynes, B.A.Araneo, T.A.Dowell, K.Huang,D.Dudley, Regulation of murine lymphokine production in vivo.III The lymphoid microenvironment exerts regulatory influences over T-helper cell function. *J.Exp.Med* 171:979(1990)

LIPOSOME MEDIATED MODULATION OF MACROPHAGE FUNCTIONS

Nico van Rooijen

Department of Cell Biology & Immunology
Vrije Universiteit, Van der Boechorststraat 7
1081 BT Amsterdam, The Netherlands

LIPOSOMES

Liposomes are artificially prepared spheres, consisting of concentric phospholipid bilayers separated by aqueous compartments. They form, when phospholipids e.g. phosphatidylcholine molecules, are dispersed in water. The phospholipid molecules will find a conformation in which their hydrophobic fatty acid chains are prevented from contact with water. For that reason, phospholipid bilayers are formed in which the relatively hydrophilic head groups are making up both of the outer parts of each bilayer, whereas the hydrophobic fatty acid groups are located directly opposed to each other in the inner side of the bilayer. Part of the aqueous solution together with hydrophilic molecules, solved in it, will be encapsulated during the formation of the liposomes. Lipophilic molecules will be associated with the phospholipid bilayers themselves. The hydrophobic parts of amphipathic molecules will be inserted in the bilayers, whereas their hydrophilic parts are extending in the aqueous compartments or are exposed on the outer surfaces of the liposomes (figure 1). Numbers of concentric phospholipid bilayers (unilamellar and multilamellar liposomes), phospholipid composition and charge of the liposomes can be varied. Targeting of the liposomes may be achieved by the insertion of target molecules (e.g. monoclonal antibodies or sugar residues) in their outer (surface) bilayer (Gregoriadis, 1988).

LIPOSOMES AND MACROPHAGES

Apart from liposomes that have been developed to avoid their uptake by macrophages (so called "stealth" liposomes), their usual fate is ingestion and digestion by macrophages. For this reason, liposomes form a suitable tool to manipulate macrophage function (Van Rooijen, 1992a). Macrophages ingest the liposomes, followed by phospholipase mediated disruption of the liposomal bilayers and intracellular release of the encapsulated and/or associated molecules. Such liposome-delivered molecules can be processed (antigens), activate the macrophage (immunomodulators) or reversely disturb the metabolism of the cell (several cytotoxic drugs). Resident macrophages can be found in most organs in the body whereas local inflammatory reactions may attract macrophages from the circulation. In several organs, liposomes cannot be targeted to macrophages, because they are not able to pass the vascular barriers formed by capillary walls. In other organs, liposomes can be targeted to defined macrophage (sub)populations provided that they are given along appropriate administration routes. Intravenous administration must be chosen when liposomes have to be targeted to macrophages in the liver (Kupffer cells) and/or spleen (Van Rooijen, 1992b). Subcutaneous administration allows targeting of the liposomes to the draining lymph nodes (Delemarre et al.1990), and intratracheal administration of liposomes causes their

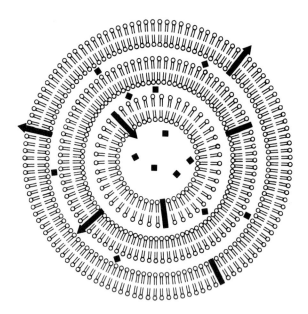

Ω = **Hydrophilic group**
∏ = **Hydrophobic fatty acid chains**

Figure 1. Schematic representation of a liposome with encapsulated hydrophilic molecules (squares) in its aqueous compartments, lipophilic molecules (bars) associated with its phospholipid bilayers, and amphipathic molecules (arrows), with their lipophilic parts in the bilayers and their hydro-philic parts (arrowheads) extending in the aqueous compartments or on the outer surfaces of the liposomes.

uptake by alveolar macrophages in the lung (Thepen et al.1989). It has been postulated that incorporation of mannose residues in the bilayers allows the liposomes to pass the blood-brain barrier (Umezawa and Eto, 1988; Huitinga et al. 1990), but other authors were not able to confirm this postulate (Micklus et al. 1992) Direct local injection of liposomes in the tissues can be used to influence macrophages in organs with a loosely woven structure such as the testes (Bergh et al. 1993). The fate of liposomes is also influenced by their characteristics. So, cholesterol "rich" and cholesterol "poor" liposomes were shown to differ with respect to their relative targeting to macrophages in spleen and liver (Patel, 1992). Contrary to many other macrophages, peritoneal macrophages recognize phosphatidylserine in apoptotic cells and may be expected to prefer liposomes with this negatively charged phospholipid in their bilayers (Fadok et al. 1992).

LIPOSOMES AS ANTIGEN CARRIERS

Several authors have shown that liposomes are responsible for a substantial enhancement of the immune response elicited against antigens which had been entrapped in their aqueous compartments or were associated with their phospholipid bilayers (Gregoriadis, 1990; Van Rooijen, 1990; Alving, 1991). Since liposomes are biodegradable and are composed of non-toxic and immunologically inert phospholipids, they have been suggested as promising carriers for haptens and as an immunoadjuvant for associated antigens. The toxicity of some antigens may be reduced by their incorporation in liposomes while at the same time their immunogenicity is increased. Furthermore, liposome entrapped allergens may be safe and effective in immunotherapy by the combination of a decreased allergic response and an increased antigenicity of the allergen (Arora and Gangal, 1992). Since liposome encapsulated antigens are masked and thus prevented from recognition by surface receptors on lymphoid cells, and liposomes are avidly phagocytosed by macrophages, phagocytosis of liposomes followed by unmasking of the encapsulated antigens seems to be a logical first step in the induction of an immune response against entrapped antigens. Several experiments have confirmed that macrophages are involved in the processing of liposome encapsulated antigens (Van Rooijen, 1992b). It is not likely, that macrophages by themselves are responsible for both processing and presentation of particulate antigens. They are postulated to be involved in the induction of humoral immunity against liposome associated antigens, by performing a (pre)processing step. In this dual accessory cell concept, processing by macrophages is followed by transfer of the processed antigens to cells which are better equipped for their presentation (Van Rooijen, 1992b). Liposomes were also demonstrated to be excellent antigen carriers for the induction of cytotoxic T-lymphocyte (CTL) responses. Arguments have been given for an "in vivo" role of macrophages in the induction of CTL responses against liposome encapsulated antigens (Huang et al. 1992; Zhou et al. 1992).

LIPOSOMES FOR MACROPHAGE DEPLETION

To obtain more insight in the role of defined macrophage subpopulations in immune and non-immune defense mechanisms, 'in vivo' studies are inevitable. Recently we have developed a new approach to study macrophage functions "in vivo". This method is based on the 'in vivo' depletion of macrophages using the liposome encapsulated drug dichloromethylene bisphosphonate (clodronate, see Van Rooijen, 1989, 1992c). The mechanism by which intracellularly released clodronate damages the macrophages, ultimately leading to their physical depletion from the tissues, is still under investigation (Van Rooijen, 1992d). The fact that these highly water soluble molecules do not easily pass phospholipid bilayers is important. As a consequence, these molecules are not easily leaking out of the liposomes, and once within the cytosol of macrophages, they tend to be accumulated because they are not able to escape from here either. Liposomal encapsulation of the drug both warrants its selective targeting into macrophages, and minimalizes its effect on non-phagocytic cells. The half life of clodronate released in the circulation from dying cells is extremely short, since the drug is rapidly removed by the kidneys (Fleisch, 1988). It is considered a safe drug which is used for treatment of osteolytic bone diseases in men, because, in a bone attached form, it affects the activities of osteoclasts. Moreover, liposomes are biodegradable and immunologically inert carriers. Thus, if any damage to non-phagocytic cells is observed, it is most probably caused by enzymes and/or other cell remnants released from dying macrophages. Macrophage (sub)populations can be successfully depleted from several organs using this liposome mediated macrophage "suicide" approach, provided that vascular barriers are absent or can be avoided by administration of the liposomes along appropriate routes (see Van Rooijen, 1992c). The new approach is used in an increasing number of studies aimed at the unfolding of macrophage functions "in vivo". The activity of macrophages with respect to inflammatory responses induced by autoimmunity or as a result of transplantation, may well have an overall negative effect on the host. As a consequence, temporary depletion of macrophages using the above macrophage "suicide" approach has shown beneficial effects in studies on experimental allergic encephalomyelitis (Huitinga et al. 1990). Also, depletion of phagocytic synovial lining cells has been shown to result in beneficial effects in experimental arthritis (Van Lent et al. 1993). Alveolar macrophages are actively involved in suppression of antibody responses by suppressing the antigen presenting cell function of pulmonary dendritic cells (Holt et al. 1993). Depletion of alveolar macrophages before intratracheal administration of antigen will, as a consequence, result in a positive effect on the pulmonary immune response (Thepen et al. 1989).

LIPOSOMES FOR MACROPHAGE ACTIVATION

Taking advance of the natural fate of liposomes, immunomodulators can be targeted to cells of the mononuclear phago-cyte system (MPS,Fidler, 1992; Phillips, 1992; Daemen, 1992). Using this approach, cells of the MPS can be activated e.g. to a tumoricidal, virocidal, bactericidal or fungicidal state. Systemic administration of liposomes containing various immunomodulators has been shown to bring about re-gression of lymph node, lung and liver metastases, and promotes effective prophylaxis of viral infections in rodents (Fidler,1992). Usually, muramyl dipeptide (MDP), a component of the bacteri-al cell wall, or MDP derivatives are used for activation of the immune system. Both hydrophi-lic MDP as well as lipophilic muramyl tripeptide phosphatidyl-ethanol-amine (MTP-PE) have potent effects on macrophages, but incorporation in liposomes is increased if the latter compound is used (Fidler, 1992). It has also be reported that IFNγ and MTP-PE, if delivered within the same liposomes, act synergistically in the destruction of a metastatic tumour burden and in the long-term survival of mice with a large metastatic tumour burden (Fidler, 1992). Another possibility to optimize the incor-poration of MDP within liposomes and their ability to activate macrophage tumoricidal activity, is to use the lipophilic prodrug MDP-glycerol dipalmitate (MDP-GDP, Phillips, 1992).

LIPOSOMES FOR MACROPHAGE BLOCKING

It has been demonstrated that liposomes without any encapsulated agent (empty liposomes) can block macrophage functions for certain periods of time (Juliano, 1982; Proffitt et al. 1983; Dave and Patel, 1986). By blocking of phagocytic and other functions of macrophages, using high doses of empty liposomes, killing of macrophages is avoided. The release in the circulation, of lysosomal enzymes and other unwanted macrophage products from dying macrophages, as a consequence of their liposome mediated "suicide" is circumvented in this way. A disadvantage, however, may be that blocking of phagocytic functions is not complete, its duration is short, and it is not yet known whether the production of soluble mediator molecules (e.g. Il1, Il6 and TNF) is also blocked. The overall effects of liposome encapsulated clodronate, liposome encapsula-ted immunomodulators and empty liposomes on immune and non-immune defense mechanisms depends on 1. The influence of the liposomes on macrophages and 2. The role of the macrophages in the particular host defense mechanism.

REFERENCES

Alving,C.R. 1991. Liposomes as carriers of antigens and adjuvants. J.Immunol. Meth. 140: 1.

Arora,N. and Gangal, S.V. 1992. Efficacy of liposome entrapped allergen in down regulation of IgE response in mice. Clin. Exp. Allergy, 22: 35.

Bergh,A.,Damber,J.E. and Van Rooijen,N. 1993. Liposome-mediated macropha-ge depletion: an experimental approach to study the role of testicular macrophages in the rat. J.Endocrinol. 136: 407.

Daemen,T. 1992. Activation of Kupffer cell tumoricidal activity by immunomodulators encapsulated in liposomes. Res.Immunol. 143: 211.

Dave,J. and Patel,H.M.1986. Differentiation in hepatic and splenic phagocytic activity during reticuloendothelial blockade with cholesterol-free and cholesterol-rich liposomes. Bioch.Bioph.Acta 888: 184.

Delemarre,F.G.A.,Kors,N.,Kraal,G., and Van Rooijen, N. 1990. Repopulation of macrophages in popliteal lymph nodes of mice after liposome mediated depletion. J. Leuk. Biol.47: 251.

Fadok,V.A.,Savill,J.S.,Haslett,C.,Bratton,D.L.,Doherty,D.E.,Campbell,P.A. and Henson,P.M. 1992. Different populations of macrophages use either the vitronectin receptor or the phosphatidylserine receptor to recognize and remove apoptotic cells. J.Immunol. 149: 4029.

Fidler,I.J.1992. Systemic macrophage activation with liposome-entrapped immunomodulators for therapy of cancer metastasis. Res.Immunol. 143: 199.

Fleisch,H. 1988. Bisphosphonates: a new class of drugs in diseases of bone and calcium metabolism. Handbook Exp. Pharmacol. 83: 441.

Gregoriadis,G.1988. Liposomes as Drug Carriers: Recent Trends and Progress, John Wiley & Sons, Chichester,UK.

Gregoriadis,G.1990. Immunological adjuvants: a role for liposomes. Immunology Today 11: 89.

Holt,P.G., Oliver,J., Bilyk,N., McMenamin,C., McMenamin,P.G., Kraal,G. and Thepen,T.1993. Downregulation of the antigen presenting cell functions of pulmonary dendritic cells in vivo by resident alveolar macrophages. J. Exp. Med. 177: 397.

Huang,L.,Reddy,R.,Nair,S.K.,Zhou,F.,Rouse,B.T.1991. Liposomal delivery of soluble protein antigens for Class I MHC mediated antigen presentation. Res.Immunol. 142: 192.

Huitinga,I.,Van Rooijen,N. ,De Groot,C.J.A., Uitdehaag,B.M.J. and Dijkstra,C.D. 1990. Suppression of experimental al-lergic encephalomyelitis in Lewis rats after elimination of macrophages. J.Exp.Med. 172: 1025.

Juliano, R.L.1982. Liposomes and the retciculoendothelial system: Interactions of Liposomes with Macrophages and Behavior of Liposomes "in vivo". In: Targeting of Drugs, NATO ASI Series A, Vol. 47, Gregoriadis,G.,Senior,J. and Trouet, A. eds. Plenum Press, New York U.S.A.

Micklus,M.J.,Greig,N.H.,Tung,J. and Rapoport,S.I. 1992. Organ distribution of liposomal formulations following intracarotid infusion of rats. Bioch. Bioph. Acta 1124: 7.

Patel,H.M. 1992. Serum opsonins and liposomes: Their interaction and opsonophagocytosis. Crit. Rev. Ther. Drug Carr. Syst. 9: 39.

Phillips,N.C. 1992. Stimulation of Kupffer cell tumoricidal activity by liposomal muramyl dipeptides. Res.Immunol. 143:205.

Proffitt, R.T., Williams, L.E., Presant, C.A., Tin, G.W., Uliana,J.A., Gamble,R.C. and Baldeschwieler,J.D. 1983. Liposomal blockade of the reticuloendothelial system: Improved tumor imaging with small unilamellar vesicles. Science 220: 502.

Thepen,T.,Van Rooijen,N. and Kraal,G.1989. Alveolar macrophage elimination in vivo is associated with an increase in pulmonary immune responses in mice. J. Exp. Med.170:499.

Umezawa,F. and Eto,Y.1988. Liposome targeting to mouse brain: mannose as a recognition marker. Bioch.Bioph.Res.Commun. 153: 1038.

Van Lent, P.L.E.M.,Van Den Bersselaar,L.,Van Den Hoek,A.E.M.,Van De Ende, M.,Van Rooijen,N. and Van Den Berg,W.B.1993. Reversible depletion of synovial lining cells after intraarticular treatment with liposome encapsulated dichloromethylene diphosphonate. Rheumat. Intern. 13: 21.

Van Rooijen,N. 1989. The liposome mediated macrophage "suicide" technique. J.Immunol.Meth. 124:1.

Van Rooijen,N. 1990. Liposomes as carrier and immunoadjuvant of vaccine antigens. Adv. Biotechnol. Proc. 13: 255.

Van Rooijen,N.1992a. Liposomes as an "in vivo" tool to study and manipulate macrophage function: 41 Forum in Immunology. Res.Immunol. 143: 177.

Van Rooijen,N. 1992b. Macrophages as accessory cells in the "in vivo" humoral immune response: From processing of particulate antigens to regulation by suppression. Sem. Immunol. 4:237.

Van Rooijen,N. 1992c. Liposome-mediated elimination of macrophages. Res.Immunol. 143: 215.

Van Rooijen,N. and Poppema,A.1992. Efficacy of various water-soluble chelator molecules in the liposome-mediated macrophage "suicide" technique. J.Pharmacol.Tox.Meth. 28: 217.

Zhou,F.,Rouse,B.T. and Huang,L. 1992. Induction of cytotoxic T lymphocytes with protein antigen entrapped in membranous vehicles. J.Immunol. 149:1599.

IN VIVO gp39-CD40 INTERACTIONS OCCUR IN THE NON-FOLLICULAR COMPARTMENTS OF THE SPLEEN AND ARE ESSENTIAL FOR THYMUS DEPENDENT ANTIBODY RESPONSES AND GERMINAL CENTER FORMATION

A.J.M. van den Eertwegh[*], M. Van Meurs[*], T.M. Foy[#], R.J. Noelle[#], W.J.A. Boersma[*] and E. Claassen[*]

[*]Dept. Immunology and Medical Microbiology, TNO-MBL, POB 5815, 2280 HV, Rijswijk, The Netherlands
[#]Dept. of Microbiology, Dartmouth School, One Medical Center drive, Lebanon, NH 03757, USA

INTRODUCTION

The initiation of thymus-dependent (TD) antibody responses requires class II-restricted antigen-specific helper T cell cognate interactions with B cells. None of the molecularly cloned cytokines, alone or in combination, can replace the contact-dependent requirement for B cell activation[1]. The molecule which mediates the contact-dependent signal is a 39 kD membrane protein which is expressed on the surface of activated T-helper (Th) cells[2,3]. This membrane protein, gp39, was identified as the ligand for the B cell membrane protein CD40. CD40, a mitogenic receptor expressed on all mature B lymphocytes[4], is a type I membrane protein and member of the TNF receptor family[5]. Evidence that CD40 is an important receptor on B cells is derived from studies that anti-CD40 mAb and cofactors such as anti-immunoglobulin (Ig) and cytokines initiate both B cell growth and differentiation[6,7].

The ligand for CD40, gp39 is a type II membrane protein which is homologous to TNF-α and -β[8,9]. It is transiently expressed on activated CD4$^+$ cells *in vitro*[3]. It was demonstrated that gp39-bearing plasma membranes (PM) from activated Th showed can activate resting B cells[10]. A soluble, CD40-Ig fusion protein and a gp39-specific monoclonal antibody (mAb) were able to block the activation of B cells by these PM[3]. After activation, the Ig-secretion of activated B cells is regulated by Th cell derived cytokines[10,11,12]. Recently, we demonstrated that gp39$^+$ cells are upregulated after immunization with TI-2 and TD antigens and are localized in juxtaposition to antigen-specific antibody-forming cells in restricted compartments of the spleen[13]. It was demonstrated that these putative gp39-CD40 interactions are critical for the development of secondary antibody responses against soluble TD antigens[14].

Germinal centers (GC) are clusters of B lymphoblastoid cells which develop after antigenic stimulation in follicles of peripheral lymphoid organs and are thought to play a major role in the generation of B cell memory[15]. GC formation is known to be TD[16], although it is not known how T cells are involved in the the induction of the GC reaction. *In vitro* studies suggested that the CD40-molecule is important for GC formation[17]. Therefore, we investigated in this study the localization of CD40-ligand bearing cells in the spleen during the formation of GC. Furthermore, the *in vivo* localization of gp39-CD40 interactions in the spleen, and their role in primary antibody responses and GC formation was assessed.

In Vivo Immunology, Edited by E. Heinen *et al.*
Plenum Press, New York, 1994

MATERIALS AND METHODS

Animals BCBA.F$_1$ (C57BL x CBA) and BALB/c mice were bred at the TNO breeding facilities, Rijswijk, The Netherlands. Animals were used at 16-24 weeks of age and were kept under a standard protocol with free access to pelleted food and acidified water (pH 3).

Chemicals Alkaline phosphatase (AP; P-6774, type VII-T, 1020 U/mg protein) 3-amino-9-ethylcarbazole (A-5754), Fast blue BB Base (F-0125), horse radish peroxidase (HRP), levamisole, naphthol AS-MX phosphate (3-hydroxy-2-naphtoic acid 2,4-dimethyl-anilide),TNP sulfonic acid (TNBS, grade I) were obtained from Sigma, St. Louis, MO, USA.

Reagents TNP-Ficoll and TNP-KLH were prepared as previously described[18]. The control hamster antibodies and ascites from the cell lines MR1 (3), a mAb directed to gp39 and RG7, a mAb specific for rat/hamster Igκ (RG-7[19]) chain were purified by means of a protein-A column. TNP-AP was prepared according to the previously described methods[18].

Experimental design BCBA.F$_1$ mice were injected i.v. with 100 μg of TNP-KLH or 20 μg of TNP-Ficoll and killed after 0, 1, 2, 3, 4, 5, 6, and 7 days. To determine the functional role of gp39$^+$ cells in TD and TI-2 antibody responses, BALB/c mice were injected i.v. with either 100 μg of TNP-KLH or 20 μg TNP-Ficoll on day 0. Subsequently, at day 0, 2, 4 mice were given 250 μg of purified anti-gp39 mAb (MR1) or 250 μg purified hamster Ig or PBS, i.p., as previously described[14]. Mice were bled at day 7 and 14, sacrificed at day 14 and serum was prepared. In all experiments spleens were removed and immediately frozen in liquid nitrogen and stored at -70°C.

Immunohistochemistry Immunohistochemistry was done as earlier described[21,22].

TNP-specific ELISA. Mouse serum TNP-specific IgM and IgG were determined by means of a direct ELISA as described earlier[23]. The isotype-specific capture ELISA was performed as described by Vos et al.[24]. The TNP-specific titer was the dilution at which 50% of the maximal absorbance was found. Titers of each isotype were related to that of control (PBS) group, which was set at 100%.

RESULTS AND DISCUSSION

Localization and kinetics of gp39$^+$ cells in lymphoid tissue. Spleen sections from immunized mice were stained for the expression of gp39[13]. Gp39$^+$ Th cells were found predominantly in the outer-periarteriolar lymphocyte sheaths (PALS) and around the terminal arterioles (TA) of the spleen (Fig. 1), but not in the follicles or marginal zone of the spleen. At day 3 and 4 after injection of TNP-KLH we observed the maximum number of gp39$^+$ cells[13]. Thereafter, the number decreased and remained stable during the next 10 days. Immunization with TNP-Ficoll, a TI type 2 antigen, resulted in an increase in the frequency of gp39$^+$ Th cells, reaching maximum frequencies 5 days after injection[13]. Similar as observed for TD antigens, in the antibody response against TNP-Ficoll gp39$^+$ cells were localized in the outer-PALS and around the TA of the spleen.

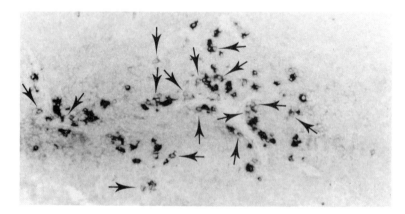

Fig. 1. Gp39+ cells (arrow) are found in close conjunction to TNP-AFC around the terminal arterioles of the spleen 4 days after immunization with TNP-KLH

Gp39+ cells co-localize with antigen-specific B cells

As gp39[+] Th cells are essential for the activation of B cells *in vitro* and *in vivo*, their anatomical localization in relation to resting and antibody-producing B cells was examined. Double immunohistochemical staining for resting B cells (membrane IgM-bearing) or B plasma blasts (cytoplasmic Ig) and gp39, revealed that the majority of gp39[+] Th cells were co-distributed amongst both B cell types in the outer-PALS and TA (data not shown). In addition, when antibody-forming B cells, specific for the immunizing antigen, were revealed, the TNP-AFC were found in close conjunction to the gp39[+] Th cells (Fig. 1). Also in the antibody response against TNP-Ficoll we observed antigen-specific B cells (TNP-AFC) co-localizing with gp39[+] T cells in the outer-PALS and around the TA (Fig. 1). These results suggest that during TI-2 as well as TD antibody responses T-B cell interactions occur in the non-follicular compartments of the spleen[13].

Anti-gp39 administration inhibits the primary IgG antibody responses to TD antigens.

In vitro studies indicated that anti-gp39 mAb blocked the Th-dependent activation of B cells[3]. We observed high frequencies of gp39[+] cells in juxtaposition to TNP-AFC at 2-4 days after TNP-KLH immunization. In order to investigate whether these putative gp39-CD40 interactions were essential for the primary antibody response against TNP-KLH mice were treated with anti-gp39 mAb after immunization. The primary anti-TNP antibody response was completely inhibited when we examined the IgG subclasses (Fig. 2). The antigen-specific IgM response was not completely inhibited after treatment with anti-gp39 mAb, confirming that this part of the response was not fully T cell (gp39)-dependent[25].

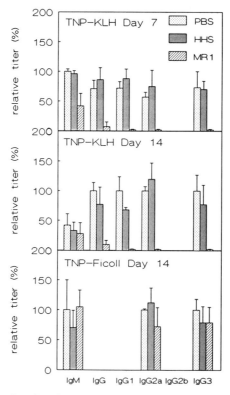

Fig. 2. Anti-gp39 antibodies (MR1) inhibit the primary antibody response against TNP-KLH

Anti-gp39 administration does not inhibit the antibody response to TI-2 antigens

We observed that gp39[+] cells were upregulated after administration of TNP-Ficoll, and localized in close conjunction to TNP-AFC, suggesting that gp39-CD40 interactions play a role in the initiation of TI-2 antibody responses. In order to address this possibility we treated TNP-Ficoll immunized mice with anti-gp39 mAb. Figure 2 demonstrates that the *in vivo* IgM, IgG2a and IgG3 antibody responses against TNP-Ficoll were not blocked by gp39-specific antibodies. These results indicate that the gp39 is not functional in the induction of TI-2 antibody responses. The gp39⁺ cells localized in juxtaposition to TNP-AFC may represent interactions between activated cytokine-producing Th cells and antigen-specific antibody-forming cells[22]. The demonstration of activated T cells in the spleen after TNP-Ficoll immunization substantiates previous reports, which showed that T cells are important for the development of antibody responses against TI-2 antigens[26,27].

Anti-gp39 administration inhibits GC formation
GC formation is a T cell dependent process. Nude mice do not develop GC upon antigenic challenge, but are able to produce GC after reconstitution with T cells[16]. To investigate whether gp39⁺ (activated) T cells play a role in GC formation we studied the influence of the anti-gp39 treatment on the formation of GC at day 14 after TNP-KLH immunization. Interestingly, anti-gp39 treatment completely inhibited GC formation. Since we demonstrated in previous reports[14] that gp39⁺ are not depleted after injection of anti-gp39, these results suggest that gp39-CD40 interactions play a role in GC formation. Gp39⁺ cells were never observed in the follicles of spleens after primary immunization, indicating that the initial B cell activation occurs outside the follicles, as was earlier suggested[28,29,30]. Apparently, after activation by gp39⁺ cells, B cells get the competence to proliferate in the microenvironment of follicles, which will lead to the development of GC.

Conclusions

Data presented and previous studies on the localization and migration of immune cells[30] suggest that during primary antibody responses, TD antigens are presented by interdigitating cells in the PALS, leading to increasing numbers of antigen-specific T cells which subsequently encounter antigen-specific B cells in the PALS, forming T-B cell conjugates. During this cognate T-B cell interaction, Th cells will be activated by antigen-presenting B cells and express the ligand for CD40. Gp39 will trigger B cell growth and differentiation. Part of the activated B cells migrates to the follicles to undergo follicular processes, such as somatic mutation and memory formation[15]. Another part of the activated B cells migrates to the TA and differentiates into antigen-specific AFC regulated by activated cytokine-producing T cells[13,30]. In conclusion, presented data suggest that the gp39-CD40 interactions which occur in the outer-PALS and around the terminal arterioles of the spleen are essential for the induction of TD antibody responses and germinal center formation.

REFERENCES

1. D.C. Parker. T cell dependent B cell activation, *Annu. Rev. Immunol.* 11:331 (1993).
2. R.J. Armitage, W.C. Fanslow, L. Strockbine, T.A. Sato, K.N. Clifford, B.M. Macduff, D.M. Anderson, S.D. Gimpel,T. Davis-Smith, C.R. Maliszewski, E.A. Clark, C.A. Smith, K.H. Grabstein, D. Cosman, and M.K. Spriggs. Molecular and biological characterization of a murine ligand for CD40, *Nature* 257:80 (1992).
3. R.J. Noelle, , M. Roy, D.M. Shepherd, I. Stamenkovic, J.A. Ledbetter, and A.A. Aruffo. A novel ligand on activated helper T cells bind CD40 and transduces the cognate activation of B cell, *Proc. Natl. Acad. Sci. USA* 89:6550 (1992).
4. E.A. Clark, and P.J. Lane. Regulation of human B-cell activation and adhesion, *Ann. Rev. Immunol.* 9:97 (1991).
5. I. Stamenkovic, E.A. Clark, and B. Seed. A B lymphocyte activation molecule related to the nerve growth factor receptor and induced by cytokines in carcinoma, *EMBO J.* 8:1403 (1989).
6. H.H. Jabara, S.M. Fu, R.S. Geha, and D. Vercelli. CD40 and IgE:Synergism between anti-CD40 monoclonal antibody and interleukin 4 in the induction of IgE synthesis by highly purified human B cells, *J. Exp. Med.* 172:1861 (1990).

7. J. Banchereau, P. De Paoli, A. Vallé, E. Garcia, and F. Rousset. Long-term human B cell lines dependent on interleukin-4 antibody to CD40, *Science* 251:70 (1991).
8. D. Hollenbaugh, Grosmaire, L.S., Kullas, C.D., Chalupny, N.J., Braesh-Andersen, Noelle, R.J., Stamenkovic, I., Ledbetter, J.A., and A. Aruffo. The human T cell antigen gp39, a member of the TNF gene family, is a ligand for the CD40 receptor: expression of a soluble form of gp39 with B cell co-stimulatory activity, *EMBO* 11:4313 (1992).
9. T. Farah, and C. A. Smith. Emerging cytokine family, *Nature* 358:26 (1992).
10. R. J. Noelle, J. Daum, W.C. Bartlett, J. McCann, and D.M. Shepherd. Cognate interactions between helper T cells and B cells; V. reconstitution of T helper cell function using purified plasma membranes from activated Th1 and Th2 T helper cells and lymphokines, *J. Immunol.* 146:1118 (1991).
11. K.H. Grabstein, Maliszewski, K. Shanebeck, T.A. Sato, M.K. Spriggs, W.C. Fanslow, and R.J. Armitage. The regulation of T cell-dependent antibody formation in vitro by CD40 ligand and IL-2, *J. Immunol.* 150:3141 (1993).
12. R.J. Armitage, B.M. Macduff, M.K. Spriggs, and W.C. Fanslow. Human B cell proliferation and Ig secretion induced by recombinant CD40 ligand are modulated by soluble cytokines, *J. Immunol.* 150:3671 (1993).
13. A.J.M Van den Eertwegh, R.J. Noelle, M. Roy, D.M. Shepherd, A. Aruffo, J. A. Ledbetter, W.J.A. Boersma and E. Claassen. *In vivo* CD40-gp39 interactions are essential for thymus dependent humoral immunity. I. *In vivo* expression of CD40 ligand, cytokines and antibody production delineates sites of cognate T-B cell interactions, *J. Exp. Med.* (in press).
14. T.M. Foy, Durie, F.H., Shepherd, D.M., Aruffo, A., Ledbetter, J.A., and R.J. Noelle. *In vivo* CD40-gp39 interactions are essential for thymus dependent humoral immunity. II. Prolonged suppression of the humoral immune response by an antibody to the ligand for CD40, gp39, *J. Exp. Med.* (in press).
15. Y. Liu, G.D. Johnson, J. Gordon, and C.M. Maclennan. Germinal centres in T-cell dependent antibody responses, *Immunol. Today* 13:17 (1992).
16. E.B. Jacobson, L.H.Caporale, and G.J. Thorbecke. Effect of thymus cell injections on germinal center formation in lymphoid tissues of nudes (thymusless) mice, *Cell. Immunol.* 13:416 (1974).
17. Y.L. Liu, D.E. Joshua, G.T. Williams, C.A. Smith, J. Gordon and I.C.M. MacLennan. 1989. Mechanism of antigen-driven selection in germinal centres, *Nature* 342:929 (1989).
18. E. Claassen, N. Kors, and N. Van Rooyen. Influence of carriers on the development and localization of anti-trinitrophenyl antibody forming cells in the murine spleen, *Eur. J. Immunol.* 16:271 (1986).
19. T.A. Springer, A. Bhattacharya, J.T. Cardoza, F. Sanchez-Madrid. Monoclonal antibodies specific for rat IgG1, IgG2a and IgG2b subclasses, and kappa chain monotypic and allotypic determinants: reagents for use with rat monoclonal antibodies, *Hybrid.* 1:257 (1982).
20. E. Claassen, and L. Adler. Sequential double immunocytochemical staining for the in situ identification of an auto-anti-allotype immune response in allotype suppressed rabbits, *J. Histochem. Cytochem.* 36:1455 (1988).
21. A.J.M. Van den Eertwegh, J.D. Laman, M.M. Schellekens, W.J.A. Boersma, and E. Claassen. Complement mediated follicular localization of T-independent type 2 antigens: the role of marginal zone macrophages revisited, *Eur. J. Immunol.* 22:719 (1992).
22. A.J.M. Van den Eertwegh, M.J. Fasbender, M.M. Schellekens, A. Van Oudenaren, W.J.A. Boersma, and E. Claassen. *In vivo* kinetics and characterization of IFN-γ-producing cells during a thymus independent immune response, *J. of Immunol.* 147:439 (1991).
23. E. Claassen E., N. Kors, and N. Van Rooijen. Immunomodulation with liposomes: The immune response elicited by liposomes with entrapped dichloromethylenediphosphonate and surface associated antigen or hapten, *Immunology* 60: 509 (1987).
24. Q. Vos, E. Claassen, and R. Benner. Substantially increased sensitivity of the spot-ELISA for the detection of anti-insulin antibody-secreting cells during a capture and enzyme-conjugated insulin, *J.Immunol. Meth.* 126:89 (1990).
25. G.Koch, and R. Benner. Differential requirement for B memory and T memory cells in adoptive antibody formation in mouse bone marrow, *Immunol.* 45:697 (1982).
26. J.J. Mond, J. Farrar, W.E. Paul, J. Fuller-Farrar, M. Schaefer, and M. Howard. 1983. T cell dependence and factor reconstitution of in vitro antibody responses to TNP-B. abortus and TNP-Ficoll: restoration of depleted responses with chromatographed fractions of a T-cell derived factor, *J. Immunol.* 131:633 (1983).
27. R. Endres, E. Kushnir, J.W. Kappler, P. Marrack, and S.C. Kinsky. A requirement for T cell help factors in antibody responses to "T-independent" antigens, *J. Immunol.* 130:781 (1983).

28. D. Gray. Recruitment of virgin B cells into an immune response is resticted to activation outside follicles, *Immunol* 65:659 (1988).
29. R.H. Vonderheide and S.V. Hunt. Immigration of thoracic duct B lymphocytes into established germinal centers in the rat, *Eur. J. Immunol.* 20:79 (1990).
30. A.J.M. Van den Eertwegh, W.J.A. Boersma, and E. Claassen. Immunological functions and *in vivo* cell-cell interactions of T-lymphocytes in the spleen, *Crit. Rev. Immunol.* 11:337 (1992).

THE ROLE OF DENDRITIC CELLS IN THE UPTAKE AND PRESENTATION OF ORAL ANTIGENS

L.M. Liu and G.G. MacPherson
Sir William Dunn School of Pathology, University of Oxford, UK

INTRODUCTION

For T cell activation, antigen has to be captured, processed and presented in association with MHC molecules by antigen presenting cells (APC). Potential antigen presenting cells (APC) in the small intestine include macrophages[1], B cells[2], epithelial cells[3] and dendritic cells (DC)[4]. DC are found in the Lamina Propria (LP)[5] and Peyer's patches (PP)[6]. In PP, DC are present under the dome area and in the T cell area[6]. Peyer's patch DC may be important in the initiation of intestinal immune responses in that IgA secretion can be induced by the interaction of B cells with a DC-T cell mixture derived from murine PP and this DC-T cell mixture can induce pre-B cells to secrete high levels of IgA[7,8].

DC acquire antigens in the periphery and transport them to lymph nodes. Bujdoso et al.[9] showed that in sheep, lymph DC draining the site of subcutaneous antigen could stimulate sensitized T cells. Macatonia et al.[10] showed that after skin painting with FITC, DC in the draining lymph node express FITC, could stimulate sensitized T cells and could sensitize a naive recipient. Crowley et al.[11] have shown that splenic DC can acquire and present intravenous antigen. DC in the gut can also acquire antigen and transport it to mesenteric lymph nodes for presentation. Thus, DC-like cells from intestinal lymph have been shown to carry *Salmonella* antigens following an intestinal infection[12] and we have shown that lymph-borne DC (L-DC) can acquire intra-intestinal antigens and present them to sensitized T cells[13].

The intestine receives a huge antigenic load. Most are dietary proteins but some are pathogens. The intestinal immune system has to generate protective immunity to pathogens but prevent hypersensitivity to dietary antigens. Oral antigen can induce both local and systemic responses and may induce local immunity but systemic tolerance[14] (oral tolerance). The mechanisms underlying these responses are not fully understood and, in particular, the role of differential antigen handling and presentation has been little investigated.

The experiments described here investigate the function of different APC in the uptake, transport and presentation of intestinal antigens.

In Vivo Immunology, Edited by E. Heinen *et al.*
Plenum Press, New York, 1994

METHODS, RESULTS AND DISCUSSION

Antigen uptake by L-DC after oral antigen administration

We have shown that L-DC can acquire intra-intestinal soluble antigens and present them to sensitized T cells in a MHC Class II and CD4 dependent manner[13]. To test whether oral antigen can also be acquired by L-DC, mesenteric lymphadenectomized (MLNX) rats were given oral OVA prior to thoracic duct cannulation[15.] L-DC collected over the next 24h were added to sensitized spleen cells and proliferation measured. Such L-DC stimulate a specific response from OVA-sensitized T cells (less than that following intra-intestinal injection) (data not shown). When, however, the ability of these L-DC to prime T cells 'in vivo' was tested, specific priming was seen with doses down to 1mg (see below). These experiments show that L-DC can acquire process, and present orally administered antigens.

Fate of antigen after intra-intestinal injection

FITC-labelled canine albumin was injected intra-intestinally and thoracic duct lymph cells were collected over the next 48h. No labelled L-DC or other cells were seen. Frozen sections of small intestine taken 1, 3, and 6 h after injection, and cell suspensions prepared from the lamina propria and Peyer's patches were stained for MHC class II or OX62[16], an antibody that labels DC and probably gamma/delta T cells, but not macrophages. Antigen was clearly present in some large MHC class II negative macrophages but was not seen in OX62[+] cells. These results suggest that only small amounts of antigen are acquired by L-DC.

'In vivo' priming of T cells in naive rats by antigen-bearing L-DC

To test the ability of antigen-bearing cells to prime naive rats, L-DC, B cells and T cells were enriched from XTDL, pulsed with OVA and injected into the footpads of naive rats. After 10 days, popliteal lymph node cells were cultured with OVA or HRP and proliferation measured. The results showed that both the L-DC and B cell fractions sensitized specifically whereas T cells were inert (Table 1). 500-2000 L-DC sufficed to sensitize whereas at least 100x more B cells were needed to initiate a similar response. The priming effect of B cells is explained by contamination with L-DC as B cells from normal TDL (containing less than 0.1% L-DC) were unable to prime (Figure 1). 'In vitro' pulsed peritoneal macrophages were also unable to prime naive rats[15].

Experiments with L-DC derived from XTDL collected 24h after oral or intra-intestinal antigen administration gave similar results. L-DC from rats challenged via both routes were effective at all doses of antigens tested (Fig 2) and intra-intestinal antigen gave rise to larger responses than oral antigen but the differences were not large. Thus, it is clear that after oral or intra-intestinal administration, DC in the wall of the intestine acquire antigen and are able to prime naive T cells in lymph node 'in vivo'. Given that only small amounts of antigen can be acquired by L-DC after intra-intestinal Ag administration (see above) and that only a small percentage of injected DC are likely to migrate to the draining lymph node[17], the process of sensitization is remarkably efficient.

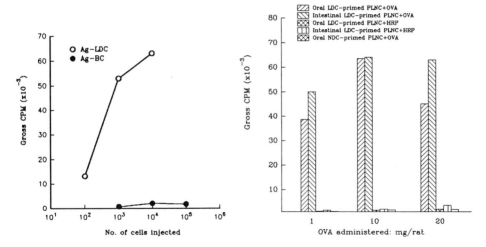

Figure 1a L-DC from MLNX rats and B cells from normal TDL were pulsed with OVA (1mg/ml) and injected into the footpads of naive rats. 10 days later, popliteal lymph node cells were prepared and cultured with OVA (50μg/ml) for 5 days and proliferation measured and expressed as gross CPM.

Figure 1b MLNX rats were cannulated and challenged with different doses of OVA (1mg, 10mg and 20mg/rat) orally or intra-intestinally. L-DC were enriched and injected into the footpad of naive PVG rats (5x10⁴/footpad). 10 days later, popliteal lymph node cells were prepared and cultured with OVA (50μg/ml) for 5 days and proliferation measured and expressed as gross CPM.

Direct antigen presentation by antigen-bearing L-DC

We have shown that antigen-bearing L-DC can prime naive T cells, but host DC might obtain antigen from donor L-DC and then present it to host T cells. To address this question, L-DC from PVG-RT1^u or congenic PVG-RT1^c rats, which differ at the MHC, were either pulsed 'in vitro' with OVA or obtained from PVG-RT1^c or PVG-RT1^u rats that had been injected with OVA intra-intestinally. These L-DC were injected into the footpads of (PVG-RT1^c x PVG-RT1^u) F1 rats. 10 days later, draining popliteal lymph nodes were depleted of B cells and MHC class II bearing cells and cultured with irradiated PVG-RT1^c or PVG-RT1^u spleen cells in the presence of OVA or HRP. The results showed that the responses were restricted to the MHC class II molecules on the immunizing L-DC (Table 2). T cells from F1 animals injected with Ag-bearing L-DC from PVG-RT1c rats only respond to OVA in the presence of PVG-RT1c spleen cells but not of PVG-RT1u spleen cells. Similarly, T cells from F1 animals injected with Ag-bearing L-DC from PVG-RT1u rats only respond to OVA in the presence of PVG-RT1u spleen cells but not of PVG-RT1c spleen cells. Experiments using Ag-L-DC pulsed 'in vivo' or 'in vitro' gave similar results. This experiment strongly suggests that Ag-bearing L-DC are presenting antigen to naive T cells directly. Inaba et al.[18] also demonstrated the direct presentation after the injection of DC, either pulsed 'in vitro' or 'in vivo', from one parental strain into F1 recipients. T cells from these recipients gave a sensitized response only to antigen presented on APC from the strain from which the injected DC were obtained.

Table 1. Priming of naive rats with 'in vitro' OVA-pulsed cells from XTDL.

Cells injected	Ag	Ag concentration in culture			
		100µg	50µg	25µg	No Ag
L-DC(2x105)	OVA	54169	35783	26708	2989
	HRP	6424	1689		
L-DC(2x104)	OVA	20039	13526		490
	HRP	916	1001		
L-DC(2x103)	OVA	13191	9789		777
	HRP	536	489		
BC(2x106)	OVA	28606	13229	12755	2912
	HRP	1618	2750	3063	
BC(2x105)	OVA	15370	7854	5541	257
	HRP	1246	1649	1744	
TC(2x106)	OVA	6649	5011	1634	838
	HRP	1381	2060	2903	
TC(2x105)	OVA	487	860	617	359
	HRP	312	769	971	

L-DC were enriched to 70% purity by centrifugation over 14.5% Metrizamide and B cells and T cells enriched by rosetting (85-90% purity for B cells; 90-92% for T cells). There were about 1-1.5% L-DC in the B cell fraction as identified by morphology and MHC Class II staining. L-DC, B cells and T cells were cultured with OVA (1mg/ml) for 3h, washed three times and injected into the footpads of naive rats. 10 days after immunization, popliteal lymph node cells were prepared and cultured with OVA or HRP in different concentrations (100µg/ml, 50µg/ml and 25µg/ml) for 120 h. 16h before harvesting, ^{3}HTdr was added into the wells. Results are expressed as gross C.P.M.

Antibody response after priming by Ag-bearing L-DC

To determine whether antigen-bearing L-DC were able to induce an antibody response, naive rats were primed with orally or intra-intestinally challenged L-DC, 'in vitro' antigen-pulsed L-DC, soluble antigens, or antigens emulsified with CFA. 10 days after priming, sera were obtained and the rats were boosted with soluble antigens subcutaneously (OVA or HRP). 10 days after boosting, rats were bled again to obtain sera. The results showed that neither 'in vitro' nor 'in vivo' antigen-pulsed L-DC, BC or peritoneal macrophages were able to induce a primary response. However, after boosting with soluble antigens, weak IgG antibody responses were present in all rats that had been primed with antigen-bearing L-DC (data not shown). Small doses of antigen tend to stimulate cell-mediated responses selectively[19] and the L-DC that induce T cell sensitization do not carry directly detectable amount of antigen (see above). Probably most antigen acquired by L-DC is processed and expressed in the form of peptides and is unable to stimulate an antibody response against whole native antigen. The weak responses observed after challenge with soluble antigen may reflect the ability of CD4+ T cells, sensitized in the primary response, to give increased levels of help to B cells.

Table 2 Ag-bearing L-DC present Ag directly to host T cells

F1 T cells	APC	Gross CPM		
		OVA	HRP	No Ag
cF1T	cAPC	15941	2360	
cF1T	uAPC	1412	214	
cF1T		600		
cF1T				630
uF1T	uAPC	16388	1848	
uF1T	cAPC	1743	263	
uF1T		1140		
uF1T				330

L-DC from rats which had been injected with OVA (10mg/ml) intra-intestinally were injected into the footpads of naive F1 rats (PVG-RT1^c x PVG-RT1^u). 10 days later, T cells were enriched from popliteal lymph node cells of those L-DC-injected rats as described in Materials and Methods and cultured with OVA or HRP in the presence of irradiated spleen cells from PVG-RT1^c or PVG-RT1^u rats for about 120 hours. ^{3}HTdr was added to the cultures 16h prior to harvesting, . The results are expressed as gross CPM. Concentration of Ag in culture: 50μg/ml. No. of spleen cells as APC: 1x10^5/well. No. of F1 T cells : 1x10^5/well. cF1T: T cells enriched from F1 rats which had been injected with Ag-pulsed L-DC from PVG-RT1^c; uF1T: T cells enriched from F1 rats which had been injected with Ag-pulsed L-DC from PVG-RT1^u; cAPC: spleen cells from PVG-RT1^c rats;   uAPC: spleen cells from PVG-RT1^u rats.

Conclusions

1, L-DC can acquire soluble protein antigens administered orally.

2, L-DC which have acquired antigens administered orally or intra-intestinally are able to prime naive T cells directly. Only L-DC in thoracic duct lymph can prime naive T cells.

3, A primary antibody response cannot be detected after priming with antigen-bearing L-DC. A small IgG response is present after a boosting injection.

4, We have developed an 'in vivo' model for the investigation of antigen presentation by intestinal antigen presenting cells. This system can be applied to many other antigens including pathogens and potential vaccines.

References

1. MacDonald T.T., and P.B. Carter. 1982. Isolation and functional characteristics of adherent phagocytic cells from mouse Peyer's patches. *Immunology*. 45:769.
2. Kammer G.M., and E.R. Unanue. 1980. Accessory cell requirement in the proliferative response of T lymphocytes to haemocyanin. *Clin. Immunol. Immunopathol*. 15:434.
3. Bland P.W., and Warren L.G. 1986. Antigen presentation by epithelial cells of the rat small intestine. II. Selective induction of suppressor T cells. *Immunology* 58:9.
4. Spalding D.M., W.J. Koopman, J.H. Eldridge, J.R. McGhee and R.M. Steinman. 1983. Accessory cells in murine Peyer's patch. I. Identification and enrichment of a functional dendritic cell. *J. Exp. Med*. 157:1646.
5. Pavli P., C.E. Woodhams, W.F. Doe, and D.A. Hume. 1990. Isolation and characterization of antigen-presenting dendritic cells from the mouse intestinal lamina propria. *Immunology*. 70:40.
6. Wilders M.M., H.A. Drexhage, E.F. Weltervreden, H. Mullink, A. Duijvestijn , and S.G.M. Meuwissen. 1983. Large mononuclear Ia-positive veiled cells in Peyer's patches. Isolation and characterization in rat, guinea pig and pig. *Immunology*. 48:453.

7. Spalding D.M., Williamson S.I., Koopman W.J. and J.R. McGhee. 1984. Preferential induction of polyclonal IgA secretion by murine Peyer's patch dendritic cell-T cell mixtures. J. Exp. Med. 160:941.
8. Spalding D.M. and J.A. Griffin. 1986. Different pathways of differentiation of pre-B cell lines are induced by dendritic cells and T cells from different lymphoid tissues. Cell. 44:507.
9. Bujdoso R., J. Hopkins, B.M. Dutia , P. Young, and I. McConnell. 1989. Characterization of sheep afferent lymph dendritic cells and their role in antigen carriage. *J. Exp. Med.* 170:1285.
10. Macatonia S.E., S.C. Knight, A.J. Edwards, S. Griffiths, and P. Fryer. 1987. Localisation of antigen on lymph node dendritic cells after exposure to the contact sensitizer fluorescein isothiocyanate. Functional and morphological studies. *J .Exp. Med.* 166:1654.
11. Crowley M., K. Inaba, & R.M. Steinman. 1990. Dendritic cells are the principal cell in mouse spleen bearing immunogenic fregments of foreign proteins. *J. Exp. Med.* 172:383.
12. Mayrhofer G., P.G. Holt, J.M. Papadimitriou. 1986. Functional characteristics of the veiled cells in afferent lymph from the rat intestine. *Immunology.* 58:379.
13. Liu L.M. and G.G. MacPherson. 1991. Lymph-borne (veiled) dendritic cells can acquire and present intestinally administered antigens. *Immunology.* 73:281.
14. Challacombe S.J., and T.B.Jr. Tomasi. 1980. Systemic tolerance and secretory immunity after oral immunization. *J. Exp. Med.* 152:1459.
15. Liu L.M. and G.G. MacPherson. 1993. Antigen acquisition by dendritic cells: intestinal dendritic cells acquire antigen administered orally and can prime naive T cells in vivo. J. Exp. Med. 177:1299.
16. Brenan M. and M. Puklavec. 1992. The MRC OX-62 antigen: a useful marker in the purification of rat veiled cells with the biochemical properties of an integrin. *J. Exp. Med.* 175:1457.
17. Fossum S. 1988. Lymph-borne dendritic leucocytes do not recirculate, but enter the lymph node paracortex to become interdigitating cells. *Scand. J. Immunol.* 27:97.
18. Inaba K., J.P. Metlay, M.T. Crowley and R.M. Steinman. 1990. Dendritic cells pulsed with protein antigens in vitro can prime antigen-specific, MHC restricted T cells in situ. *J. Exp. Med.* 172:631.
19. Lamont A.G., A.M. Mowat, and D.M. Parrott. 1989. Priming of systemic and local delayed-type hypersensitivity response by feeding low doses of ovalbumin to mice. *Immunology.* 66:595.

BLOCKAGE OF THYMIC MEDULLARY EPITHELIAL CELL ACTIVATION: IN

VIVO CONSEQUENCES

E.F. Potworowski[1], C. Beauchemin[1], D. Flipo[2], and M. Fournier[2]

[1]Institut Armand-Frappier, P.O. Box 100, Laval, QC, Canada, H7N 4Z3
[2]Département des Sciences Biologiques, Université du Québec à Montréal

INTRODUCTION

The orderly interactions between thymocytes at discrete stages of their differentiation and particular stromal elements generate a predictable phenotypic profile of thymocyte subsets (Scollay and Shortman, 1986). Interference with such interactions by the *in vivo* injection of selected monoclonal antibodies, has made it possible to delineate both the developmental relationships existing between various thymocyte subsets as well as the function of particular lympho-stromal complexes (MacDonald et al., 1988; McDuffie et al., 1986; Kruisbeek et al., 1985; Kyewski et al., 1989).

We have developed an *in vitro* system of thymic medullary epithelial cells (E-5) forming complexes with thymocytes (Potworowski et al., 1989). It is unique in that complex formation resulted in the activation, not of thymocytes, but of epithelial cells: tyrosine phosphorylation was indeed observed on an epithelial gp90, after contact with thymocytes through the gp23/45 ligand (Couture et al., 1990, 1992). Such an epithelial activation could not be achieved by cross-linking a monoclonal antibody to the 23kD chain of the ligand; this antibody (C3C12) however, when placed in the co-culture of thymocytes and epithelial cells, prevented complex formation and the ensuing epithelial gp90 phosphorylation (Couture et al., 1992).

As the formation of this complex resulted in neither proliferation, phenotype modification nor apoptosis of the complexed thymocytes, it became pertinent to gain an insight into the role of this particular lympho-stromal interaction within the wider context of the complete thymic microenvironment.

METHODS

Time-pregnant C57BL/6 mice were obtained from Charles River Canada, St. Constant, QC. They were kept one per cage for the duration of the experiment. Monoclonal antibody C3C12, an IgG2a was raised in LOU rats against the glycoprotein fraction of C57BL/6 mouse thymic medullary epithelial cells of the E-5 line (Couture et al., 1990). It reacts

In Vivo Immunology, Edited by E. Heinen *et al.*
Plenum Press, New York, 1994

specifically with the gp23 chain of the gp 23/45 epithelial adhesion molecule of E-5 cells, and with some medullary epithelial cells in frozen thymus sections. Ascites were prepared in AO x LOU rats and the IgG fraction was purified on a T-Gel purification kit (Pierce, Rockford, IL. USA). The antibody was concentrated on a PM-10 membrane (Amicon, Beverly, MA. USA) to between 4.0 and 5.0 mg/mL. Gravid mice were injected daily from day 16 of gestation until parturition with 0.5 mg antibody administered intraperitoneally.

Control mice routinely received an equivalent volume of PBS, once it had been established that an irrelevant isotype-matched antibody was ineffective. Cytofluorometric analysis was carried out on thymocytes of newborn mice using a FACSCAN (Beckton-Dickinson). Anti-CD8 (Clone 53-6.7) antibody conjugated to FITC (Beckton-Dickinson) and to phycoerythrin (Boehringer-Mannheim, Mannheim, Germany) was used respectively with phycoerythrin-conjugated anti-CD4 (clone GK1.5, Beckton-Dickinson) and FITC conjugated anti-CD3 (clone 145-2C11, Pharmingen, San Diego, CA, USA) in dual fluorescence analyses. Small lymphocytes and blasts were gated on the basis of forward light scatter to allow separate analysis of these populations as well as of the entire thymocyte population.

RESULTS AND DISCUSSION

Co-analysis of CD4 and CD8 yielded similar results for the group of newborn mice whose mothers had received the C3C12 mAb ("experimental group") and those whose mothers had received PBS ("control group"). Total cell analysis gave values of approximately 4% for the single positive CD4$^+$ cells, 83% for the double positive cells, 11% for the double negative cells and 3% for the single positive CD8$^+$ cells, which is compatible with data obtained by other groups on neotates (Ceredig et al., 1983).

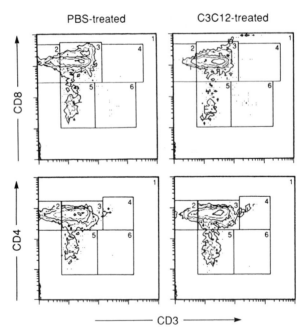

Figure 1. Cytofluorometric analysis of thymocytes from newborn mice whose mothers were treated either with PBS (left quadrants) or C3C12 antibody (right quadrants). Note that window #2 in the C3C12 groups is clearly depleted of cells.

Table 1. Population shifts of newborns' thymocytes[1] after C3C12 administration to mothers

Gating	Group	CD8^{++}CD3^{-}[2]	CD8^{++}CD3$^{\pm}$[3]
All thymocytes	PBS	14.85 ± 1.52	68.59 ± 2.75
	C3C12	7.25 ± 0.66	75.48 ± 1.89
Small thymocytes	PBS	18.06 ± 1.56	79.49 ± 2.42
	C3C12	9.98 ± 0.02	87.84 ± 0.49
Blasts	PBS	10.20 ± 1.67	52.30 ± 3.01
	C3C12	3.37 ± 0.06	56.43 ± 0.51

Gating	Group	CD4^{++}CD3^{-}	CD4^{++}CD3$^{\pm}$
All thymocytes	PBS	19.23 ± 1.99	62.28 ± 0.75
	C3C12	11.74 ± 0.41	67.80 ± 1.03
Small thymocytes	PBS	25.47 ± 0.59	69.98 ± 1.71
	C3C12	18.81 ± 1.68	74.80 ± 1.23
Blasts	PBS	14.81 ± 0.45	40.82 ± 1.71
	C3C12	9.33 ± 0.65	41.55 ± 0.11

1   n= 3-5 newborn thymuses from at least 2 litters
2   Window 2 on cytofluorogram
3   Window 3 on cytofluorogram

For the co-analysis of CD4 and CD3 and of CD8 and CD3, windows were placed around CD4^{++} CD3^{-}, CD4^{++} CD3$^{\pm}$, CD4^{++} CD3^{+}, CD4^{+} CD3$^{\pm}$, and CD4^{+} CD3^{+}. Other combinations had negligible quantities of cells (Fig 1). There was a markedly lower proportion of CD4^{++} CD3^{-} in the antibody-treated group; this was compensated mostly by a larger proportion of CD4^{++} CD3$^{\pm}$ cells in that group. This difference was evident both when all thymocytes were analysed together (Fig 1 and Table 1), as well as in small lymphocytes. Among blasts, the lower value in the CD4^{++} CD3^{-} population seemed to be compensated mostly by a relative increase among the CD4^{+} CD3$^{\pm}$ cells.

Similarly, the percentage of CD8^{++} CD3^{-} cells in the antibody-treated group was about half that found in the PBS-treated group. This was also the case when small lymphocytes were analysed separately. In the case of blasts, the antibody-treated mice had approximately two thirds less cells of this phenotype. In all three cases a corresponding increase was noted mainly in the CD8^{++} CD3$^{\pm}$ population.

Antibody treatment brought about a marked depletion of CD3$^-$ cells, both among CD4^{++} and CD8^{++} thymocytes, and a corresponding increase in CD3$^\pm$ expression among the same CD4^{++} and CD8^{++} cells. While simultaneous detection of CD3, CD4 and CD8 by three-colour fluorescence was not done, it is well-known that the CD3$^-$ and CD3$^\pm$ phenotypes are found only in association with double negative or double positive CD4/CD8 thymocytes (reviewed in Boyd and Hugo, 1991). It is safe, therefore, to conclude that C3C12 antibody treatment causes an accumulation of CD4^{++}CD8^{++}CD3$^\pm$, and a depletion of CD4^{++}CD8^{++}CD3$^-$ thymocytes. Since single positive CD4 and CD8 cells appear to be unaffected, one is clearly not dealing with a differentiation *blockage*, which would affect all downstream populations.   The key observation in this work is that the affected populations are cortical thymocytes which have yet several steps to undergo before they make contact with medullary epithelial cells. This leads to the inevitable conclusion that contact-induced activation of medullary epithelial cells triggers the secretion of a soluble factor whose ultimate target is "upstream" among the populations which have been disturbed by C3C12 antibody treatment.   This interpretation would corroborate a number of previous observations both from our laboratory and that of others.   First, thymocytes adhering in vitro to E-5 epithelial cells do not undergo differentiation, activation (Couture et al., 1992) nor do they increase their base-line reactivity to PHA (Hugo et al., 1990), whereas thymocytes present in the same culture but not participating in the complex, had their responsiveness to that mitogen significantly increased, suggesting the participation of a soluble factor (Potworowski et al., 1989). Second, thymocyte-induced upregulation of IL-1 secretion has been documented in primary cultures of human thymic epithelial cells (Le et al., 1990).   The target cells of IL-1 would likely be cortical thymocytes.   Our preliminary data, however, indicate that neither IL-1α, IL-1-ß nor indeed IL-6 are secreted after E-5 activation (in preparation). One cannot at this stage dismiss the possibilities that cells of the E-5 clone have lost the ability to secrete IL-1 in vitro (either constitutively as reported for medullary epithelial cells by Farr et al., 1989 or as a result of activation as reported by Le et al., 1990), or that new cytokines are secreted by activated E-5 cells, and by their in vivo counterpart (Kasai and Hirokawa, 1991). If such is indeed the case, injection of a mAb which prevents medullary epithelial activation and the ensuing cytokine secretion would no doubt have repercussions on the target cells of such cytokines.

While the mediators in the signalling pathway between medullary epithelial cells and cortical thymocytes remain to be identified, the evidence presented here argues in favor of the existence of such a pathway.   In order to ensure the maintenance of thymic homeostasis, one could easily envisage a mechanism whereby mature medullary thymocytes, about to leave the thymus, should send a proliferating signal to the cortex.

ACKNOWLEDGMENTS

Supported by the Medical Research Council of Canada. We thank Mr. Marcel Desrosiers for flow cytometry.

BIBLIOGRAPHY

Boyd, R.L. and Hugo, P., 1991, Towards an integrated view of thymopoiesis. *Immunol. Today* 12:71.

Ceredig, R., MacDonald, H.R. and Jenkinson, E.J., 1983, Flow microfluorometric analysis of mouse thymus development in vivo and in vitro. *Eur. J. Immunol.* 13:185.

Couture, C., Amarante-Mendes, G. and Potworowski, E.F., 1992, Tyrosine kinase activation in thymic epithelial cells: necessity of thymocyte contact through the gp23/45/90 adhesion complex. *Eur. J. Immunol.* 22:2579.

Couture, C., Patel, P.C. and Potworowski, E.F., 1990, A novel thymic epithelial adhesion molecule. *Eur. J. Immunol.* 20:2769.

Farr, A.G., Hosier, S., Braddy, S.C., Anderson, S.K., Eisenhardt, D.J., Yan, Z.J. and Robles, C.P., 1989, Medullary epithelial cell lines from murine thymus constitutively secrete IL-1 and hematopoietic growth factors and express class II antigens in response to recombinant Inteferon-γ. *Cell. Immunol.* 119:427.

Hugo P. and Potworowski, E.F., 1990, Selection of CD4⁺CD8⁺ thymocytes by complex formation with medulla-derived epithelial cells. *Cell. Immunol.* 126:143.

Kasai, M. and Hirokawa, K., 1991, A novel cofactor produced by a thymic epithelial cell line: promotion of proliferation of immature thymic lymphocytes by the presence of interleukin-1 and various mitogens. *Cell. Immunol.* 132, 377.

Kruisbeek, A.M., Bridges, S., Carmen, J., Longo, D.L. and Mond, J.J., 1985, *In vivo* treatment of neonatal mice with anti-I-A antibodies interferes with the development of the class I, class II, and Mls-reactive proliferating T cell subset. *J. Immunol.* 134:3597.

Kruisbeek, A.M., Mond, J., Fowlkes, B., Carmen, J., Bridges, S. and Longo, D., 1985, Absence of Ly-2⁻, L3T4⁺ lineage of T cells in mice treated neonatally with anti-AI correlates with absence of intrathymic I-A bearing antigen presenting function. *J. Exp. Med.* 161:1029.

Kyewski, B.A., Schirmacher, V. and Allison, J.P., 1989, Antibodies against the T cell receptor/CD3 complex interfere with distinct intra-thymic cell-cell interactions *in vivo*: correlation with arrest of T cell differentiation. *Eur. J. Immunol.* 19:857.

MacDonald, H.R., Hengartner, H. and Pedrazzini, T., 1988, Intrathymic deletion of self-reactive cells prevented by neonatal anti-CD4 antibody treatment. *Nature* 335:174.

McDuffie, M., Born, W., Marrack, P. and Kappler, J., 1986, The role of the T cell receptor in thymocyte maturation: Effets *in vivo* of anti-receptor antibody. *Proc. Natl. Acad. Sci. USA.* 83:8728.

Le, P.T., Wollger, L.W., Haynes, B.F. and Singer, K.H., 1990, Ligand binding to the LFA-3 cell adhesion molecule induces IL-1 production by human thymic epithelial cells. *J. Immunol.* 144:4541.

Potworowski, E.F., Hugo, P. and Couture, C., 1989, Binding of cortical thymocytes to a medullary epithelial cell line: A brief review. *Thymus* 13:237.

Scollay, R. and Shortman, K., 1985, Identification of early stages of T lymphocyte development in the thymus cortex and medulla. *J. Immunol.* 134:3632.

HALF-LIVES OF ANTIGEN/MHC CLASS II COMPLEXES DIFFER BETWEEN DISTINCT ORGAN MICROENVIRONMENTS

Klaus-Peter Müller and Bruno A. Kyewski

Tumor Immunology Programme, German Cancer Research Centre
Im Neuenheimer Feld 280, D 69 120 Heidelberg, FRG

INTRODUCTION

Antigen presentation is central to two processes: establishment of self tolerance in primary lymphoid organs requires presentation of self antigens[1], whereas initiation of immune responses in peripheral (secondary) lymphoid organs requires presentation of foreign antigens. While the molecular mechanism of antigen presentation in both instances is probably the same, tolerance induction proceeds continuously, whereas induction of an immune response against a particular foreign antigen is usually transient. T cells are generated throughout life and they need to be tolerized against an unknown array of self peptides. It is assumed that the spectrum of tolerizing self antigens within the thymus remains constant during adult life. In contrast, the spectrum of foreign antigens in peripheral lymphoid organs varies with time depending on antigenic exposure. This different homeostasis of antigen presentation in both processes is primarily regulated by availability of antigen (self *versus* foreign), but may also be influenced by other parameters, *e. g.* the half-lives of antigen presentation in the respective microenvironments.

Half-lives of antigen/MHC complexes *in vivo* may be subject to complex regulation, *e. g.* by the rate of synthesis and recycling of MHC molecules in different cell types, which in turn may depend on their state of differentiation *in situ*. In addition, the local availability of antigen and the turnover rate of antigen presenting cells (APC) in distinct organ microenvironments will influence the half-lives *in vivo*. Little is known to date to which extent these parameters dictate the half-lives of immunogenic or tolerogenic peptide/MHC complexes in different organs. Here, we present estimates of half-lives of murine peptide/MHC class II complexes in various microenvironments *in vivo*, which differ from the respective half-lives *in vitro*.

In Vivo Immunology, Edited by E. Heinen *et al.*
Plenum Press, New York, 1994

MATERIALS AND METHODS

Animals and Reagents

Female BALB/c mice (H-2^d) 3-5 weeks of age were used throughout these studies and were obtained from the Zentrale Versuchstieranstalt, Hannover, FRG. The Mgb specific T-T hybridoma 13.26.8 (generously supplied by Dr. A. Livingstone, Basel), recognizes the peptide aa 132-147 (sequence: NKALELFRKDIAAKYK) in the context of I-E^d as previously described[2]. The internal peptide has been synthesized on an Applied Biosystems peptide synthesizer (model 4318).

Antigen pulse *in vivo*

Sperm whale myoglobin, Mgb (Serva, Heidelberg, FRG) or an internal peptide thereof were dissolved in sterile PBS and each mouse received 1 mg Mgb or 60 µg peptide per g body weight i. v. in a volume of 200 µl. Various time intervals after antigen pulse, APC were isolated from different organs and assayed *in vitro*. Alternatively, APC were isolated 2 h after the antigen pulse *in vivo* and assayed at various time intervals after culture *in vitro*.

Isolation of APC

Unseparated splenocytes, lymph node and bone marrow cells were prepared according to standard procedures. For each time point thymocyte rosettes (T-ROS) and thymic nurse cells (TNC) were isolated and purified from 40 pooled thymi and splenic rosettes (Spl-ROS) from 10 pooled spleens as described previously[3]. T-ROS and TNC were enriched to a degree such that cross-contamination was < 5 %.

Antigen presentation assay

Graded concentrations of various freshly isolated APC populations were cocultured with a Mgb specific T-T hybridoma (50 000 cells/well) in triplicates in flat bottom 96 well plates (Costar, Dannstadt, FRG) for 24 h in Iscove's modified Dulbecco's medium supplemented with 10 % FCS, 5 x 10^{-5} M 2-ME, 10 mM Hepes, 2 mM glutamine and penicillin/streptomycin. Parallel cultures were set up with and without addition of 100 µg/ml Mgb or 50 µg/ml peptide. IL-2 production by the T-T hybridoma was quantitated by culturing the IL-2 dependent T cell clone CTLL (5000 cells/well) in the presence of 100 µl of the culture supernatant for another 24 h. The proliferation of the indicator cell line was measured by addition of [^{3}H] dTdR (1 µCi/well, Amersham Buchler, Braunschweig, FRG) during the last 4 h of incubation. Incorporation of [^{3}H] dTdR was determined according to standard procedures using a betaplate counter (Pharmacia, Freiburg, FRG).

Calculation of half-life of peptide/MHC complexes

Values in the linear range of the titration curves of APC isolated from mice at different time intervals after antigen pulse were used to calculate the time-dependent loss of antigen presentation by plotting the ratio of IL-2 production/APC *versus* time (Figure 1B and 1D), as previously described[4]. Half-lives were calculated using a curve fitting computer software with the assumption of an exponential decay.

RESULTS AND DISCUSSION

Antigen half-lives *in vivo* and *in vitro*

BALB/c mice were pulsed with sperm whale myoglobin (Mgb) i. v. and after 2, 12, 24, and 36 h APC from various organs were isolated and cocultured with a Mgb-specific T-T-hybridoma *in vitro*. Six APC populations were compared: unseparated splenocytes, highly enriched splenic APC (*i.e.* Spl-ROS), whole bone marrow and lymph node cells, thymic cortical epithelial cells (*i.e.* thymic nurse cells, TNC), and thymic medullary dendritic cells (i.e. thymocyte rosettes, T-ROS). Previous studies had shown that TNC represent resident cortical epithelial cells more than 90 % of which express MHC class II antigens and markers specific for cortical epithelial cells such as CDR1 and TR-4 (for review see ref. 5). T-ROS represent lymphostromal complexes between immature thymocytes and thymic macrophages (MØ) or dendritic cells (DC). Within T-ROS strong MHC class II expression and MHC class II-restricted antigen presentation segregate with non-adherent DC-type cells. More than 85 % of MHC class II positive stromal cells within T-ROS coexpress the CD11c antigen detected by the mAb N418 (ref. 6), hence APC activity by T-ROS is ascribed to thymic DC. Likewise splenic ROS are highly enriched for cells expressing the N 418 epitope (> 90 % Spl-ROS are positive as compared to 1 % cells in whole spleen, data not shown).

As shown in Table 1, antigen half-life *in vivo* differed considerably among organs. Peripheral APC (spleen, lymph node and bone marrow) displayed short half-lives (3-10 h) when compared to thymic APC, the latter showing half-lives between 13 and 22 h. Enrichment of APC cannot account for this difference between thymic and splenic half-lives, since enriched (~ 100 times) splenic DC (Spl-ROS) revealed a similar short half-life as unseparated spleen. While the results for thymic APC are compatible with a constant clearance of antigenic complexes over the period examined, the data for splenic APC suggest a biphasic clearance with a rapid loss within the first 24 h followed by a slower decline thereafter (Figure 1C).

Next we analyzed whether the half-life of antigen presentation *in vivo* is influenced by the processing capacity of the different APC subsets. Instead of whole Mgb, mice received a Mgb peptide (an internal 16mer, aa 132-147) which is recognized by the T-T hybridoma 13.26.8 (see ref. 2). Although half-life values for peptide presentation did vary from those for intact Mgb, there was no consistent change, *i.e.* reduction or augmentation, when the different APC sources were compared (Table 1).

In order to assess whether there was a correlation between the half-life of antigenic complexes and the availability of the antigen *in vivo*, we determined the blood half-life of Mgb and peptide. Both antigenic forms were injected after labeling with ^{131}I and the clearance of radioactivity from blood, spleen, thymus, kidney and liver was monitored between 5 and 120 min after injection Half-lives for Mgb and peptide in blood and organs were shorter (< 60 min) than those of cell-associated MHC/peptide complexes. It is thus unlikely that the differences in half-lives result from local trapping of antigen.

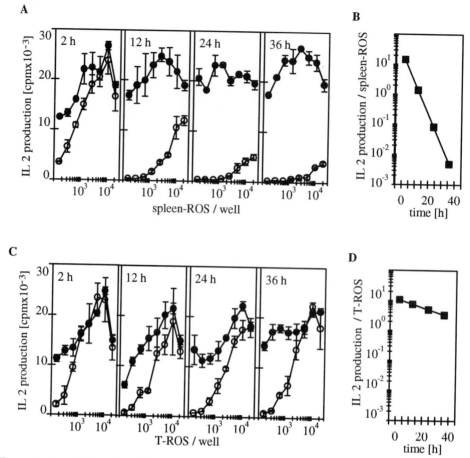

Figure 1. Presentation of myoglobin peptide by enriched splenic (A,B) and thymic (C,D) dendritic cells. Time-dependent presentation of a myoglobin specific peptide by splenic (A) and thymic dendritic cells (C) *ex vivo*. The linear range of the titration curve was used for calculation of half-lives (see part B and D). Presentation after loading *in vivo* (O) is compared with additional peptide loading *in vitro* (●). Semi-logarithmic plot of IL-2 production per APC versus time for splenic (B) and thymic (D) dendritic cells. Half-lives were calculated from these curves.

The stability of peptide/MHC class II complexes has been determined for different APC populations of human and mouse origin. The half-life values range from 20-50 h for human cells (EBV-transformed B cells and T cells, ref. 4) and from 60 min to 5 h for mouse B cell lymphomas or peritoneal MØ, respectively[7]. In order to assess whether the intra- and interorgan differences of half-lives *in vivo* reflect intrinsic properties of the specific APC subsets or the *in vivo* microenvironment (*e.g.* tissue kinetics), we determined the *in vitro* half-lives of the same APC subsets after an antigen pulse *in vivo*. The *in vitro* half-lives were considerably longer than the respective values *in vivo* (Table 1) except for thymic DC, which displayed the longest antigen retention *in vivo*. There was no correlation between half-lives *in vivo* and *in vitro* for a particular APC type and no correlation between the requirement for processing and the stability of peptide/MHC complexes for a given APC subset. Our data suggest that the APC subsets isolated *ex vivo* in this study do not rapidly exchange peptide due to recycling of MHC class II antigens as reported for the B lymphoma line TA3 (ref. 7).

Table 1. Half-life of antigen/I-E^d complexes *in vivo* and *in vitro*.

	in vivo		*in vitro*	
	myoglobin	peptide	myoglobin	peptide
thymic medullary dendritic cells (T-Ros)	a)22	20	19.7	22.3
thymic cortical epithelial cells (TNC)	13.1	17	17.9	25.6
splenocytes	8.6	5.9	31.3	21.3
splenic dendritic cells (Spl-ROS)	5.6	2.9	18.5	24.1
bone marrow cells	4.8	7	42.6	26.9
mesenteric lymph node cells	11	12	n.d.	n.d.

a) values in hours; for details of calculation of half-lives see Material and Methods section and Figure 1

n.d. = not done

An intriguing observation of this study is the relatively long half-life of antigen MHC class II complexes within the thymus. Moreover, within the thymus bone marrow-derived, medullary DC retain antigen longer than resident cortical epithelial cells. In contrast, stimulatory antigen/MHC complexes have considerably shorter half-lives in spleen or bone marrow. This difference is not a matter of enrichment of relevant APC subsets, since Spl-ROS, which are even more potent stimulators than T-ROS, display a similar short half-life as whole splenocytes. The values are independent of the particular peptide/MHC combination, since preliminary studies with an I-A^b restricted self peptide yield similar results. Assuming DC to be the main stimulator cells within T-ROS and splenocytes the results reveal yet another difference in this cell lineage between different organs. Thymic and splenic DC display differences in their phenotype[8,9] and their ontogeny[3,10].

Half-lives *in vivo* were generally shorter than the respective half-lives *in vitro*. Several parameters determine the half-life of antigen/MHC complexes *in vivo*; (a) the rate of MHC class II-synthesis, (b) the rate of MHC-recycling[7], (c) the stability of membrane-bound peptide/MHC complexes[4], and (d) the turnover rate of APC in various organ microenvironments. Little is known about the regulation of these parameters in the local microenvironments.

Studies with Langerhans cells (LC) for instance have shown that the rate of MHC class II synthesis may vary with the state of activation, *i.e.* tissue location of APC. Whereas freshly isolated LC show a high rate of MHC class II synthesis and are very efficient in antigen processing, culture *in vitro* leads to a rapid and specific downregulation of MHC class II synthesis and concomitant loss of antigen processing capacity[11,12]. The turnover rate of APC *in situ* may be yet another determinant of variations in half-life. Splenic DC are thought to be a fast turning over population[13] with an estimated replacement rate of 10 % per day[14]. A rapid turnover of splenic DC is furthermore inferred from radiation chimeras in which highly radiosensitive DC are fully replaced within 2 weeks[3]. Such a turnover rate, however, could not solely account for the half-life of antigen/MHC complexes in the range of 3-8 h. Thymic DC are known to be rapidly replaced after radiation or cortisone-mediated depletion. In non-radiation chimeras without prior ablation of hemopoietic cells a steady state chimerism is attained within 2-3 weeks, compatible with a daily replacement rate of about 5 % (ref. 3,15). In the absence of precise determination of the tissue half-life of APC in the various organs, it is open whether the tissue kinetics directly correlate with the half-lives observed. The observation that resident thymic epithelial cells display shorter half-lives than thymic DC, which are continuously replaced, would argue against such a simple correlation.

The difference between the *in vivo* half-life of peptide/MHC complexes in thymus and peripheral lymphoid organs is intriguing in view of the different role antigen presentation plays in these microenvironments. In the thymus antigen presentation to immature thymocytes induces antigen specific tolerance, it is worth noting that both cortical epithelial cells and medullary DC capture and process extrathymic antigens. Tolerance induction is a continuous process and thus necessitates the continuous presentation of self peptides to developing thymocytes. A relative long half-life of self peptide/MHC complexes within the thymus would contribute to a stable spectrum of tolerizing complexes. This consideration may apply in particular to self antigens whose physiological concentration varies with time, *e.g.* hormones or acute phase proteins. When intrathymic compartments are compared, medullary DC are more easily accessible to circulating antigens *in situ* (unpublished data), more efficient in deleting self antigen specific thymocytes *in vitro*[16], and they retain antigen longer *in vivo* when compared to cortical epithelial cells. The thymic medulla is thus a favorable site for (self) antigen presentation. In contrast, antigen presentation in peripheral lymphoid organs is central to the induction of an immune response, which usually is transient. In case of limited supply of antigen, the rapid removal of peptide/MHC complexes from the site of T cell induction could be an important mechanism to downregulate the response.

ACKNOWLEDGEMENTS

We thank Dr. Alexandra Livingstone, Basel for generous supply of reagents, Dr. Robert Busch for critical comments, the EMBL protein group for peptide synthesis and Prof. Volker Schirrmacher for continuous support. The technical assistance of Sonja Höflinger is gratefully acknowledged. This study has been supported by a grant of the BMFT Schwerpunkt "Autoimmunität" and the German Cancer Research Centre.

REFERENCES

1. Kappler, J. W., N. Roehm, and P. Marrack. 1987. T cell tolerance by clonal elimination in the thymus. *Cell* 49:273.
2. Ruberti, G. , K. S. Sellins, C. M. Hill, R. N. Germain, C. G. Fathman, and A. Livingstone. 1992. Presentation of antigen by mixed isotype class II molecule in normal H-2^d mice. *J. Exp. Med.* 175:157.
3. Kyewski, B. A., C. G. Fathman, and R. V. Rouse. 1986. Intrathymic presentation of circulating non MHC antigens by medullary dendritic cells. *J. Exp. Med.* 163:231.
4. Lanzavecchia, A. , P. A. Reid, and C. Watts. 1992. Irreversible association of peptides with class II MHC molecules in living cells. *Nature* 357:249.
5. Kyewski, B. A. 1986. Thymic nurse cells: possible sites of T-cell selection. *Immunol. Today* 7(12):374.

6. Metlay, J. P., M. D. Witmer Pack, R. Agger, M. T. Crowley, D. Lawless, and R. M. Steinman. 1990. The distinct leukocyte integrins of mouse spleen dendritic cells as identified with new hamster monoclonal antibodies. *J. Exp. Med.* 171:1753.

7. Harding, C. V., R. W. Roof, and E. R. Unanue. 1989. Turnover of Ia-peptide complexes is facilitated in viable antigen-presenting cells: biosynthetic turnover of Ia vs. peptide exchange. *Proc. Natl. Acad. Sci. U. S. A.* 86:4230.

8. Crowley, M., K. Inaba, M. Witmer-Pack, and R. M. Steinman. 1989. The cell surface of mouse dendritic cells: FACS analysis of dendritic cells from different tissues including thymus. *Cell. Immunol.* 118:108.

9. Ardavin, C. and K. Shortman. 1992. Cell surface marker analysis of mouse thymic dendritic cells. *Eur. J. Immunol.* 22:859.

10. Kyewski, B. A. 1987. Seeding of thymic microenvironments defined by distinct thymocyte- stromal cell interactions is developmentally controlled. *J. Exp. Med.* 166:520.

11. Pure, E., K. Inaba, M. T. Crowley, L. Tardelli, M. D. Witmer Pack, G. Ruberti, G. Fathman, and R. M. Steinman. 1990. Antigen processing by epidermal Langerhans cells correlates with the level of biosynthesis of major histocompatibility complex class II molecules and expression of invariant chain. *J. Exp. Med.* 172:1459.

12. Kämpgen, E., N. Koch, F. Koch, P. Stöger, C. Heufler, G. Schuler, and N. Romani. 1991. Class II major histocompatibility complex molecules of murine dendritic cells: synthesis, sialylation of invariant chain, and antigen processing capacity are down-regulated upon culture. *Proc. Natl. Acad. Sci. U. S. A.* 88:3014.

13. Kupiec-Weglinski, J. W., J. M. Austyn, and P. J. Morris. 1988. Migration patterns of dendritic cells in the mouse. Traffic from the blood, and T cell-dependent and -independent entry to lymphoid tissues. *J. Exp. Med.* 167:632.

14. Steinman, R. M., D. S. Lustig, and Z. A. Cohn. 1974. Identification of a novell cell type in peripheral lymphoid organs of mice. III. Functional properties in vivo. *J. Exp. Med.* 139:1431.

15. Kampinga, J., P. Nieuwenhuis, B. Roser, and R. Aspinall. 1990. Differences in turnover between thymic medullary dendritic cells and a subset of cortical macrophages. *J. Immunol.* 145:1659.

16. Pircher, H., K. Brduscha, U. Steinhoff, M. Kasai, T. Mizuochi, R. M. Zinkernagel, H. Hengartner, B. Kyewski, and K. -P. Müller. 1993. Tolerance induction by clonal deletion of CD4[+]8[+] thymocytes *in vitro* does not require dedicated antigen-presenting cells. *Eur. J. Immunol.* 23:669.

REGULATION OF NEURAL AND PERIPHERAL CYTOKINE PRODUCTION BY BENZODIAZEPINES AND ENDOGENOUS ANXIOGENIC PEPTIDES

Véronique Taupin[1], Sylvie Toulmond[2], Jesus Benavides[2], Jean Gogusev[3], Béatrice Descamps-Latscha[1] and Flora Zavala[1]

[1]INSERM U25, Hôpital Necker, Paris, France
[2]Synthelabo LERS, Bagneux, France
[3]INSERM U90, Hôpital Necker, Paris, France

INTRODUCTION

Our search to understand the molecular links between immune and nervous systems has led us to propose that central benzodiazepine receptors (CBR) and peripheral benzodiazepine receptors (PBR) could represent an integrative network whereby endogenous ligands could modulate anxiety as well as immune functions [1].

Among the molecular messengers that are involved not only in communication within cells of the immune system but also in information exchange between several integrated systems and particularly with the nervous system, are the cytokines. Benzodiazepine ligands modulate the production of cytokines and this interaction can take place at the periphery as well as within brain. In the present paper, we demonstrate that picomolar concentrations of triakontatetraneuropeptide (TTN), the major processing form of diazepam binding inhibitor (DBI), an endogenous peptide ligand of the benzodiazepine receptor, is able to modulate the gene expression of several pro-inflammatory cytokines by human monocytes[2]. Furthermore, an *in vivo* injection of a pharmacological ligand specific for the peripheral receptor significantly modulates the cytokine levels induced by fluid percussion trauma in rat brain[3].

In Vivo Immunology, Edited by E. Heinen *et al.*
Plenum Press, New York, 1994

RESULTS AND DISCUSSION

Triakontatetrapeptide (TTN), the Major Processing Form of Diazepam Binding Inhibitor (DBI) Increases mRNA Levels of Cytokines in LPS-treated Human Monocytes

Human PBMC were isolated by centrifugation on a Ficoll-Paque density gradient from heparinized blood of healthy donors, who had not taken benzodiazepines for at least 3 months. After 1 hr of adherence in flat-bottomed six-well microtiter plates, adherent cells (approximately 90% monocytes) were incubated at 2×10^6 cells per well, in RPMI 1640 medium supplemented with 5% heat-inactivated fetal calf serum, 100 units/ml penicillin, 100 µg/ml streptomycin, and 2 mM L-glutamine, in the presence or absence of LPS (1 µg/ml) and/or TTN (10^{-11}M) at 37°C for 4 hr. To extract total RNA, cells were directly lysed in the wells with 400 µl of 4M guanidinium isothiocyanate and Northern analysis was performed as described [2].

As shown on Figure 1, unstimulated cells cultured in the presence of serum contained low levels of TNFα, IL1β, GM-CSF, IL6 and IL8 mRNAs. TTN alone had no detectable

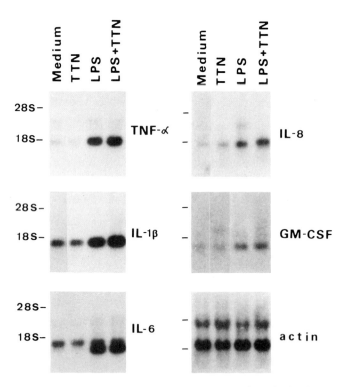

Figure 1. Effect of TTN on cytokine mRNA accumulation in LPS-stimulated human monocytes. Total cellular RNA was extracted from adherent mononuclear cells after 4 h of incubation without LPS (control medium), with TTN alone (10^{-11}M), with LPS (1 µg/ml), with both LPS and TTN and hybridized with specific ^{32}P-labeled cDNA probes for TNFα, IL1β, IL6, IL8, GM-CSF and β-actin.. (From ref.2, reprinted by permission from Mol. Pharmacol..)

enhancing effect on mRNA expression, whereas LPS increased TNFα, IL1β, GM-CSF, IL6 and IL8 mRNA accumulation approximately 2-3 fold. TTN (10^{-11}M) increased LPS-induced TNFα and IL1β mRNA expression by about 60% and GM-CSF, IL6, IL8 mRNA expression by 30%. Under the same conditions, Northern blot analysis of actin were unaffected by LPS alone and with TTN.

This is the first demonstration that a specific endogenous benzodiazepine receptor ligand, at picomolar concentrations, interferes with cytokine production at the level of gene expression. Whether TTN augments transcription or rather increases mRNA stabilization remains to be determined.

DBI, the endogenous ligand of BZD receptors has been shown to displace diazepam from CBR and from PBR. It is produced both in brain and in peripheral tissues where PBR are densely expressed. TTN, the most abundant biologically active processing product of DBI preferentially interacts at PBR and its anxiogenic action can be blocked by PK11195, the PBR antagonist but not by Ro15-1788, the CBR antagonist. Its anxiogenic activity is thought to be mediated by its stimulatory effect on the synthesis of neurosteroids that affect GABA affinity at GABA$_A$ receptors.

The fact that TTN exerted cytokine modulation at picomolar concentrations correlates well with its binding affinity for the Ro5-4864 subsite of PBR, which is expressed on human monocytes.

The endogenous BZD receptor ligand DBI has been suggested to play a role in the pathogenesis of both severe depression and hepatic encephalopathy, based on its levels in cerebrospinal fluid. All the cytokines modulated by TTN have been shown to favour the development of a pro-inflammatory reaction where they have a mutually stimulatory effect and act in synergy. The possibility that DBI or TTN could be involved in the physiological regulation of the inflammatory response appears an interesting hypothesis to investigate.

A Peripheral Benzodiazepine Ligand Stimulates the Production of Cytokines Induced in Brain by Fluid Percussion Trauma

We decided to investigate the possible effect of a pharmacological specific PBR ligand, Ro5-4864, on an *in vivo* model of inflammatory reaction that takes place within brain. PBR is expressed on brain astrocytes and microglia and PBR binding has been used as an index of glial cell proliferation

A potential role of cytokines in the response of brain tissue injury has been suggested by studies demonstrating that the concentrations of several of these mediators is greatly elevated in experimental brain lesion. Cytokines such as IL1, TNFα and IL6 not only participate in the process that leads to the formation of glial scar but may also act directly or indirectly as trophic factors and favour the regeneration of the neuronal network.

Traumatic lesions of the rat brain were performed by fluid percussion Rats were killed by decapitation at different times after surgery and brain structures were dissected, frozen in dry ice and stored at -80°C. For the detection of the levels of cytokines, brain structures were homogenized in PBS by polytron, centrifuged at 10 000 g for 15 min at 4°C and supernatants filtered. Cytokines were measured on the basis of their biological activity neutralized by specific antibodies [2].

In the cortex and hippocampus of control and sham-operated rats, the levels of these cytokines were very low and constant. IL-6 and IL-1 levels in the ipsilateral cortex increased rapidly following trauma to reach a maximum 8h after the lesion, remained elevated until 18h and decreased thereafter to basal values. TNF levels were maximally elevated at 3h and 8h and returned to basal values by 18h. Similar changes, but with 25-80 fold smaller amplitude, were seen in the contralateral cortex and in the ipsi-and contralateral hippocampus. The levels of IL-6 in the plasma of sham-operated and lesioned rats were only slightly elevated whereas IL-1 and TNF were undetectable.

The administration of Ro5 4864 (0.5 mg/kg i.p.), a specific PBR ligand , did not result in any significant effect on the levels of IL-6, IL-1 or TNF in the brain of control or sham-operated animals. However, when administered 24h before or 15 min after trauma, this benzodiazepine enhanced the increase of these cytokines by 2-4 folds in the ipsilateral cortex (Table 1). Ro5 4864 had no effect on IL-6 levels in the plasma of lesioned rats.

Table 1. Influence of a pre- or post-traumatic treatment with Ro5-4864 on cytokine levels in ipsilateral cortex at various times after trauma.

	Measuring Time after trauma	Treatment 24 h before trauma with		Treatment 15 min post trauma with	
		Excipient[1]	Ro5-4864[2]	Excipient[1]	Ro5-4864[2]
IL6	3 h	44 ± 29[3]	53 ± 10	N.D.	N.D.
	8 h	315 ± 88	252 ± 63	289 ± 77	603 ± 49**
	18 h	104 ± 23	521 ± 75**	193 ± 88	481 ± 77**
IL1	3 h	8 ± 1	7 ± 2	N.D.	N.D.
	8 h	14 ± 3	11 ± 1	21 ± 2	35 ± 3**
	18 h	8 ± 0	18 ± 4**	16 ± 2	33 ± 4**
TNF	3 h	12 ± 0	20 ± 8*	N.D.	N.D.
	8 h	12 ± 1	38 ± 8**	7 ± 3	18 ± 3*
	18 h	3 ± 1	3 ± 2	2 ± 0	2 ± 0

[1] Excipent was 1% EtOH in saline
[2] Ro5-4864 was injected i.p. at 0.5 mg/kg in 1% EtOH in saline
[3] Results are expressed as mean $\pm$ SEM, 6 rats per group
   Statistical significance was assessed using Student's t-test (*, $p<0.05$, **, $p<0.02$)

The fact that Ro5-4864 enhances the increase in IL1, IL6 and TNFα induced by fluid percussion trauma but does not affect basal production of these cytokines in brain or in the periphery suggests that this compound exerts a priming effect on cytokine producing cells. Furthermore, the fact that Ro5-4864 does not modulate significantly the cytokine production measured in the plasma after trauma supports the hypothesis of an activation of cytokine producing cells at the site of brain injury. These cells may correspond to the invading neutrophils observed by histochemistry at the time of cytokine production as well as to local glial cells.

These results suggest that PBR ligands may modulate the glial reaction that results from the inflammatory reaction at the site of brain injury. The glial reaction as well as an elevated level of cytokines are a constant feature of a high number of human neurodegenerative processes including Alzheimer's disease, AIDS, multiple sclerosis, Parkinson's disease and Huntington chorea as well as acute brain injury in stroke and trauma.

The modulation by a PBR ligand of cytokine production in the injured brain may open the way to the pharmacological control of the inflammatory reaction to brain injury. Whether the endogenous peptide ligand DBI and its processing products play a physiological role in development and repair processes in brain will be interesting to investigate.

CONCLUSION

BZD ligands are thus able to modulate cytokine production and may influence the development of an inflammatory reaction, in the periphery as well as within brain.

The endogenous precursor ligand DBI can be differentially processed leading to peptides that exert their anxiogenic properties by interacting at CBR but also, like TTN, by binding preferentially to PBR. Most pharmacological ligands exhibit this mixed type profile. The mutual influence of BZD ligands as neuropeptides and of cytokines in the immune system may therefore represent the molecular basis of a novel neuroimmune network.

REFERENCES

1. V. Taupin, A. Herbelin, B. Descamps-Latscha, and F. Zavala, Endogenous anxiogenic peptide, ODN-diazepam binding inhibitor, and benzodiazepine influence monokine production, *in*: "Lymphatic Tissues and In Vivo Immune Response", B.A. Imhof, S. Berrih-Aknin and S. Ezine, eds., Marcel Dekker, Inc., New York (1991)
2. V. Taupin, J. Gogusev, B. Descamps-Latscha, and F. Zavala, Modulation of TNFα, IL1β, IL6, IL8 and GM-CSF expression in human monocytes by an endogenous anxiogenic benzodiazepine ligand, triakonta-tetraneuropeptide: evidence for a role of prostaglandins. *Mol. Pharmacol.* 43:64 (1993)
3. V. Taupin, S. Toulmond, A. Serrano, J. Benavides and F. Zavala; Increase in IL-6, IL-1 and TNF levels in rat brain following traumatic lesion. Influence of pre- and post-traumatic treatment with Ro5-4864, a peripheral type (*p* site) benzodiazepine ligand. *J. Neuroimmunol.* 42:177 (1993)

COULD ACTH BE OF PRIME IMPORTANCE IN RAPIDLY
ALTERING THE THYMOCYTE COMPOSITION IN THE THYMUS?

Marion D. Kendall[1], Helen D. Loxley,[2] Michael R. Dashwood,[3] Sukwinder
Singh,[2] Richard Stebbings[1] and Julia C. Buckingham[2]

[1]Thymus Laboratory, IAPGR, Cambridge & Rayne Institute, UMDS
[2]Pharmacology, Charing Cross & Westminster Medical School
[3]Physiology, Royal Free Hospital Medical School, London

INTRODUCTION

Communication between the neuroendocrine and immune system is crucial to host
defence in both health and disease for it provides a means whereby the central nervous
system may fine tune the immune system and thereby bring to bear the influence of a
variety of physical, emotional and environmental factors. Several lines of evidence now
suggest that humoral factors originating within the immune system (e.g. cytokines,
ecosanoids and peptides) exert specific regulatory actions within the brain and pituitary
gland, whilst neural and endocrine factors contribute to the control of immunological
activity (Weigent and Blalock, 1987). Central to this communication are the thymic
hormones, thymulin, thymosin$_\alpha$1 and thymopoietin which provide the basis of the humoral
link between the thymus and the hypothalamo-pituitary complex and are themselves subject
to regulation by hormones derived from the pituitary gland and peripheral endocrine
organs (Millington and Buckingham, 1992).

The potential involvement of thymulin, a highly conserved nonapeptide, in the process
of thymocyte development has received scant attention probably because the peptide is not
strongly implicated in the development of the T-cell receptor. However, thymulin is
released at sites of prothymocyte activity (subcapsular cortex) and in the medulla where
single positive CD4 or CD8 thymocytes and recirculating T cells are found. Moreover,
flow cytometric analyses have shown that the phenotypic composition of thymocytes is
modified within hours of an injection of physiological doses of thymulin (Kendall et al.,
1992) and that changes persist for several weeks (Dardenne et al., 1978).

There is now widespread evidence that the secretion of thymulin is regulated both by
local factors and by hormones derived from the pituitary gland and peripheral endocrine
organs (Dardenne and Savino, 1990; Millington and Buckingham, 1992). Studies in man
have revealed a striking correlation between the plasma profiles of cortisol and thymulin
both over the 24 hr cycle, and following cardiac surgery (Kendall et al., 1991) while in
the rat, we have observed increases in thymulin release *in vivo* in conditions associated
with hypersecretion of ACTH and *in vitro* following ACTH challenge (Buckingham et al.,
1992). These data strongly suggest that the ACTH, which is released in response to
stressful stimuli, plays an important role in the control of thymulin release. In order to
provide some insight to the site of ACTH action in the thymus, we have examined the

In Vivo Immunology, Edited by E. Heinen *et al.*
Plenum Press, New York, 1994

distribution of specific ACTH binding sites (receptors) by autoradiographic methods and investigated the influence of the peptide on early gene expression (c-fos) using immunocytochemistry (full paper, Kendall et al., in preparation).

MATERIALS AND METHODS

Autoradiography was conducted in London and immunostaining in Cambridge. At both sites particular care was taken to minimise stress in the animals employed. Rats were moved to a quiet room with controlled lighting and temperature approximately 2 weeks before the experiments commenced and handled regularly thereafter. Food and water were available *ad libitum*.

Tissue for *in vitro* autoradiography was removed *post mortem* from 45 day old Sprague-Dawley rats between 09.00-11.00h and frozen on solid CO_2. Sections (20 μm) were cut from frozen tissue, thaw mounted onto gelatinized microscope slides and stored at -70°C until required. Sections were preincubated for 15 min at 20°C in 50mM Tris buffer (pH 7.4), containing 0.2% bovine serum albumin, 100 KIU/ml aprotinin and 5mM $MgCl_2$ in order to reduce endogenous peptide levels. In initial experiments, the sections (n = 6/group) were transferred to buffer containing graded concentrations of ^{125}I-ACTH (5-600pM) so as to establish the concentration of ACTH needed for maximum binding (100pM). This concentration was used in subsequent displacement experiments in which the degree of non-specific binding was established by incubation of the sections with ^{125}I-ACTH and in the presence of unlabelled $ACTH_{1-24}$ or $ACTH_{1-39}$ (0.06-35μM). Sections were then washed twice in Tris buffer for 5 mins at 4°C, blotted and dried on a heated plate. Low- and high-resolution autoradiography were then performed as described by Moody et al. (1990). After generating autoradiograms, underlying tissue was stained with Mayer's haematoxylin for histology. Sections and autoradiograms were viewed under dark- and bright-field illumination and photographed where appropriate.

For the studies of activation of early gene expression, the polyclonal antibody c-fos (Ab-2) (Cambridge Biosciences) was used. This reacts against residues 4-17 of human Fos (DeTogni et al., 1988) and is reactive on rodent tissues. Ten Porton Wistar rats were used in 2 groups of 5, each group being injected subcutaneously with 1μg $ACTH_{1-24}$ (Synacthen, Ciba) or saline. The rats were sacrificed after 90 mins, and blocks of thymus tissue rapidly frozen in iso-pentane cooled with liquid nitrogen and stored at -80°C until used. Sections (20μm and 40μm) were reacted with a rabbit anti-human polyclonal antibody to c-fos protein at optimal dilution (1/1,000) overnight at 4°C, washed in phospate buffered saline and incubated overnight (4°C) with donkey anti-rabbit Ig/HRP (1/500) (Amersham, UK) and then visualised using an immunoperoxidase diaminobenzidine method with nickel enhancement.

RESULTS

The autoradiographic studies demonstrated the presence of specific (i.e. displaceable with $ACTH_{1-24}$ and $ACTH_{1-39}$) binding-sites in the thymic tissue. The binding sites were particularly abundant in the cortex but also evident in the medulla (Figure 1).

The c-fos gene product was detected in the nuclei of cells situated mainly at the cortico-medullary junction of the thymus, to a lesser extent in the medulla and occasionally in cells scattered in the cortex. Positively stained nuclei (3-4 μm diam.) were located in small rounded mononuclear cells of lymphoid morphology. The number of c-fos positive cells were greatly increased, particularly in the medulla after ACTH treatment (Figure 2). However, the c-fos protein was not detected in the thymic epithelial cells of either control or ACTH-treated rats.

1-24

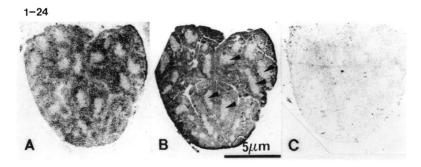

A B 5μm C

Figure 1 (i). Autoradiograms showing ^{125}I-ACTH$_{1-24}$ binding to the thymus.
Left: autoradiograms from sections incubated in ^{125}I-ACTH alone (total binding).
Left to Right; concentrations-dependent reduction in binding in the presence of increasing concentrations of unlabelled ACTH$_{1-24}$.
(ii) and (iii) Autoradiograms showing ^{125}I-ACTH$_{1-24}$ binding associated with the cortex (ii) and adrenal cortex (iii) in the rat. A = binding to a section incubated in ^{125}I-ACTH$_{1-24}$ alone (total binding). B = Haematoxylin stained tissue underlying A. C) = binding to a section, incubated as in A, in the presence of unlabelled ACTH$_{1-39}$ (non-specific binding).

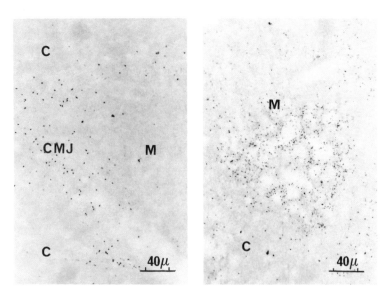

Figure 2. Fos protein at the corticomedullary junction in a saline injected rat (left), and in an ACTH-injected rat (right). C = cortex, M = medulla and CMJ = corticomedullary junction.

DISCUSSION

The results presented add further support to the concept that ACTH plays a significant role in the regulation of thymic function, for they not only demonstrate the presence of specific ACTH binding sites within the cortex and medulla, but also show that ACTH has the ability to increase the intra-thymic expression of the early gene, c-fos, over a time course which complements the ACTH-induced increase in thymulin release (Buckingham et al., 1992).

The low-resolution autoradiographic studies do not permit identification of the cell types on which the receptors lie but, the pattern of binding we observed indicates that ACTH receptors are located primarily, although not necessarily exclusively, in the cortex. These findings raise the possibility that ACTH may fulfil a more diverse role in the regulation of thymic function than has been envisaged to date, but provide little insight as to the locus of ACTH action with respect to thymulin release. It is possible that ACTH acts directly on the epithelial cells to effect thymulin release and, in this context, data from our preliminary high-resolution study suggest that ACTH receptors are indeed present on some epithelial cells. On the other hand, the data we obtained from the immunocytochemical study do not accord with the view that the early actions of ACTH on the thymus are effected directly at the level of epithelial cells for the increase in c-fos expression induced by the peptide was evident only within a small mononuclear population in the region in which mature recirculating lymphoid cells are found. Of course it is possible that the ACTH-driven increase in thymulin release we have reported previously (Buckingham et al., 1992) is not associated with alterations in early gene-expression. However, a more plausible explanation may be that hypersecretion of thymulin is effected by a paracrine mechanism and thus dependent upon the release of a chemical mediator (e.g. a cytokine) from an ACTH-sensitive sub-population of lymphocytes or thymocytes. These possibilities are now being examined.

ACKNOWLEDGEMENTS

Financial support is gratefully acknowledged by MDK from Volkswagen Stiftung, The Anatomical Society of GB and Ireland (for RS), and The Welton Foundation; and by MRD from the British Heart Foundation.

REFERENCES

Buckingham, J.C., Safieh, B., Singh, S., Arduino, L.A., Cover, P.O. and Kendall, M.D., 1992, Interactions between the hypothalamo-pituitary adrenal axis and the thymus in the rat: a role for corticotrophin in the control of thymulin release. *J. Neuroendocrinol.* 4:295-301.

Dardenne M., Charreire, J. and Bach, J.F., 1978, Alterations in thymocyte surface markers after *in vivo* treatment by serum thymic factor. *Cell. Immunol.* 39:47-54.

Dardenne, M. and Savino, W., 1990, Neuroendocrine control of the thymic epithelium: modulation of thymic endocrine function, cytokine expression and cell proliferation by hormones and peptides. *Prog. NeuroEndocrinImmunol.* 3:18-25.

DeTogni, P., Niman, H., Raymond, V., Sawchenko, P. and Verma, I.M. 1988, Detection of *fos* protein during osteogenesis by monoclonal antibodies. *Mol. Cell Biol.* 8:2251-2256.

Kendall, M.D., Safieh, B., Sareen, A., Venn, G., Matheson, L. and Ritter, M., 1991, Thymulin secreting cells in man: distribution, LM histochemistry and plasma thymulin levels, *in* Lymphatic Tissues and *in vivo* Immune Responses," B.A. Imhof, S. Berrih-Aknin and S. Ezine, Dekker New York.

Kendall, M.D., Safieh, B., Buckingham, J.C. and Ritter, M.A., 1992, A rise in plasma thymulin alters thymocyte phenotype. Neuroimmunomodulation in Pharmacology 2nd Course of the Fed. Europ. Pharmacol. Socs., Paris, Feb. 5-7.

Moody, C., Dashwood, M.R., Sykes, R.M. et al., 1990, Functional and autoradiographic evidence for endothelin receptors on human and rat cardiac myocytes: comparison with single smooth muscle cells. *Circ. Res.* 67:764-769.

Millington, G. and Buckingham, J.C., 1992, Thymic peptides and neuroendocrine-immune communication. *Curr. Sep.* 10:Abs 41, 98-99.

Weigent D. and Blalock E., 1987, Interactions between the neuroendocrine and immune systems: common hormones and recptors. *Immunol. Rev.* 100:79-108.

ADRENERGIC AND CHOLINERGIC REGULATION OF APOPTOSIS AND DIFFERENTIATION OF THYMIC LYMPHOCYTES

Ingo Rinner,[1] Tania Kukulansky,[2] Elisabeth Skreiner,[1] Amiela Globerson,[2] Michiyuki Kasai,[3] Katsuiko Hirokawa,[3] and Konrad Schauenstein[1]

[1]Institute of General and Experimental Pathology, University of Graz, Austria, [2]Department of Cell Biology, Weizmann institute of Science, Rehovot, Israel, [3]Department of Immunopathology, Tokyo Metropolitan Institute of Gerontology, Tokyo, Japan

INTRODUCTION

We have recently shown that in vivo treatment of rats with adrenergic or cholinergic agonists/antagonists leads to consistent changes in lymphocyte functions, and interferes with the signalling of the activated immune system to the brain [1,2]. Here we summarize experimental evidence that the adrenergic/cholinergic balance exerts regulatory influences also on thymic differentiation and selection processes.

MATERIALS AND METHODS

In vivo treatment

Female Sprague Dawley rats (150 g) were treated for 24 hrs with s.c. implanted pellets containing adrenaline (output 1.3 mg) either alone, or together with the beta blocker propranolol (output 14.2 mg) or the alpha blocker regitine (output 1.3 mg)[1]. Furthermore, rats were treated for 2 weeks with physostigmine (daily output 0.012 mg) or atropine (daily output 1.2 mg)[2]. The animals were killed after treatment and thymocyte suspensions were analyzed by flow cytometry immediately and after 24 hrs at culture conditions.

In Vivo Immunology, Edited by E. Heinen *et al.*
Plenum Press, New York, 1994

Coculture of murine thymic epithelial (TEC) lines with fetal thymic lobes

The TEC 1.4 (cortical) and TEC 2.3. (medullary) cell lines were prepared from thymus of C57BL/6 mice[3].TEC cells (5 x 10^4) of either line were seeded on Nucleopore filters, resting on gelatine sponges. After 24 hours four thymus lobes prepared from 15 day C57BL/6J embryos (FT)[4] were placed on top of each TEC layer. Cultures were incubated in RPMI supplemented with 10% fetal calf serum. Noradrenaline or carbachol at concentrations from 10^{-6} to 10^{-8} M were daily added to the cultures. After seven days the thymocytes were collected for flow cytometry.

Flow cytometry

Analysis of CD4/CD8 subsets was performed with a Becton-Dickinson FACScan cytometer using anti-Lyt2 (CD8) FITC and anti-L3T4 (CD4) phycoerythrin conjugates. Apoptotic cells were recognized by low DNA staining with acridine orange[5].

RESULTS

In vivo data in the rat model

In vivo treatment with adrenaline plus propranolol led to an increase of apoptosis in thymocytes after 24 hrs culture, whereas adrenaline alone (not shown) or together with regitine had no effect (Fig. 1 a). Treatment with atropine strongly increased the number of apoptotic cells already in fresh thymocyte suspensions. Physostigmine had no effect (Fig. 1 b).

Carbachol antagonizes in vitro effects of a murine cortical TEC line

Both TEC lines enhanced apoptosis in cells of cocultivated FT, the effect being more pronounced with the cortical TEC line 1.4 (Fig. 2 a). Treatment with 10^{-8} M carbachol suppressed significantly the effect of TEC 1.4, but not of TEC 2.3. Other concentrations were ineffective (not shown), as was noradrenaline at either concentration. No effect was observed on FT cultures in the absence of TEC lines. TEC 1.4 exhibited also a decreasing effect on CD4+CD8+ cells in cocultured FT (Fig. 2 b). Carbachol significantly antagonized also this effect of TEC 1.4. The CD4-CD8- subset was influenced in the opposite way (not shown). Other concentrations were again ineffective, as was noradrenaline at either concentration.

CONCLUSIONS

The in vivo data in rats indicate that the endogenous cholinergic tonus may protect thymocytes from programmed cell death. This notion is supported by the in vitro findings in

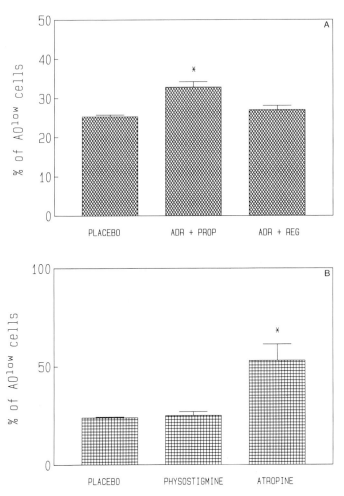

Figure 1. Effect of in vivo treatment with adrenergic (A) and cholinergic (B) agonists/antagonists on the number of apoptotic (AO^{low}) rat thymus cells. (ADR=adrenaline, PROP=propranolol, REG=regitine). For details see text.*significantly different from placebo according to ANOVA

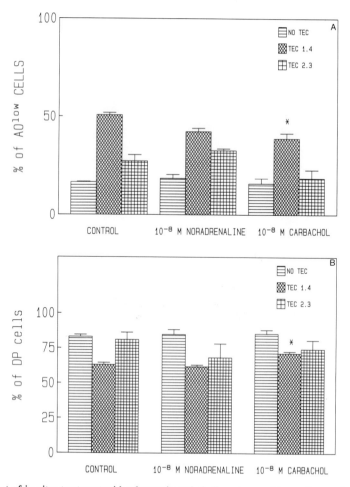

Figure 2. Effect of in vitro treatment with adrenergic and cholinergic agonists on the number of apoptotic (AO^{low}) (A) and CD4+CD8+ (DP) (B) cells in murine fetal thymus cocultured with cortical (TEC 1.4) or medullary (TEC 2.3) epithelial cell lines. For details see text. *significantly different from controls according to ANOVA.

murine fetal thymus lobes. It appears that the thymus epithelium is the primary cholinergic target, as no effect was seen in FT in absence of TEC lines. Carbachol also antagonized the decreasing effect of the cortical TEC line on the CD4+CD8+ fraction of thymocytes. Cholinergic stimulation of the thymus epithelium in vivo could be provided by innervation and/or - as recently shown by us - by thymic lymphocytes themselves[6]. Although in the present experiments the medullary TEC line was resistent to cholinergic influence, it needs to be further examined if cortex and medulla are indeed differently sensitive to cholinergic signals. No effect of adrenergic stimulation was noted in the in vitro experiments with murine fetal thymus. The observed in vivo effects in the rat may be due to mechanisms secondarily elicited by α-adrenergic stimulation. Studies are underway to clarify this issue, as well as the question if adrenergic stimuli may counteract cholinergic effects on thymus cell differentiation.

Acknowledgments

Supported by the Jubiläumsfonds der Oesterreichischen Nationalbank, Project Nr. 4349, and by the Austrian Science Foundation, Project 7509

REFERENCES

1. P.Felsner, D.Hofer, I.Rinner, H.Mangge, M.Gruber, and K.Schauenstein, Continuous in vivo treatment with catecholamines suppresses in vitro reactivity of rat peripheral blood T-lymphocytes via α-mediated mechanisms, *J.Neuroimmunol.* 37:47 (1992)

2. I.Rinner and K.Schauenstein, The parasympathetic nervous system takes part in the immune-neuroendocrine dialogue, *J.Neuroimmunol.* 34:165 (1991)

3. M.Kasai and K.Hirokawa, A novel cofactor produced by a thymic epithelial cell line: promotion of immature thymic lymphocytes by the presence of interleukin and various mitogens, *Cell.Immunol.* 132:377 (1991)

4. R.Eren, D.Zharhary, L.Abel, and A.Globerson, Age related changes in the capacity of bone marrow cells to differentiate in thymic organ cultures, *Cell.Immunol.* 112:449 (1988)

5. M.M.Compton, J.S.Haskill, and J.A.Cidlowski, Analysis of glucocorticoid actions on rat thymocyte desoxyribonucleic acid by fluorescence-activated flow cytometry, *Endocrinology* 122:158 (1988)

6. I.Rinner and K.Schauenstein, Detection of choline-acetyltransferase activity in lymphocytes, *J.Neurosci. Res.* 35:188 (1993)

CELL TRAFFIC

AUTOIMMUNE *lpr* AND *gld* MICE: MODELS OF ABNORMAL ADHESION MOLECULE REGULATION AND DEFECTIVE LYMPHOCYTE TRAFFIC

Morris O. Dailey and Robert Jensen

University of Iowa College of Medicine
Departments of Pathology and Microbiology
365 MRC
Iowa City, IA 52242-1182

INTRODUCTION

Mice of the MRL-*lpr/lpr* strain develop at several months of age a massive generalized lymphadenopathy and severe SLE-like autoimmune disease with autoantibody production and glomerulonephritis. The *lpr* gene has been bred into other mouse strains and, when homozygous, leads to similar lymphoproliferation but a somewhat attenuated autoimmunity. The genetically unrelated *gld* mutation causes a nearly identical autoimmune and lymphoproliferative syndrome.[1] The *lpr* genetic defect has recently been identified as the *fas* gene, which is involved with the regulation of programmed cell death in lymphocytes.[2] The *gld* gene has not yet been identified, although it is genetically linked to the gene coding for murine L-selectin (I. Weissman, personal communication). In both *lpr* and *gld* mice, the cells that accumulate are abnormal T cells that are relatively anergic and have the same unusual phenotype. The majority of them express both the Thy-1 and B220 antigens and are CD4⁻ and CD8⁻, but several other minor populations of defective cells are also present, as are some residual normal B and T cells. These abnormal *lpr* and *gld* cells proliferate very slowly in lymphoid tissues, but in the case of *lpr* mice, the cells replicate rapidly in the liver.[3] One remarkable feature of both *lpr* and *gld* mice is that the lymphoproliferative disorder involves primarily the lymph nodes, while Peyer's patches and the lamina propria are virtually unaffected. This is similar to the distribution of cells observed with certain LN-homing lymphomas which also spare PP. These lymphomas express L-selectin, the lymph node homing receptor, which facilitates the entry of normal or malignant cells from the bloodstream into the LN parenchyma.

In the present studies, we examined the tissue localization, homing pattern, and expression and regulation of cell surface adhesion molecules by *lpr* and *gld* cells. We found that *lpr* and *gld* lymphocytes actually home to LN less well than do normal cells, so that the massive lymphadenopathy is not explained by selective cell migration. As a further paradox, although these cells migrate poorly to LN, they express a high level of L-selectin and adhere well to high endothelial venules (HEV) *in vitro*. These findings, together with the observation that L-selectin is abnormally regulated in these cells, suggests that a post-adhesion defect in transendothelial migration is responsible for their inability to traffic to LN *in vivo*.

In Vivo Immunology, Edited by E. Heinen *et al.*
Plenum Press, New York, 1994

MATERIALS AND METHODS

Mice

Adult MRL-+/+, MRL-*lpr/lpr*, MRL-*gld/gld*, AKR/J, and C3H/J mice were bred in our colony or were obtained from Jackson Laboratories.

Flow Cytometry

LN cells (1×10^6) were stained with MEL-14-PE, anti-Thy-1-biotin/Texas red-avidin, and FITC-conjugated antibodies to Pgp-1 (CD44), LFA-1, $\alpha4$ integrin (mAb R1-2), ICAM-1, and $\beta7$ integrin and B220. They were analyzed on a FACS 440 using 4 decade log amplification. Abnormal *lpr* and *gld* cells were identified as the Thy-1+B220+ cells.

In Vivo Homing Assay

Suspensions of *lpr* and *gld* LN cells (Thy-1.2) were mixed with normal control cells and injected iv into AKR/J (Thy-1.1) mice. At various times thereafter, LN, spleen, and PP were harvested and suspensions stained with anti-Thy-1.2 and anti-B220. The number of donor abnormal DP cells homing to an organ was determined from the proportion of Thy-1.2+6B2+ cells, while the homing of the normal T cells was quantitated by the number of Thy-1.2+B220- cells. The results are expressed as the relative localization ratio (RLR), the ratio of homing of abnormal DP cells to that of normal T cells.

HEV Binding Assay

The ability of test cells to adhere to HEV in frozen sections of lymph nodes was determined as previously described.[4] Results are expressed as the relative adherence ratio (RAR), the ratio of binding of test cells to that of normal T cells.

RESULTS

Mice homozygous for either the *lpr* or *gld* gene mutation develop by two months of age a progressively severe lymphoproliferative disease. Interestingly, this proliferation results in massively enlarged LN while the PP remain of normal size (Figure 1). The majority of the cells in these LN are T cells that express both the B cell antigen B220 and the T cell marker Thy-1 and hence are referred to as double positive (DP) cells. (Note that > 90% of these cells are also CD4-CD8- and are therefore frequently referred to in the literature as *double negative* lymphocytes.) One possible explanation for the selective LN involvement is that the DP lymphocytes express high levels of surface adhesion molecules that would increase their homing to LN, but not to PP. We therefore performed flow cytometric analysis to determine the adhesion and molecule phenotype of these cells. As shown in Figure 2, the DP lymphocytes in C3H-*lpr/lpr* mice express high levels of L-selectin, the LN homing receptor, compared to the expression by normal T cells in

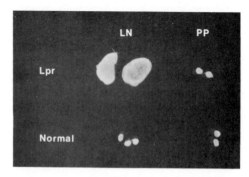

Figure 1. Lymphoid tissue from a 6-month-old C3H-*lpr/lpr* and a normal C3H-+/+ mice. The lymph nodes from the *lpr* mouse are markedly enlarged, while the Peyer's patches are of normal size.

C3H-+/+ animals. These cells are also CD44-high. In contrast, expression of LFA-1 is approximately equal on the DP and normal T cells (Figure 2), as is the LPAM-1 (VLA-4α) antigen and ICAM-1 (data not shown). The adhesion molecules expressed by DP cells are similar in young mice, as soon as the DP cells can be detected, and old animals and are virtually identical in both *lpr* and *gld* mutant animals.

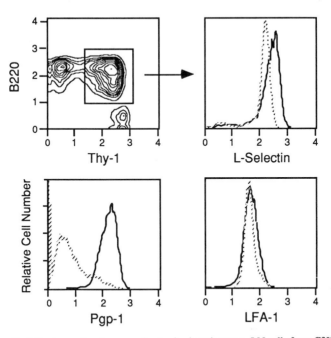

Figure 2. Adhesion molecule expression by *lpr* lymphocytes. LN cells from C3H-*lpr/lpr* mice were stained with anti-B220, Thy-1, and various adhesion molecules. Histograms of CD44, L-selectin, and LFA-1 intensity are gated on the double positive cells as shown. Adhesion molecule expression by normal T cells is also shown (dotted line).

The high level of L-selectin on DP cells suggests that they should home very well to LN *in vivo*. Surprisingly, however, when *lpr* cells are injected iv into normal recipients, the proportion of cells homing to LN is approximately 75% less than that of normal cells (Figure 3). In contrast, these cells home well to PP and spleen, ruling out a generalized defect in cell migration. DP cells from *gld* animals also traffic poorly to LN. These experiments demonstrate that selective homing of cells to LN does not explain why they are preferentially enlarged in *lpr* and *gld* diseased animals.

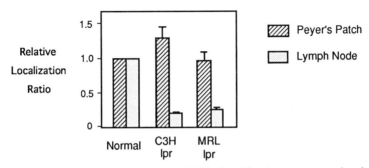

Figure 3. Homing of *lpr* lymphocytes 2 hours after iv injection. The data are expressed as the ratio of the localization of test cells to normal control cells.

121

Since these DP lymphocytes do not follow the usual pattern that L-selectin[+] cells home well to LN, we examined whether this adhesion molecule is somehow functionally defective by determining the ability of these cells to adhere to HEV endothelium *in vitro*. As shown in Figure 4, MRL-*lpr/lpr* cells actually adhere better to LN HEV than do normal cells.

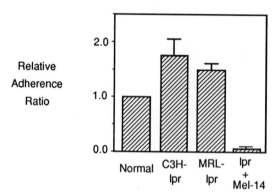

Figure 4. Adhesion of C3H-*lpr/lpr* lymphocytes to LN HEV in frozen sections. The data are shown as the ratio of binding of test cells to that of normal T cells.

We are thus left with a set of paradoxes. Both *gld* and *lpr* DP cells are strongly L-selectin[+] and adhere very well to HEV *in vitro*. However, these cells do not migrate well to LN *in vivo*, implying that there may be some defect in cell adhesion or motility after the initial leukocyte-endothelium binding event. We therefore examined whether DP T cells abnormally regulate surface L-selectin. We previously showed that, in normal T cells, protein kinase C (PKC) regulates the expression of L-selectin.[5] Agents that activate PKC cause the rapid proteolytic cleavage and shedding of the cell surface L-selectin molecule. Figure 5 shows the results of a typical experiment in which lymphocytes from normal or *lpr* mice were treated *in vitro* with PMA for 60 minutes and then stained for 3-color FACS analysis with antibodies to B220, Thy-1, and L-selectin. Normal T cells completely down regulate L-selectin whereas *lpr* DP T cells retain most of the receptor, even at high concentrations of PMA. Similar results are obtained with *gld* cells as well as with other, minor populations of abnormal *lpr* cells, such as the small B220[+] CD4[+] subset (data not shown). Thus, cells affected by the *lpr* and *gld* mutations are resistant to PKC-mediated receptor proteolysis and down regulation.

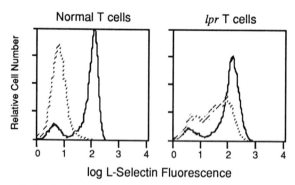

Figure 5. L-selectin expression after treatment with PMA. Normal and *lpr/lpr* LN cells were treated with 8 ng/ml PMA for one hour, followed by staining with the MEL-14 monoclonal antibody conjugated to phycoerythrin. Solid line: untreated cells; dotted line: PMA-treated.

DISCUSSION

The recirculation of cells from the bloodstream, through HEV into LN and PP, to efferent lymph, and then back into the blood is important in maintaining normal immune surveillance and in the dissemination of immunologic memory. The major site of regulating this process is at the surface of HEV at which lymphocyte surface homing receptors mediate the adhesion of the leukocyte to the vascular endothelium. Cells which express the LN-specific homing receptor, L-selectin, generally home to LN and, conversely, cells that do not express L-selection cannot recirculate through LN.

In addition to their autoimmunity, homozygous *lpr* and *gld* mice present an interesting system of abnormal lymphocyte migration. The experiments presented herein demonstrate some paradoxical findings. First, the severe lymph node involvement by the lymphoproliferative process is not explainable on the basis of selective homing of cells, but rather must involve some property of the LN microenvironment that promotes the *retention* of these cells locally. It is not clear what this factor is or why it is characteristic of LN but not PP, to which cells do migrate but apparently do not remain or accumulate. The second paradoxal observation is that while double positive T cells express high levels of homing receptors and adhere well to HEV *in vitro*, they nevertheless home poorly to LN *in vivo*. This suggests that these lymphocytes can adhere to the luminal surface of HEV *in vivo*, but that they are deficient in their ability to traverse through the endothelium and into the parenchyma of the LN. The passage of leukocytes through an endothelial barrier is a poorly understood process, but involves changes in both cell motility and adhesiveness.

The activation of lymphocyte PKC, either with PMA[5] or through the TCR/CD3 complex (manuscript in preparation) results in the activation of a cell surface protease which then cleaves L-selectin close to the plasma membrane, releasing a receptor fragment that retains ligand binding activity. It has been suggested that receptor cleavage might be required for normal cell migration, perhaps being necessary for lymphocyte passage between the endothelial cells or by facilitating the de-adhesion of lymphocytes from the endothelium at the abluminal side of the vessel.[5] Such receptor shedding could be induced by the interaction of L-selectin with its endothelial ligand.[6] The abnormal resistance of *lpr* and *gld* cells to receptor proteolysis and shedding could therefore inhibit their traffic to LN by interfering with the normal process of receptor shedding and transendothelial migration. The mechanism responsible for defective receptor proteolysis is unknown, but could be related to the numerous signaling abnormalities previously described in these cells.

ACKNOWLEDGMENT

This work was supported by NIH Grant R01-AI22730.

REFERENCES

1. Roths, J. B., E. D. Murphy, and E. M. Eicher. 1984. A new mutation, gld, that produces lymphoproliferation and autoimmunity in C3H/HeJ mice. *J. Exp. Med.* 159:1.

2. Watanabe-Fukunaga, R., C. I. Brannan, N. G. Copeland, N. A. Jenkins, and S. Nagata. 1992. Lymphoproliferation disorder in mice explained by defects in Fas antigen that mediates apoptosis. *Nature* 356:314.

3. Ohteki, T., S. Seki, T. Abo, and K. Kumagai. 1990. Liver is a possible site for the proliferation of abnormal CD3+4-8- double-negative lymphocytes in autoimmune MRL-lpr/lpr mice. *J. Exp. Med.* 172:7.

4. Jung, T. M., W. M. Gallatin, I. L. Weissman, and M. O. Dailey. 1988. Down-regulation of homing receptors after T cell activation. *J. Immunol.* 141:4110.

5. Jung, T. M. and M. O. Dailey. 1990. Rapid modulation of homing receptors (gp90^{MEL-14}) induced by activators of protein kinase C. Receptor shedding due to accelerated proteolytic cleavage at the cell surface. *J. Immunol.* 144:3130.

6. Palecanda, A., B. Walcheck, D. K. Bishop, and M. A. Jutila. 1992. Rapid activation-independent shedding of leukocyte L-selectin induced by cross-linking of the surface antigen. *Eur. J. Immunol.* 22:1279.

VASCULAR ADDRESSIN EXPRESSION IN PEYER'S PATCHES: AN *IN VIVO* STUDY OF SITE-ASSOCIATED REGULATION

Astrid G. S. van Halteren[1], Reina E. Mebius[2] and Georg Kraal[1]

[1] Department of Cell Biology, Vrije Universiteit Amsterdam, The Netherlands
[2] Department of Pathology, Stanford University, U.S.A.

INTRODUCTION

Peyer's patches (PP), together with mesenteric lymph nodes (MLN) and tonsils, belong to the MALT (Mucosa Associated Lymphoid Tissue). Here, plasma cell precursors are generated that will produce protective sIgA antibodies after maturation in the epithelia of the respiratory, alimentary and genito-urinary tracts. PP are known to generate plasma and memory cells of the IgA isotype upon stimulation by gut-derived antigens, while MLN are more involved in the generation of plasma cells of the IgG or IgE isotype upon stimulation with villi-derived antigens.

Lymphocytes enter these lymphoid organs from the blood via specific adhesive interactions between their surface receptors and ligands on specialized high endothelial venules (HEV). In the mouse, these endothelium-specific ligands, vascular addressins, can be distinguished by two different monoclonal antibodies: MECA-367[1] and MECA-79[2]. The mucosal vascular addressin (MAdCAM) is recognized by MECA-367, the peripheral vascular addressin is recognized by MECA-79. Adult peripheral lymph nodes (PLN) exclusively express the MECA-79 antigen on their HEV, while HEV in adult PP usually express MECA-367 only, but HEV are sometimes slightly MECA-79 positive as well. In adult MLN however, HEV are always positive for both MECA-367 and MECA-79. This differential expression of addressins on the HEV of adult lymphoid organs may result from local environmental factors, thereby influencing the specific entrance of lymphocyte subsets via these HEV. Eventually, this distinct migration process will determine the overall composition and the immune reactivity of these organs.

Previously, we have established that the vascular addressin expression in murine PLN and MLN is determined around birth and that ectopic transplantation of adult lymphoid tissue (mucosal versus peripheral sites) is of little consequence for this expression[3]. Because PP are so uniquely positioned in the intestinal wall, having distinct immune reactivity as well, we wished to determine whether transplantation of PP into a peripheral site would have an effect on the addressin expression, the lymphocyte composition and the ability to evoke IgA mediated immune responses. Using immuno-histochemistry and the ELIspot assay, the results of transplanted PP were compared to control transplantations of mesenteric and popliteal lymph nodes (PLN) and control non-operated PP, PLN or MLN.

MATERIALS AND METHODS

Animals

Female BALB/c mice (8-12 weeks) were either purchased at Bomholtgard (Ry, Denmark) or at Harlan/Centrale Proefdier Bedrijf (Zeist, The Netherlands). All animals were kept under routine laboratory conditions.

Transplantation procedure

This method has been described previously[3]. Briefly, donor mice were sacrificed and their PP or MLN were collected and kept on ice in RPMI 1640 medium (Gibco Life Technologies, Breda, The Netherlands) until the organs were transplanted. Recipients were anaesthetized intra-peritoneally with 1 μl/gram body weight of a 4:3 mixture of Aescocet (Aesculaap N.V., Gent, Belgium) and Rompun (Bayer, Leverkussen, Germany) respectively. The recipient's popliteal lymph node was removed (or disconnected from blood and lymph supply in case of control transplantations) and donor MLN, PP or PLN were placed in the popliteal fossa or in the mesentery. The incisions were closed with 0.5 metric 7-0 monofil suture material (Ethicon, Johnson and Johnson, Amersfoort, The Netherlands).

At different timepoints after transplantation mice were killed and donor and non-operated contra-lateral popliteal lymphoid tissue was collected. Approximately thirty minutes before sacrifice, succesful restoration of afferent lymphatics onto the donor lymphoid organs was verified by injection of 10 μl of a 10% India ink solution into the corresponding and contra-lateral footpad. Restoration was assessed by the presence of ink particles in cryostat sections of the draining transplanted and control non-operated lymph nodes. Additionally, the skin of the hind legs was painted with the hapten Rhodamin B isothiocyanate twenty four hours before sacrifice. Cryostate sections of the draining transplanted lymphoid organs and contra-lateral PLN were analyzed for the presence of Rhodamin bearing dendritic cells in the paracortical areas by the use of a fluorescence microscope[4].

Immuno-histochemical staining of the transplanted lymph nodes or Peyer's patches

Acetone fixed (10 min at RT) and air-dried cryostat sections (6-8μm) were incubated for one hour with the following rat anti-mouse monoclonal antibodies: MECA-367 and MECA-79 (vascular addressins), Thy-1 (Pan T cells), 187-1 (anti kappa light chain; B cells) and MOMA-1 (subcapsular sinus macrophages). After washing thoroughly in 0.01M PBS, the sections were incubated with peroxidase-conjugated second stage antibody, containing 1% normal mouse serum (either goat anti-rat IgG/IgM, Jackson Immuno Research, San Fransisco, CA or rabbit anti-rat Ig, Dako, Glostrup, Denmark) for another hour at room temperature. All antibodies were diluted in 0.01M PBS containing 0.5% bovine serum albumin (Boseral, Organon Tecknika, Boxtel, The Netherlands). Again after thorougly washing, the sections were stained for peroxidase activity with 3,3' diaminobenzidine tetrahydrochloride (Sigma, St. Louis, MO) in 0.5 mg/ml Tris-HCl buffer (pH 7.6) containing 0.01% H_2O_2. Finally, the sections were counterstained with haematoxylin.

ELIspot assay

To determine the number of anti-TNP plasma cells in transplanted PP, MLN and PLN after TNP-KLH immunization, we used the spot-ELISA method originally described elsewere[5]. Briefly, single-cell suspensions of transplanted and control PLN were prepared and incubated for two hours at 37°C in 96 wells microtiter plates coated with 5 μg/ml trinitrophenylated ovalbumin. After washing the plates with 0.01M PBS containing 0.1% Tween 20, the plates were incubated for two hours at 37°C with the following alkaline phosphatase conjugated antibodies: goat-anti-mouse IgG, IgM and IgA (Sanbio, Uden, The Netherlands). Secreted anti-TNP antibodies were visualized with the alkaline phosphatase substrate 5-bromo-4-chloro-3-indoly phosphate (5-BCIP, Sigma Chemical Co., St. Louis, Missouri U.S.A.) diluted in AMP buffer (Sigma, St. Louis, U.S.A.) added in agarose. Spots were counted by the use of an inverted microscope.

RESULTS

Compared to MLN and PLN, transplantation of PP into the popliteal fossa was found to be rather difficult. While ingrowth of new blood and lymphatic vessels occured within two weeks in transplantend MLN or PLN, this was usually not the case for PP. Transplanted PP showed either transplant failure or transplants with flat walled HEV, that were weakly positive for both MECA-367 and MECA-79.

Situated in the intestinal wall, PP are covered by follicle-associated epithelium, which probably interferes with the restoration of blood and lymph supply. In order to facilitate the ingrowth of new vessels, we decided to bisect PP just before the implantation into the popliteal fossa. This procedure did not improve the results, as these PP showed the same characteristics compared to intact PP at different timepoints after transplantation (data not shown).

As PP are known to be much smaller in germ-free mice[6], the lack of continuous antigenic stimulation after transplantation might influence the morphology of the PP and hereby the transplant survival as well. In order to improve our transplantation protocol, we tried to stimulate the transplanted PP by subcutaneous injections of TNP-KLH in complete Freund's adjuvans in the corresponding footpad. Again, transplant survival was not found to be improved. We therefore concluded that the results were not due to our transplantation procedure itself, since control transplantations of PLN were always successful.

After these first critical three weeks and up to five weeks, successful transplanted PP clearly expressed both MECA-367 and MECA-79 positive HEV, which seemed to be functionally active according to their high walled morphology (figure 1 and 2). At seven weeks after transplantation, transplanted PP slowly started to transform into a more peripheral lymphoid organ, characterized by a shift from MECA-367 positive HEV into MECA-79 positive HEV (figure 1 and 2). Together with this altered vascular addressin expression we observed a change in cellular composition as well. While under normal conditions PP contain about 25% T-cells and 75% B cells, in the transplanted PP at five weeks after transplantation, only a small majority of the lymphocytes was positive for Thy-1, while at seven weeks most of the lymphocytes were clearly expressing the Thy-1 antigen. Although B-cells were present, we were never able to find plasma cells upon immunization with TNP-KLH at different timepoints after transplantation (Table 1).

Transplanted mice were studied up to twelve weeks after transplantation, at which timepoint the PP were almost completely transformed into a lymphoid organ with peripheral lymph node phenotype, characterized by an altered lymphocyte composition and HEV with only MECA-79 expression. However, the population of subcapsular sinus macrophages was never completely present and a situation of non-responsiveness to TNP-KLH was found at least nine weeks after transplantation. Strikingly, even when only a few subcapsular macrophages were presesent, Rhodamin positive dendritic cells could be detected in the transplanted PP after skin painting. Sometimes however, ink particles could be found in the absence of subcapsular sinus macrophages, indicating that some restoration of lymphatic vessels had occured.

Control PLN or MLN, transplanted into the mesentery or in the popliteal fossa, always showed their characteristic morphology, irrespective of the transplantation site. Compared to transplanted PP at twelve weeks after transplantation, subcapsular sinus macrophages were completely present in transplanted PLN at five to seven weeks after transplantation, in correlation with functional afferent lymphatics, as shown by the influx of Rhodamin positive dendritic cells in the paracortex after skin painting and India ink particles in the subcapsular sinus. Additionally, transplanted PLN showed many TNP-specific plasma cells after immunization with TNP-KLH. These results indicate that transplanted PLN appear to have the same function and characteristics as control non-transplanted PLN.

Table 1. Anti-TNP specific plasma cells (PC) per 1×10^6 cells in transplanted PP, MLN, PLN and in control non-transplanted PLN upon immunization with TNP-KLH in complete Freund's adjuvans. Mice were immunized at 5 weeks after transplantation at day 0 with 50 μg TNP-KLH in CFA and boostered at day 14 with 50 μg TNP-KLH. At day 18 mice were sacrificed and transplanted organs of at least 2 mice were pooled to prepare a single-cell suspension.

	anti-TNP PC (IgA)	anti-TNP PC (IgG)	anti-TNP PC (IgM)
control PLN	-	100	10-20
transplanted PP	-	-	-
transplanted MLN	-	-	8-10
transplanted PLN	-	50-100	10-20

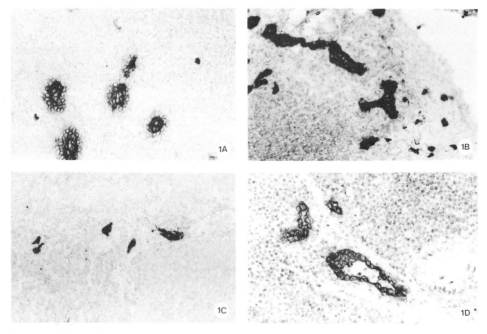

Figure 1. MECA-367 expression in control and transplanted PP. A-C: transplanted PP at 5,7 and 12 weeks after transplantation respectively. D: control PP (magnifications 40x).

In contrast with our previous studies on MLN and PLN transplantations to either peripheral or mesenteric sites[3], PP transplantations into the popliteal fossa were found to be less successful. Although control transplantations clearly demonstrate that transplant failure of PP is not due to the procedure itself, as transplanted PLN and MLN are perfectly able to survive in the popliteal fossa, it is concluded that the mucosa-associated PP is not able to maintain its functional characteristics in a peripheral local environment. It remains speculative which factors are responsible for this transplantation failure.

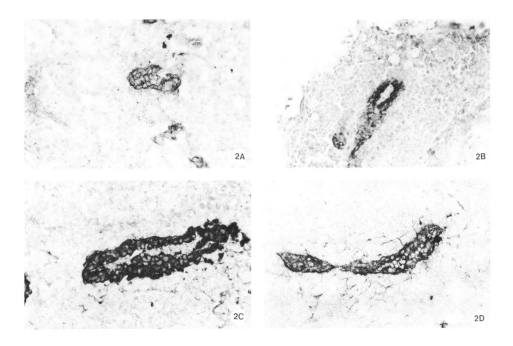

Figure 2. MECA-79 expression in control PLN and transplanted PP. A-C: transplanted PP at 5,7 and 12 weeks after transplantation. D: control PLN (magnifications 40x).

DISCUSSION

Summarizing the transplantation results, the take of PP after transplantation into the popliteal fossa was found to be a transient phenomenon, whereby at best, the PP as such will function approximately seven to nine weeks. After this period, or much earlier when the organ is less well taken, a transition to a more PLN-like organ is found. This coincides with a loss of MAdCAM expression and a change in lymphocyte composition. Such development of a PLN is not seen when the popliteal lymph node is only removed and not replaced by any other lymphoid organ (unpublished data). This indicates that elements of the PP, such as reticular stromal cells, can form a substrate for the formation of a new PLN.

Interestingly, this transition, with loss of MAdCAM expression, is not seen after transplantation of the MLN[3]. In this study we observed a normal MAdCAM expression after transplantion of MLN into the popliteal fossa. This indicates that MAdCAM expression can be maintained at a peripheral site and suggests essential differences in the organisation between lymph nodes and Peyer's patches.

REFERENCES

1. P.R. Streeter, E.L. Berg, B.T.N. Rouse, R.F. Bargatze and E.C. Butcher, A tissue-specific endothelial cell molecule involved in lymphocyte homing, *Nature* 331:41 (1988a).

2. P.R. Streeter, B.T.N. Rouse and E.C. Butcher, Immunohistologic and functional characterization of a vascular addressin involved in lymphocyte homing into peripheral lymph nodes, *J. Cell Biol.* 107:1853 (1988b).

3. R.E. Mebius, J. Brevé, G. Kraal and P.R. Streeter, Developmental regulation of vascular addressin expression: a possible role for site-associated environments, *International Immunology* Vol.5, No.5:443 (1993).

4. E.J.G. van Wilsem, J. Brevé and G. Kraal, Antigen bearing Langerhans cells in skin draining lymph nodes. Phenotype and kinetics of migration, *submitted*.

5. J.D. Sedgwick and P.G. Holt, A solid-phase immunoenzymatic technique for the enumaration of specific antibody-secreting cells, *J. Immunol. Methods* 57:301 (1983).

6. H.A. Gordon and E. Bruckner-Kardoss, Effects of the normal microbial flora on various tissue elements of the small intestine, *Acta. Anat.* 44:210 (1961).

DOMAIN 5 OF THE INTERCELLULAR ADHESION MOLECULE-1 (ICAM-1) IS INVOLVED IN ADHESION OF B-CELLS AND FOLLICULAR DENDRITIC CELLS

Piet Joling[1], Saskia Boom[2], Judith Johnson[3], Marjoleine E.M. Dekker[1], Jan G. van den Tweel[1], Henk-Jan Schuurman[4] and Andries C. Bloem[2]

[1]Department of Pathology and [2]Department of Immunology
University Hospital, 3508 GA Utrecht, The Netherlands
[3]Institute of Immunology, Munich, Germany
[4]Sandoz, Basel, Switzerland

INTRODUCTION

Intercellular adhesion molecule 1 (ICAM-1; CD54) is an adhesion molecule, that participates in a variety of cell-cell adhesion phenomena[1]. It serves as a ligand for the leucocyte integrins LFA-1 and Mac-1 [2,3] and as a receptor for different pathogens[4,5]. ICAM-1 is constitutively expressed in vivo on cells of the high endothelial venules and on germinal centre cells in lymph node[6,7], whereas its expression is readily induced on leucocytes and different types of adherent cells. ICAM-1 is especially present in areas of inflammation, where its expression of mRNA and protein has been induced by inflammatory mediators, such as lipopolysaccharide, IFNγ, IL-1 and , TNF[8].

Here the role of ICAM-1 in cell interactions between follicular dendritic cells (FDC) and B-lymphocytes will be discussed. FDC form a network in the lymphoid follicles. They trap antigen in the form of antigen-antibody complex, allowing these cells to participate in antigen driven selection of B cells to plasma cells and memory cells[9]. Two adhesion pathways are recently reported to participate in the interaction between B-cells and FDC i.e. the LFA-1/ICAM-1 and the VLA-4/VCAM-1 pathways [10]. In this study we provide evidence for a third independent pathway between FDC and B cells, in which domain 5 of the ICAM-1 molecule participates.

MATERIALS AND METHODS

Antibodies. Monoclonal antibodies used in this study were P3.58-BA11 (IgG1), P3.58-BA14 (IgG2b) and F10.2 (IgG1) all directed to ICAM-1[11,12]; CD11a mAb F8.8

(IgG1)[13]; VLA-4 mAb HP2/1 (Immunotech, Marseille, France); VCAM-1 mAb 4B9 (Dr. Harlan, Seattle, USA); W6/32 (IgG2a) specific for a non-polymorphic determinant of HLA-ABC (Dako, Glostrup, Denmark); CD35 (IgG1) reactive with C3b receptor (CR1).

Cells. Human follicular dendritic cells were isolated from tonsils obtained at tonsillectomy of children[14]. Tonsils were minced in small fragments and the leucocytes were removed by washing. After collagenase digestion (15 U/ml) 1xg sedimentation was done on a discontinuous gradient of bovine serum albumin (BSA). The interphase between 2.5 and 5% BSA was harvested, and layered on a discontinuous Percoll (Pharmacia, Uppsala, Sweden) gradient of 1.030, 1.060 and 1.070 mg/ml, respectively. The FDC-enriched population was harvested from the 1.030-1.060 interphase. Cytocentrifuge preparations stained by May Grünwald-Giemsa showed cells with the morphology of FDC (30 -40%). FDC appeared as solitary cells clustered with lymphoid cells. Lymphoid cells were mainly B-lymphocytes and cells with a macrophage-like cytology were almost absent.

Adhesion assay. Homotypic B-B cell adhesion: cells (10^5) of EBV transfected B cells were seeded in 96 wells flat bottom culture plates and incubated in the presence of mAb at 37°C. After 1 h spontaneously formed aggregates were measured.

FDC-B cell adhesion: isolated FDC were suspended in Hepes buffered RPMI-1640 (Gibco Laboratories, Gaithersburg, MD) containing 10% FCS. In 96-well flat-bottomed microtiter plates, 2 x 10^5 isolated FDC/well were seeded in triplicate with mAb, titrated for optimal inhibitory effect, and incubated at 37°C. Spontaneous aggregation of FDC and the B-lymphocytes, that were present in the enriched fraction, was measured. After three hours the FDC-B aggregation was measured in a semiquantitative manner as described by Koopman et al[10].

RESULTS AND DISCUSSION

MAb P3.58-BA11 and P3.58-BA14 were raised against a 89 kD cell surface glycoprotein of human melanocytes (P3.58 antigen). Recently P3.58 has been shown to be identical to ICAM-1[11]. The epitopes recognized by mAb BA11 and BA14 were mapped to domain 5 of the ICAM-1 molecule by binding analysis of the mAb to COS cells transfected with ICAM-1 mutant cDNA[15]. These data confirm and extend previously published data on binding studies with recombinant ICAM-1 fragments expressed in E. coli, that mapped the epitopes of BA11 and BA14 on domain 4 or 5 of the ICAM-1 molecule[16].

Binding of the CD54 mAb BA11, BA14 and F10.2 was determined together with CD11a mAb F8.8 to tonsil lymphocytes, EBV-transfected B-lymphocytes and ICAM-1 transfected MOP8 cells using flow cytometry. These experiments show that domain 5 mAb BA11 and BA14 exert comparable binding to these three cell types as domain 1 mAb F10.2.

In Table 1 results are shown how different ICAM-1 mAb interfere in the spontaneous homotypic B cell adhesion of the EBV transformed B cell line and the heterotypic adhesion between tonsil B cells and FDC. ICAM-1 domain1 mAb F10.2 1 inhibits both the homotypic B-B cell interaction and the aggregation between FDC and B cells. This agrees with previously published data showing that both processes depend on the LFA-1/ICAM-1 interaction[10,12]. Control mAb W6/32 and CD35 gave equal results as the control without mAb, Also VLA-4 mAb HP2/1 and VCAM-1 mAb 4B9 inhibits the adhesion between B cells and FDC. The domain 5 mAb BA11 and BA14 inhibits the interaction between B cells and FDC showing no effect on the homotypic B-B cell adhesion. Therefore the domain 5 mAb seems to operate through a different pathway than the LFA-1/ICAM-1 one. In the binding between B cells and FDC at least two adhesion pathways are involved: LFA-1/ICAM-1 and VLA-4/VCAM-1[10]. Blocking antibodies against these two pathways only partly inhibit the B cell-FDC interaction. Therefore, it seems likely that other, yet unidentified, adhesion pathways participate in this interaction.

Table 1. The influence of adhesion mAb on homotypic aggregation of EBV transfected B cells and heterotypic aggregation of FDC and B cells.

Antibody	Antigen	Homotypic B—cell	Heterotypic FDC/B cell
Control	—	+ + +[1]	+ + +
F8.8	LFA-1	+	+
F10.2	ICAM-1 d.1	+/—	+
P3.58—BA11	ICAM-1 d.5	+ + +	+
P3.58—BA14	ICAM-1 d.5	+ + +	+
HP2/1	VLA-4	nt	+ +
4B9	VCAM-1	nt	+
W6/32	HLA-ABC	nt	+ + +
CD35	CR1	nt	+ + +

[1] Aggregation after treatment with mAb was compared to the control value without mAb or mAb W6/32 and CD35. Control gave >50% aggregation scored as + + +, while the other mAb gave aggregation ranging from 50 to <5% scored as —. nt: not tested.

Combinations of BA14 (domain 5 ICAM-1) with blocking mAb directed against domain 1 of ICAM-1 (F10.2), LFA-1 (F8.8), VLA-4 (HP2/1) or VCAM-1 (4B9) gave an additive inhibitory effect on the B cell-FDC interaction (Figure 1). Combination of mAb directed against the antigens of the same pathway, F10.2/F8.8 (LFA-1/ICAM-1 domain 1) and HP2/1/4B9 (VLA-4/VCAM-1) did not give additive inhibition of the adhesion as could be expected (data not shown).

ICAM-1 is readily detected on follicular B cells [17] and FDC Dustin et al.[7] ICAM-1 expression as shown by staining with domain 1 and domain 5 mAb are comparable, which indicates that the epitopes on domain 5 are readily accessible for the mAb and for their putative ligand. This ligand is most likely not expressed on B cells. mAb to CD11a and domain 1 of ICAM-1 inhibited the homotypic B cell adhesion, while domain 5 mAb showed no effect on homotypic B cells aggregation of B cells from the cell line Lisette, or PMA induced homotypic adhesion of tonsillar B cells. Consequently, since domain 5 mAb do inhibit FDC-B cell interactions, the putative ligand must be expressed on the FDC. In this adhesion process LFA-1/ICAM-1 interaction participates, together with a yet undefined second adhesion pathway.

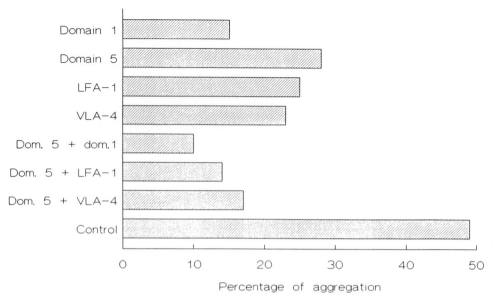

Figure 1.   Combination of adhesion mAb tested in adhesion of B-lymphocytes and follicular dendritic cells. The influence of individual mAb and combinations of mAb were compared to the aggregation observed in the control without mAb ($\pm 50\%$).

Germinal centres are important for selection of B cells by antigen presented by FDC. Furthermore selection of high affinity B cells generated by the somatic mutation and as a consequence apoptosis of many cells, probably cells with low affinity, in the germinal centres occur[9]. In the area with apoptosis, the basal light zone, a high expression of ICAM-1 is found. Adhesion molecules are essential in the selection processes since they allow the different cells to interact and communicate. Therefore studies on adhesion pathways involved in the interaction of B cells and FDC are of great importance, since they are critically involved in the physiological processes within secondary lymphoid organs.

REFERENCES

1.   Hogg, N., P.A. Bates, and J. Harvey. 1991. Structure and function of intercellular adhesion molecule-1. In: Chemical Immunology Vol 50; Integrins and ICAM-1 in immune responses. Eds. K. Ishizaka, P.J. Lachmann, B.H. Waksman. Karger, Basel, pp 98
2.   Marlin, S.D., and T.A. Springer. 1987. Purified intercellular adhesion molecule-1 (ICAM-1) a ligand for lymphocyte function-associated antigen-1 (LFA-1). *Cell 51:813.*
3.   Diamond M.S., D.E. Staunton, S.D. Marlin, and T.A. Springer 1991. Binding of the integrin Mac-1 (CD11b/CD18) to the third immunoglobulin-like domain of ICAM-1 (cd54) and its regulation by glycosylation. *Cell Biol. 111:3129.*
4.   Greve, J.M., G. Davis, A.M. Meyer, C.P. Forte, S.C. Yost, C.W. Marlor, M.E. Kamarck, and A. McClelland. 1989. The major human rhinovirus receptor is ICAM-1. *Cell 56:839.*
5.   Berendt, A.R., D.L. Simmons, J. Tansey, C.I. Newbold, and K. Marsh. 1989. Intercellular adhesion molecule-1 is an endothelial cell adhesion receptor for *Plasmodium falciparum. Nature 341:57.*
6.   Holzmann, B., J.M. Lehmann, H.W. Ziegler-Heitbrock, I. Funke, G. Riethmüller, and J.P. Johnson. 1988. Glycoprotein P3.58, associated with tumour progression in malignant melanoma, is a novel leucocyte activation antigen. *Int. J. Cancer 41:542-547.*

7. Dustin, M.L., R. Rothlein, A.K. Bahn. C.A. Dinarello, and T.A. Springer. 1986. Induction by IL 1 and interferon-γ: tissue distribution, biochemistry, and function of a natural adherence molecule (ICAM-1). *J. Immunol. 137:245.*

8. Rothlein R., M. Czajkowski,and T.K. Kishimoto. 1991. Intercellular adhesion molecule-1 in the inflammatory response. In: Chemical Immunology Vol 50; Integrins and ICAM-1 in immune responses. Eds. K. Ishizaka, P.J. Lachmann, B.H. Waksman. Karger, Basel, pp 135

9. Liu, Y-J., G.D. Johnson, J. Gordon, and I.C.M. MacLennan. 1992. Germinal centres in T-cell-dependent antibody responses. *Immunol. Today 13:17*

10. Koopman, G., H.K. Parmentier, H-J. Schuurman, W. Newman, C.J.L.M. Meijer, and S.T. Pals. 1991. *J. Exp. Med. 173:1297.*

11. Johnson, J.P., B.G. Stade, U. Hupke, B. Holzmann, and G. Riethmüller. 1988. The melanoma progression-associated antigen P3.58 is identical to the intercellular adhesion molecule, ICAM-1. *Immunobiol. 178:275.*

12. Bloemen, P., G. Moldenhauer, M. Van Dijk, H-J. Schuurman, and A.C. Bloem. 1992. Multiple ICAM-1 (CD54) epitopes are involved in homotypic B-cell adhesion. *Scand. J. Immunol. 35:517.*

13. Ahsmann, E.J.M., H.M. Lokhorst, A.W. Dekker, and A.C. Bloem. 1992. Lymphocyte-associated antigen-1 expression on plasma cells correlates with tumor growth in multiple myeloma. *Blood 79:2068.*

14. Parmentier H.K., J.A. van der Linden, J. Krijnen, D.F. van Wichen, L.H.P.M. Rademakers, A.C. Bloem, and H.-J. Schuurman. 1991. Human follicular dendritic cells: isolation and characteristics in situ and in suspension. *Scand. J. Immunol. 33:441.*

15. Joling, P., S. Boom, J. Johnson, M.E.M. Dekker, J.G. van Den Tweel, H-J. Schuurman, and A.C. Bloem. 1993. Domain 5 of ICAM-1 is involved in adhesion of B lymphocytes and follicular dendritic cells. *J. Immunol. submitted for publication.*

16. Mölgg M., W. Schwaeble, J.P. Johnson, M.P. Dierich. 1991. Generation of recombinant, carbohydrate-free intercellular adhesion molecule-1 (ICAM-1) and ICAM-1 fragments in Escherichia coli and mapping of epitopes recognized by anti-ICAM-1 monoclonal antibodies. *Immunol. Lett., 28:237.*

17. Schriever F., A.S. Freedman, G. Freeman, E. Messner, G. Lee, J. Daley, and L.M. Nadler. 1989. Isolated human Follicular Dendritic Cells display a unique antigenic phenotype. *J. Exp. Med.*169:2043.

MODIFICATIONS OF THE EXPRESSION OF HOMING AND ADHESION

MOLECULES IN INFILTRATED ISLETS OF LANGERHANS IN NOD MICE

Christelle Faveeuw, Marie-Claude Gagnerault, and Françoise Lepault

CNRS URA 1461
Hôpital Necker
Paris, FRANCE

INTRODUCTION

The NOD mouse is an experimental model for human autoimmune type I diabetes, in which lymphocyte infiltration (insulitis) into the islets of Langerhans develops from 3-5 weeks of age in both sexes while overt diabetes occurs predominantly in females from 12 weeks of age[1]. The central role of T cells in insulin-secreting beta cell destruction has been widely documented [2-5]. However, the mechanisms of lymphocyte infiltration are still unclear.

The migration of lymphocytes into peripheral lymphoid organs involves their adhesion to the post-capillary high endothelium venules (HEV). Homing receptors are involved in tissue-specific HEV recognition. In the mouse, Mab Mel-14 recognizes the lymph node-specific lymphocyte homing receptor[6], and R1.2, the Peyer's patch-specific homing receptor (LPAM)[7]. Other molecules, such as LFA-1 and Pgp-1, play an accessory role for the entry of lymphocytes into lymphoid organs[8,9]. HEV express tissue-specific lymphocyte adhesion molecules, the so-called vascular addressins. In mice, two monoclonal antibodies, Meca-79 and Meca-367, recognize addressins present on HEV of peripheral lymph nodes (pLN) and mucosal organs, respectively[10].

Expression of pLN and mucosal addressins in areas of lymphocyte infiltration create abnormal lymphocyte migration pathways contributing to the pathogenesis of chronic inflammatory diseases. However, other adhesion systems may play prominent roles in lymphocyte extravasation during inflammation: these include ICAM-1, a ligand for LFA-1, and VCAM-1, a ligand for VLA-4[11].

The present work was undertaken to better define the role of adhesion molecules in IDDM, aiming at studying, in the NOD mouse pancreas, the expression of adhesion molecules on infiltrating lymphocytes and on EC.

In Vivo Immunology, Edited by E. Heinen *et al.*
Plenum Press, New York, 1994

MATERIALS AND METHODS

Antibodies

Monoclonal antibodies to LFA-1 (35-89.9), Pgp-1 (IM7), and the lymphocyte homing receptor (Mel-14) were obtained from ascites. Monoclonal antibody to LPAM-1 α chain (R1.2) was a kind gift from I.L. Weissman (Stanford University, CA, USA). Anti-ICAM-1 was generously given by G. Kraal (Vrije University, Amsterdam, Netherlands). Meca-79 and Meca-367 were kindly provided by E.C. Butcher (Stanford University, CA, USA). These Mab were used purified or conjugated to FITC or biotin. Biotin-conjugated anti-mouse early activation marker mAb, CD69 (H1.2F3),was purchased from PharMingen (San Diego, CA, USA).

Preparation of cell suspension

For isolation of islet-derived mononuclear cells, pancreases were minced and then digested by a collagenase P solution. Islets were hand-picked under binocular lenses. Then islets were pressed through a 100μm metal sieve and the cell suspension was successively filtered through a 40μm and a 20μm nylon screen.

Immunoperoxidase staining

Sections were incubated with purified or biotinylated mAb in PBS for 30 min. Biotin-conjugated mouse anti-rat IgG or anti-rat IgM was applied, followed by an avidin-biotin horseradish peroxidase-complex. Peroxidase activity was detected using 3 amino 9 ethyl carbazole (AEC) as a substrate. Sections were counterstained with hematoxylin.

Immunofluorescence staining

Lymphocytes were stained with a mixture of two antibodies at an appropriate concentration, one being conjugated to FITC and the other biotinylated or conjugated to PE. After a 30 min incubation on ice, PE-streptavidin was added when needed and cells were incubated for another 30 min. Cells were analysed using a FACScan.

RESULTS

Immunohistochemical analysis of adhesion molecule expression in the pancreas of NOD mice

This study was performed on frozen sections of pancreas of NOD mice aged 14-17 weeks. ICAM-1 was expressed on blood vessels in the exocrine pancreas of control mice (Fig. 1a). Expression of ICAM-1 was hardly detectable on pancreatic beta cells and EC in islets of control mice and in healthy islets of NOD mice. However, in infiltrated islets ICAM-1 was highly expressed only by EC and dendritic cells present in the infiltrates. This staining was higher than on lymphocytes (Fig.1b). As previously described by E.C. Butcher et al, we confirmed the presence of the pLN and mucosal addressins, recognized by Meca-79 (Fig. 1c) and Meca-367 (Fig.1d), respectively, on HEV-like structures in infiltrated islets of Langerhans. EC present in healthy islets and in the exocrine pancreas of NOD and control mice were not labeled with these two antibodies (data not shown). VCAM was not observed in any situation (data not shown). Islet-infiltrating lymphocytes expressed the molecule Pgp-1 (Fig.1e), and Mel-14 antigen (Fig1f).

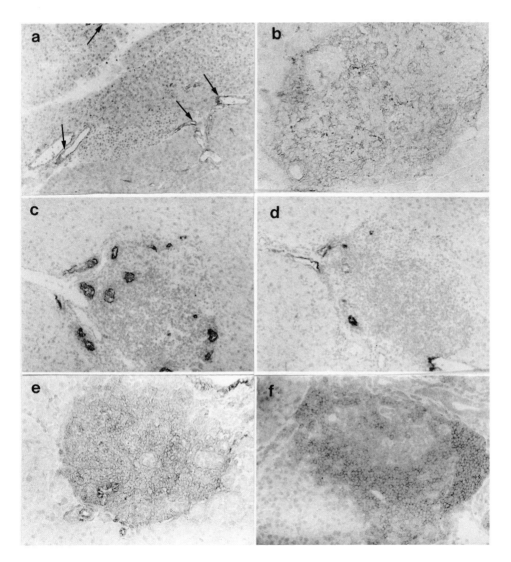

Figure 1. Adhesion molecules on frozen sections of pancreases from 14-17-week-old NOD mice. (a) ICAM-1 is expressed by blood vessels (arrows) in the exocrine pancreas of C57BL/6 and (b) in the inflamed islets of NOD mice. HEV-like structures expressed addressins recognized by Meca-79 (c) and Meca-367 (d) in inflamed islets of NOD mice. Islet-infiltrating cells expressed the molecule Pgp-1 (e), and Mel-14 antigen (f).

Adhesion molecule expression on pancreatic CD4, CD8 and B lymphocytes

Using two-color FACS analysis, we determined whether pancreatic lymphocyte subpopulations have a characteristic pattern of adhesion molecule expression as compared to peripheral lymphocytes. As shown on Fig.2A, the vast majority of CD4 and CD8 cells

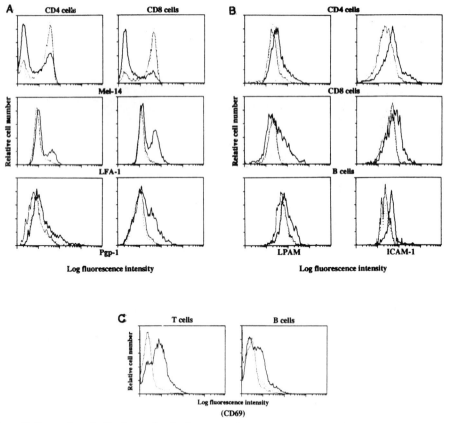

Figure 2. Expression of adhesion molecules by pancreatic CD4, CD8 and B lymphocytes, in comparison with pLN and spleen lymphocyte subpopulations. Cells were stained as described in materials and methods. CD4 and CD8 cells from islet (——), spleen (-----) , and pLN (· · · ·) were gated and analysed for (A) Mel-14, LFA-1, Pgp-1, (B) LPAM, ICAM-1, and for (C) CD69 expression. B cells were analysed for (B) LPAM, ICAM-1 and for (C) CD69 expression

in the pancreas did not express Mel-14 antigen, whereas in the spleen and pLN most CD4 and CD8 cells were Mel-14+. About 30 to 40% of pancreatic CD4 and CD8 cells were Mel-14+, as compared to 70-80% in peripheral organs. As in the periphery, all T cells were LFA-1 but the proportion of CD4 and CD8 cells expressing high levels of LFA-1 was increased in the pancreas (Fig.2A). Similar results were obtained for Pgp-1 (Fig. 2A). It is interesting to note that the proportion of Pgp-1 hi (and LFA-1 hi) lymphocytes in the islets varied from one experiment to another. 25 to 45% of the total hematopoietic population in the pancreas were Pgp-1 hi (and LFA-1 hi) as compared to 11 and 14% in pLN and spleen, respectively (data not shown). In addition, a subset of CD4 and CD8 cells in the pancreas expressed high levels of LPAM an ICAM-1 (Fig.2B).

No major differences were observed in the expression of Mel-14 antigen, LFA-1 and Pgp-1 on pancreatic B lymphocytes as compared to peripheral B cells (data not shown). However, in the pancreas B cells exhibited a weak up-regulation of LPAM and ICAM-1 (Fig.2B).

These results are consistent with the presence of activated lymphocytes in the islet of Langerhans, whose percentage probably varies among mice. This is supported by the staining with anti-CD69, which recognizes an early activation marker. While few T and B lymphocytes in pLN and spleen expressed CD69, the vast majority of T cells in the pancreas were CD69$^+$ (Fig.2C). Some B lymphocytes expressed the CD69 molecule.

DISCUSSION

In order to investigate the potential role of adhesion molecules in the pathogenesis of diabetes, the expression of some of these molecules in the pancreas of NOD mice, a relevant model for insulin-dependent-diabetes mellitus (IDDM) was analyzed.

Immunohistologic study demonstrated that the ICAM-1 molecule is constitutively expressed by blood vessels in the exocrine pancreas. In infiltrated islets of 14-17 week-old NOD mice, ICAM-1 was expressed by endothelial and dendritic cells within the infiltrate but absent from healthy areas. These cells stained more strongly than lymphocytes. In addition, as previously described by E.C. Butcher et al., we confirm the presence of HEV-like structures in inflamed islets. VCAM-1 was not observed in any situation. A recent study performed on the human diabetic pancreas showed hyperexpression of ICAM-1 on EC in inflamed islets and on the endothelium of some vessels in the exocrine pancreas, and the authors conclude that endothelial cells are likely to mediate inflammatory cell adhesion and extravasation into the pancreas during diabetic insulitis, at least in part, by regulating expression of this adhesion molecule [12]. In our study performed in prediabetic NOD mice, ICAM-1 is up regulated on EC in infiltrated islets and this result suggests that ICAM-1 may be involved in the migration of lymphocytes into islets of Langerhans during the prediabetic period. In addition, the presence of HEV-like structures expressing addressins contributes to the transendothelial migration of lymphocytes into the islets, and so participates in the development of insulitis. Futher, our results imply that expression of VCAM on the vascular endothelium is not needed for mononuclear cell infiltration into pancreatic islets.

Using two-color FACS analysis, we studied the level of expression of different adhesion molecules on lymphocyte subpopulations. The proportion of CD4 and CD8 cells which expressed Mel-14 was decreased in the pancreas as compared to peripheral organs, whereas a subset of CD4 and CD8 cells expressed high levels of LFA-1, Pgp-1, LPAM and ICAM-1. The expression of Mel-14, LFA-1 and Pgp-1 on pancreatic B lymphocytes was similar to that of peripheral B cells. However, pancreatic B cells exhibited weak upregulation of LPAM and ICAM-1. These results indicate that islet-infiltrating cells contain higher concentrations of activated T and B cells than peripheral lymphoid organs. This was supported by the increase in CD69$^+$ T and B cells in the islets. The presence of activated lymphocytes in the islets can be interpretated as a consequence of either selective recruitment of these cells from the periphery into the islet, or the acquisition of the activated phenotype after infiltration. Moreover, upregulation of ICAM-1 on B lymphocytes and expression of ICAM-1 by dendritic cells could be important for antigen presentation and induction of cytokine release in autoimmune diabetes [13].

We believe that these findings are important for research targeting the mechanisms of insulin-secreting beta cells destruction, and that specific blocking of adhesion molecules has a therapeutic potential in these inflammatory disorders.

REFERENCES

1. S. Makino, K. Kunimoto, Y. Muraoka, Y. Mizushima, K. Katagiri and Y. Tochino, Breeding of a non-obese, diabetic strain of mice, *Exp. Anim.* 29 : 1 (1980).
2. A. Miyazaki, T. Hanafusa, K. Yamada, J. Miyagawa, H. Fujino-Kurihara, H. Nakajima, K. Nonaka and S. Tarui, Predominance of T lymphocytes in pancreatic islets and spleen of pre-diabetic non-obese diabetic (NOD) mice : a longitudinal study, *Clin. Exp. Immunol.* 60 : 622 (1985).
3. M. Ogawa, T. Maruyama and T. Hasegawa, The inhibitory effect of neonatal thymectomy on the incidence of insulitis in non-obese diabetic (NOD) mice, *Biomed. Res.* 6 : 103 (1985).
4. Y. Mori, M. Suko and H. Odudaira, Preventive effects of cyclosporin on diabetes in NOD mice, *Diabetologia* 29 : 244 (1986).
5. A. Bendelac, C. Carnaud, C. Boitard and J.F. Bach, Syngeneic transfer of autoimmune diabetes from diabetic NOD mice to healthy neonates. Requirement for both L3T4+ and Lyt-2+ T cells, *J. Exp. Med.* 166 : 823 (1987).
6. W.M. Gallatin, I.L. Weissman and E.C. Butcher, A cell surface molecule involved in organ-specific homing of lymphocytes, *Nature* 304 : 30 (1983).
7. B. Holzmann, B.W. Mc Intyre, and I.L. Weissman, Identification of a murine Peyer's patch-specific lymphocyte homing as an integrin molecule with an alpha chain homologous to human VLA-4 alpha, *Cell* 56 : 37 (1989).
8. A. Hamann, D. Jablonskli-Westrich, A. Duijvestijin, E.C. Butcher, H. Baisch, R. Harder and H. Tiele, Evidence for an accessory role of LFA-1 in lymphocyte-high endothelium interaction during homing, *J. Immunol.* 140 : 693 (1988).
9. S. Jalkanen, R.F. Bargatze, J. de Los Togos and E.C. Butcher, Lymphocyte recognition of high endothelium : antibodies to distinct epitopes of an 85-95-kD glycoprotein in antigen differentially inhibit lymphocyte binding to lymph node, mucosal, or synovial endothelial cells, *J. Cell. Biol.* 105 : 983 (1987).
10. P.R. Streeter, B.T.N. Rouse and E.C. Butcher, Immunohistologic and functional characterization of a vascular addressin involved in lymphocyte homing into peripheral lymph nodes, *J. Cell. Biol.* 107 : 1853 (1988).
11. Y. Shimisu, W. Newman, Y. Tanaka and S. Shaw, Lymphocyte interactions with endothelial cells, *Immunol. Today* 13 : 106 (1992).
12. A. Hänninen, S. Jalkanen, M. Salmi, S. Toikkanen, G. Nikolakaros and O. Simell, Macrophages, T cell receptor usage, and endothelial cell activation in the pancreas at the onset of insulin-dependent diabetes mellitus, *J. Clin. Invest.* 90 : 1901 (1992).
13. M. Patarroyo, Leukocyte adhesion in host defense and tissue injury, *Clin. Immunol. Immunopathol.* 60: 333 (1991).

CHARACTERIZATION OF GIANT PERIVASCULAR SPACES IN THE THYMUS

OF THE NONOBESE DIABETIC MOUSE

Wilson Savino [1,3], Claude Carnaud [2], and Mireille Dardenne [1]

[1] CNRS URA 1461 - Hôpital Necker - Paris - France
[2] INSERM U25 - Hôpital Necker - Paris - France
[3] Department of Immunology, Institute Oswaldo Cruz - Rio de Janeiro -
Brazil

INTRODUCTION

The nonobese diabetic (NOD) mouse spontaneously develops insulin-dependent diabetes mellitus as a result of autoimmune destruction of β-cells in the pancreatic islets of Langerhans. It is thus widely accepted as a relevant experimental model for human type I diabetes [1-3]. Clinically-defined disease occurs more predominantly in females and can be observed from the age of 3 months. Insulitis always precedes the onset of diabetes, but appears in both males and females from the age of 3-4 weeks[4-5].

A large series of experiments demonstrated the direct involvement of T lymphocytes in the pathogeny of the disease in the NOD mouse. Converging data strongly suggest the participation of both CD4 and CD8 subsets [6-7].

The role of the thymus in modulating diabetes in the NOD mouse was shown by experiments in which neonatal thymectomy prevented the appearance of diabetes[8] whereas thymectomy at weaning accelerated it[9].

More recently we showed that the thymus of the NOD mouse is also a target organ, undergoing a number of alterations in both the lymphoid and microenvironmental compartments. We evidenced changes in thymic epithelial cells (TEC), reflected by abnormal distribution of monoclonal antibody-defined TEC subsets as well as by a precocious decline in the production of thymulin, a chemically-defined thymic hormone[10].

GENERAL FEATURES OF GIANT PERIVASCULAR SPACES IN THE NOD THYMUS

In addition to the epithelial abnormalities, a striking observation in the NOD mouse thymus was the existence of intralobular giant perivascular spaces (PVS), containing an extracellular matrix (ECM) network, intermingled with larger numbers of lymphocytes[10].

Such giant PVS occur in both males and females, and their size increases with age. Using image computer analysis, we recently demonstrated that the area of these structures can reach 100 times that of PVS in normal age-matched animals. It should be pointed out that such giant structures were not seen in a variety of other autoimmune mouse strains, including the *db/db* mouse, that also develops a type II diabetes.

Interestingly, we noted that the external basement membrane surrounding giant-PVS in the NOD mouse thymus exhibited some ruptures which were contiguous to those observed in the adjacent epithelial layer [10].

In Vivo Immunology, Edited by E. Heinen *et al.*
Plenum Press, New York, 1994

The intra-PVS ECM-bearing network contains laminin, fibronectin and type IV collagen. Additionally, we detected immunoglobulins co-localizing with the ECM-network, thus suggesting that in the NOD thymus, giant PVS are a target for B cell autoreactivity.

PHENOTYPING INTRA-PVS LYMPHOCYTES IN THE NOD MOUSE THYMUS

One of the first aspects we studied in the NOD thymus giant PVS was its lymphocytic composition. Most of intra-PVS cells are T lymphocytes, but some clusters of B cells were also found. These intra-PVS T cells were initially defined by the expression of the Thy1 marker. Furthermore, *in situ* double-labeling experiments revealed both CD4[+] and CD8[+] cells, expressing the CD3 complex[10].

WHAT IS THE ORIGIN OF INTRA-PVS T LYMPHOCYTES ?

In view of these data, it appeared worthwhile to further characterize the origin of intra-PVS T cells, that is whether they represent medullary thymic lymphocytes or are peripheral cells abnormally entering the thymus. We initially showed that giant-PVS persisted after two experimental procedures known to elicit thymic atrophy, sublethal irradiation and pharmacological doses of glucocorticoid hormones[11]. This suggested a rather mature phenotype of the lymphocytes.

We thus analysed cycling of intra-PVS lymphocytes following different *in vivo* pulse chase with bromodeoxyuridine BrdUrd. In all experiments, the numbers of BrdUrd[+] cells were equivalent to those found in the adjacent medullary region, thus pointing to a thymic origin of intra-PVS T cells. This notion was further supported by transfer experiments in mice congenic for the Thy1. molecule. Thus, when congenic Thy1.2[+] cells were transferred to irradiated adult Thy 1.1 recipients, donor's lymphocytes initially appeared in the subcapsular layer of the thymic lobules and reached the PVS region later, again with a kinetics similar to what was occurring in the whole medulla[11].

CONCLUSIONS AND PERSPECTIVES

It is thus apparent that intra-PVS T cells in the NOD mouse thymus are of thymic origin. To further support this notion, we are presently performing long term BrdUrd pulse chase, attempting to evidence accumulation of labeled cells within PVS.

The mechanism (s) responsible for such accumulations remain(s) to be determined. Abnormal expression of adhesion molecules is possible and since intra-PVS T cells are intermingled with an ECM-containing network, it seems worthwhile to analyse the expression of distinct ECM-receptors by these cells.

ACKNOWLEDGEMENTS

This work was partially supported with grants from CNPq (Brazil), INSERM (France) and CEC (Belgium).

REFERENCES

1. J.F. Bach, and C. Boitard, Experimental models of type-I diabetes. *Pathol. Immunopathol. Res.* 5:384 (1986)
2. H. Kolb, Mouse models of insulin-dependent diabetes: low-dose streptozotocin-induced diabetes and nonobese diabetic (NOD) mice. *Diabetes Metab. Rev.* 3:751 (1987)
3. E.H. Leiter, M. Prochaska, and D.L. Coleman, The non-obese diabetic (NOD) mouse. *Am. J. Pathol.* 128:380 (1987)
4. S. Makino, K. Kunimoto, Y. Muraoka, Y. Mizushima, K. Katagiri, and Y. Tochino. Breeding of a non-obese, diabetic strain of mice. *Exp. Anim.* 29:1 (1980)
5. E.F. Lampeter, A. Signore, E.A. Gale, and P. Pozzilli. Lessons from the NOD mouse for the pathogenesis and immunotherapy of human type 1 (insulin-dependent) diabetes mellitus. *Diabetologia* 32:703 (1989)
6. L.S. Wicker, B.J. Miller, and Y. Mullen. Transfer of autoimmune diabetes mellitus with splenocytes from onobese diabetic (NOD) mice. *Diabetes* 35:855 (1986)

7. A. Bendelac, C. Carnaud, C. Boitard, and J.F.Bach. Syngeneic transfer of autoimmune diabetes from diabetic NOD mice to healthy neonates. Requiement for both L3T4+ and Lyt-2+ T-cells. *J. Exp. Med.* 166:823 (1987)
8. M. Ogawa, T. Maruyama, T. Hasegawa, T. Kanaya, F. Kobayashi, Y. Tochino, and H. Uda. The inhibitory effect of neonatal thymectomy on theincidence of insulitis in non-obese diabetic (NOD) mice. *Biomed. Res* 6:103 (1985)
9. M. Dardenne, F. Lepault, A. Bendelac, and J.F.Bach. Acceleration of the onset of diabetes in NOD mice by thymectomy at weaning. *Eur. J. Immunol.* 19:889 (1989)
10. W. Savino, C. Boitard, J.F.Bach, and M. Dardenne. Studies on the thymus in nonobese diabetic mouse. I. Changes in the microenvironmental compartments. *Lab. Invest.* 64:405 (1991)
11. W. Savino, C. Carnaud, J.J. Luan, J.F. Bach, and M. Dardenne. Characterization of the extracellular matrix-containing giant perivascular spaces in the NOD mouse thymus. *Diabetes* 42:134 (1993)

ADHESION MOLECULE PECAM-1/CD31 IS EXPRESSED ON DEFINED SUBSETS OF MURINE LAK CELLS

Luca Piali, Beat A. Imhof and Roland H. Gisler

Basel Institute for Immunology (*)
487 Grenzacherstrasse
CH-4005 Basel 5 (Switzerland)

INTRODUCTION

Platelet-Endothelial Cell Adhesion Molecule (PECAM-1/CD31) is a member of the immunoglobulin gene superfamily [1]. It consists of six extracellular C2-like immunoglobulin domains and reveals extensive homology with Carcino-Embryonic Antigen (CEA) and Intracellular Cell Adhesion Molecule-1 (ICAM-1) [1]. It is a type I transmembrane protein, carrying an 118aa cytoplasmic tail. PECAM-1 /CD31 is present not only on platelets and endothelia but also on monocytes, granulocytes and lymphocytes, predominantly of the naive phenotype [1-7]. It stabilizes cell-cell contacts between endothelial cells, activates high affinity states of integrins on lymphocytes [3, 7], and participates in the sequential adhesive events leading to arrest and extravasation of blood-borne cells into tissues [5]. Here, we describe the distribution of PECAM-1/CD31 on different subsets of murine LAK cells using the monoclonal antibody EA-3. LAK cells, a heterogeneous mixture of

*The Basel Institute for Immunology was founded and is supported by
F. Hoffmann-LaRoche&Co. Ltd., CH-4005, Switzerland

IL-2 activated T- and NK-like cells, have been shown to reduce the number of metastases [8-10] and to infiltrate into sites of lesions of established metastases [11, 12]. On LAK cells, PECAM-1/CD31 has been shown to participate in the activation of high-affinity states of the integrin LFA-1 [13]. It is therefore conceivable that CD31+ LAK cells have advantages in infiltrating tumorous tissues.

MATERIALS AND METHODS

Preparation of LAK Cells

For the preparation of LAK cells, 10 to 14 week old, female C57BL/6 mice were used. They were prepared as described elsewhere [14]. Briefly, erythrocytes in single spleen cell suspensions were lysed by incubation with 140mM ammonium-chloride- potassium buffer. Subsequently, the cells were washed twice with RPMI 1640 (Gibco, Paisley, Scotland), and resuspended in 50 ml RPMI 1640 medium supplemented with 10% FCS (Boehringer Mannheim, Germany), non- essential amino acids, 1mM sodium pyruvate, 100U/ml Penicillin, 100μg/ml Streptomycin (all Gibco) and $5X10^{-5}M$ 2-ME (hereafter referred to as complete medium). Then the cells were transferred to a $162cm^2$ tissue culture flask (Costar, Cambridge, MA). Supernatant of IL-2 producing X63/0 BCMG Neo cells [15] was added to the cultures at a final concentration of 1000 IU/ml. After three days of incubation at 37°C and 5% CO_2, non- adherent spleen cells were removed and the flask washed twice with prewarmed (37°C) medium to remove non-attached cells. Fifty milliliters of fresh complete medium, supplemented as described above, were added and the cells were cultured for an additional three days. Cells were then harvested after a short treatment with 0,02% EDTA and washed twice in the appropriate buffer before use.

Reagents and Antibodies

Different monoclonal antibodies against murine cell-surface antigens were used either fluorescein-conjugated (FITC) or biotin-conjugated (BIOT). The following antibodies were used: anti PECAM-1/CD31 was developed in our laboratory [13] (EA-3FITC and BIOT). anti CD3ε (500A2BIOT), anti pan TCRαβ (H57-597FITC) (American Type Culture Collection, Rockville, MD), and anti NK1.1 (PK136BIOT) (Pharmingen, San Diego, CA), anti pan TCRγδ (GL3FITC) from Dr. Ronald Palacios, Dept. of Immunology, MD Anderson Cancer Center, Houston, TX. The developing reagent for biotin-conjugated antibodies was phycoerythrin-conjugated streptavidin (Jackson Immunosearch, West Grove, PA).

Cytofluorometry

The cells were harvested as described above and resuspended at 3×10^5 cells per well in V-bottom 96- well plates (Costar, Cambridge, MA) in 100µl FACS buffer (PBS, 1%BSA) on ice. After centrifugation, antibodies were added to the cell pellet and incubated for 30 min on ice. Thereafter the cells were washed twice and incubated with the streptavidin for an additional 30 min on ice. Then, the cells were suspended in 100µl FACS® buffer and flow cytometric analysis was performed using a FACScan® (Becton Dickinson FACS® Systems, Sunnydale, CA) with logarithmic amplification. The cell sorter is equipped with the LYSYS® data handling system.

RESULTS AND DISCUSSION

The LAK Cell Population Contains T- and NK-Like Cells

LAK cells were analyzed for the expression of lymphoid cell markers. The cells were completely negative for surface-immunoglobulin and markers for monocytes (data not shown). All cells were positive for Thy 1, CD2, CD45, CD71, MHC class I, CD44 and LFA-1 (data not shown). The cells were further analyzed for the expression of T-cell markers. Indeed, about 50% of the cells were positive for CD3 (Fig. 1 a-c). Half of these T-cells carried αβ T-cell receptors, half were positive for γδ T-cell receptors (Fig. 1 a and b). The cells positive for TCRαβ were also positive for CD8α (Fig. 1 c and data not shown). LAK cells have been reported to consist mainly of natural-killer-like cells [16, 17]. In the mouse, the lectin-like molecule NK1.1 serves as a marker for NK cells [18]. Indeed, about 70% of freshly prepared LAK cells are positive for this marker. The expression overlaps with cells of the TCRαβ lineage and cells of the TCRγδ lineage (Fig. 1 d and e).

PECAM-1/CD31 Is Predominantly Expressed on NK-Like LAK Cells

CD31 expression was analyzed on T- and NK- like cells within the LAK cell population. The expression of CD31 is very limited on T-cells. Only about 4% were positive (Fig. 1 i). The majority of the CD31 positive T-cells are of the TCRγδ+ type (Fig. 1 f and g). Interestingly, the expression of CD8α and CD31 never overlaps (Fig. 1 h and ref.13). Most of the CD31+ LAK cells were of the NK-like type (Fig. 1 k). CD31 expression on LAK cell subsets is summarized in Figure 2.

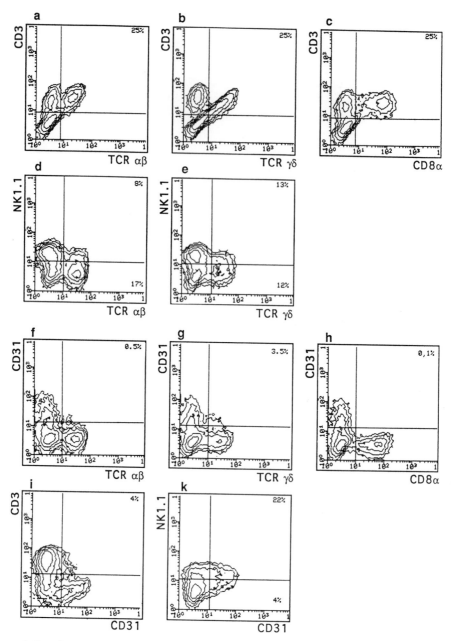

Figure 1. Cytofluorometric analysis of LAK-cell subsets. LAK cells incubated for six days in IL-2 were stained with FITC-labelled H57-597 (anti panTCRαβ), GL-3 (anti panTCRγδ), 53-6.7 (anti CD8α), or EA-3 (anti CD31) and biotin-labelled 500A2 (anti CD3ε), PK136 (anti NK1.1), or EA-3 (anti CD31), followed by phycoerythrin conjugated streptavidin. Percentages of positive cells are given in the corresponding quadrants. Percentages were determined using LYSYS® software. One representative of three experiments is shown.

The reciprocally exclusive expression of CD8 and CD31 is in contrast to peripheral lymphocytes which express both molecules together[5]. It could be that CD31 is gradually lost during in vitro culture (as for example L-Selectin, for which LAK cells are completely negative [13]). In the mouse, all freshly prepared splenocytes are positive for CD31 (data not shown). If this holds true, the total amount of cells positive for CD31 could be increased by shorter incubation times. Since CD31 is thought to be implicated in the homing of LAK cells to tumor lesions, cells incubated for shorter periods should be more effective. Indeed, LAK cells cultured for only five days in IL-2 were found to have higher infiltration capacities (P. Basse, personal communication).

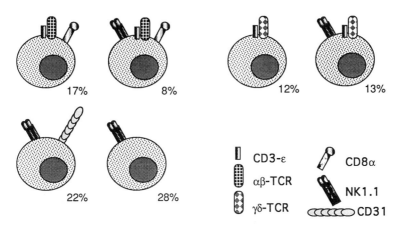

17%   8%   12%   13%

22%   28%   CD3-ε   CD8α   αβ-TCR   NK1.1   γδ-TCR   CD31

Figure 2. Relative proportions of the major LAK cell subtypes as determined by cytofluorometric analysis.

Moreover, the percentage of T-cells and NK-cells was comparable if LAK cell populations from animals of the same litter were analyzed. In contrast, we observed considerable variations between LAK cells from animals of different litters. Thus the proportion of CD3+ cells may decrease to 25%, and the NK1.1+CD3- cell subset would then increase. Under these circumstances, however, there was no change in the distribution of CD31+ cells to the different subsets (data not shown). The reason for these fluctuations between mouse litters is currently unknown. Great care was taken to use the same serum batch and IL-2 enriched supernatants when comparing LAK cell subpopulations. Age-differences of up to six weeks had no influence on the overall composition of the LAK cell population (data not shown).

Clearly, the following experiments should include a complete analysis of the capacity of LAK-cell subsets to infiltrate tumor metastases and also to lyse tumor target cells. Depending on the outcome it may be relevant to assess human LAK cell populations in order to design optimal adoptive immunotherapy protocols.

Acknowledgments

We thank Dr. Marie Kosco-Vilbois for critically reading and improving the manuscript, Philippe Hammel and Barbara Ecabert for excellent technical assistance, Marc Dessing and Stefan Meyer for help with FACS® analysis.

REFERENCES

1. Newman, P. J., Berndt, M. C., Gorski, J., White, G. C., Lyman, S., Paddock, C. and Muller, W. A., PECAM-1 (CD31) cloning and relation to adhesion molecules of the immunoglobulin gene superfamily, *Science* 247: 1219 (1990)

2. Stockinger, H., Gadd, S. J., Eher, R., Majdic, O., Schreiber, W., Kasinrerk, W., Strass, B., Schnabl, E. and Knapp, W., Molecular characterization and functional analysis of the leukocyte surface protein CD31, *J. Immunol* 145: 3889 (1990)

3. Albelda, S. M., Oliver, P. D., Romer, L. H. and Buck, C. A., EndoCAM: A Novel Endothelial Cell-Cell Adhesion Molecule, *J. Cell Biol.* 110: 1227 (1990)

4. Torimoto, Y., Rothstein, D. M., Dang, N. H., Schlossman, S. F. and Morimoto, C., CD31, a novel cell surface marker for CD4 cells of suppressor lineage, unaltered by state of activation, *J Immunol* 148: 388 (1992)

5. Tanaka, Y., Albelda, S. M., Horgan, K. J., van Seventer, G., Shimizu, Y., Newman, W., Hallam, J., Newman, P. J., Buck, C. A. and Shaw, S., CD31 expressed on distinctive T cell subsets is a preferential amplifier of β1 integrin-mediated adhesion, *J Exp Med* 176: 245 (1992)

6. Cabañas, C., Sanchez- Madrid, F., Bellon, T., Figdor, C. G., Te Velde, M., Fernandez, M., Acevedo, A. and Barnabeu, C., Characterization of a novel myeloid antigen regulated during differentiation of monocytic cells, *Eur. J. Immunol.* 19: 1373 (1989)

7. Albelda, S. M., Muller, W. A., Buck, C. A. and Newman, P. J., Molecular and cellular properties of PECAM-1 (endoCAM/CD31): a novel vascular cell-cell adhesion molecule, *J Cell Biol* 114: 1059 (1991)

8. Mazumder, A. and Rosenberg, S. A., Successful Immunotherapy of Natural Killer-Resistant Established Pulmonary Melanoma Metastases by the Intravenous Adoptive Transfer of Syngeneic Lymphocytes Activated in vitro by Interleukin-2, *J. Exp. Med.* 159: 495 (1984)

9. Rosenberg, S. A., Lotze, M. T., Muul, L. M., Chang, A. E., Avis, F. P., Leitman, S., Linehan, W. M., Robertson, C. N., Lee, R. E., Rubin, J. T., Seipp, C. A., Simpson, C. G. and White, D. E., A Progress Report on the Treatment of 157 Patients with advanced Cancer using Lymphokine-Activated Killer Cells and Interleukin-2 or high-dose Interlukin-2 alone, *N. Engl. J. Med.* 316: 889 (1987)

10. Schwarz, R. E., Vujanovic, N. L. and Hiserodt, J. C., Enhanced Antimetastatic Activity of Lymphokine-activated Killer Cells Purified and Expanded by Their Adherence to Plastic, *Cancer Res.* 49: 1441 (1989)

11. Basse, P. H., Nannmark, U., Johansson, B. R., Herberman, R. B. and Goldfarb, R. H., Establishment of Cell-to-Cell Contact by Adoptively Transferred Adherent Lymphokine-Activated Killer Cells With Metastatic Murine Melanoma Cells, *J. Natl. Cancer Inst.* 83: 944 (1991)

12. Basse, P., Herberman, R. B., Nannmark, U., Johansson, B. R., Hokland, M., Wasserman, K. and Goldfarb, R. H., Accumulation of Adoptively Transferred Adherent, Lymphokine-activated Killer Cells in Murine Metastases, *J. Exp. Med.* 174: 479 (1991)

13. Piali, L., Albelda, S. M., Baldwin, H.S., Hammel, P., Gisler, R.H. and Imhof, B. A., Murine Platelet Endothelial Cell Adhesion Molecule (PECAM-1)/CD31 modulates β2 Integrins on Lymphokine-Activated Killer Cells, *Eur. J. Immunol.* in press: (1993)

14. Gunji, Y., Vujanovic, N. L., Hiserodt, J. C., Herberman, R. B. and Gorelik, E., Generation and Characterization of Purified Adherent Lymphokine-Activated Killer Cells in Mice, *J. Immunol.* 142: 1748 (1989)

15. Karasuyama, H., Kudo, A. and Melchers, F., The Proteins Encoded by the VpreB and λ5 Pre-B Cell-specific Genes Can Associate with Each Other and with μ Heavy Chain, *J. Exp. Med.* 172: 969 (1990)

16. Herberman, R. B., Lymphokine-activated killer cell activity, *Immunol. Today* 8: 178 (1987)

17. Yang, J. C., Mulé, J. J. and Rosenberg, S. A., Murine Lymphokine-Activated Killer (LAK) Cells; Phenotypic characterization of the Precursor and Effector cells, *J. Immunol.* 137: 715 (1986)

18. Seaman, W. E., Sleisenger, M., Eriksson, E. and Koo, G. C., Depletion of Natural Killer Cells in Mice by Monoclonal Antibody to NK-1.1, *J. Immunol.* 138: 4539 (1987)

INTRATHYMIC GAP JUNCTION-MEDIATED COMMUNICATION

Luiz A. Alves[1], Antonio C. Campos de Carvalho [2], L. Parreira-Martins [2], Mireille Dardenne[3], and Wilson Savino[1]

[1] Department of Immunology, Institute Oswaldo Cruz - Rio de Janeiro - Brazil
[2] Dept. Biomechanics and Circulation, Institute of Biophysics, Federal University of Rio de Janeiro - Rio de Janeiro - Brazil
[3] CNRS URA 1461 - Hôpital Necker - Paris - France

INTRODUCTION

Intrathymic T cell differentiation comprises a complex series of events, eventually leading to migration of mature thymocytes to the T-dependent areas of peripheral lymphoid organs[1]. Key events in this process are driven by the influence of the thymic microenvironment[2], a tridimentional network composed of distinct cell types, including (among others) epithelial and dendritic cells.

Thymic epithelial cells (TEC) can influence intrathymic T cell differentiation via secretion of a variety of polypeptides such as thymic hormones and interleukins 1, 3 and 6, among others [3-5]. Additionally, cell-cell interactions occur between thymocytes and the cells of the thymic microenvironment. One involves the class I and class II MHC gene products expressed by TEC, and that interact with the T cell receptor in the context of CD8 and CD4 complexes respectively[2]. Moreover, TEC/thymocyte interactions can mediated by adhesion molecules such as LFA-3 and ICAM-1, expressed by TEC, and that respectively bind to CD2 and LFA-1 complexes existing on thymocyte membranes[6]. More recently, we demonstrated that TEC/thymocyte interactions are also mediated by extracellular matrix ligands and receptors[7]. Nonetheless, very little is known about interactions involving direct cell-cell communication among thymic cells. Such bidirectional cellular interations are essentially performed by gap junctions, which allow direct electronic coupling as well as passage of small polypeptides and second messenger molecules between adjacent cells [8,9].

Gap junctions are formed by the connexin protein family. Originally postulated by Wekerle et al.[10] studying thymic nurse cell (TNC) complexes, gap junctions between thymic cells have not been fully demonstrated.

CHARACTERIZATION OF GAP JUNCTIONS BETWEEN THYMIC EPITHELIAL CELLS

We initially showed communicating junctions in vitro, in both human and murine TEC, by lucifer yellow microinjection and patch clamp experiments (Fig. 1). Furthermore, the number of coupled TEC per injected cells varied in the cultures, as depicted in figure 2. Importantly, dye diffusion among adjacent cells could be prevented if TEC cultures were previously treated with octanol, known to inhibit gap junctions.

Immunocytochemical labeling, together with immunoblotting and northern blotting of TEC samples, demonstrated that connexin 43 is the protein involved in the formation of

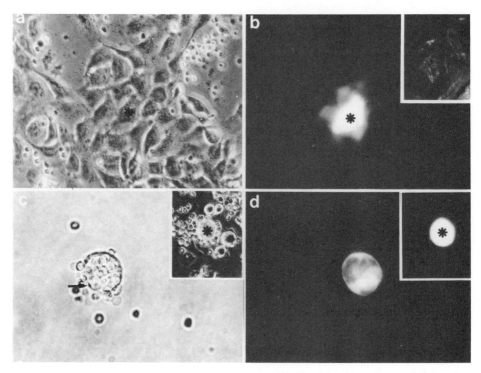

Figure 1. Dye injection experiments in cultured thymic cells. Panels a and b show the mouse TEC line in phase contrast (a) and in fluorescence after lucifer yellow transfer (b). In panels c and d TNC was injected (arrow) and two lymphocytes were labeled. The inserts show a -TR-C rosetting with thymocytes, that remained unlabeled after dye injection.

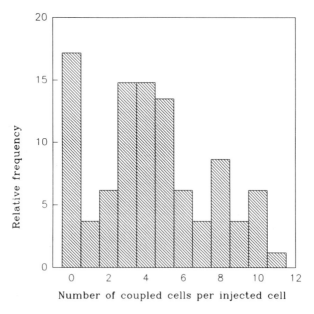

Figure 2. Relative frequency of coupled cells after 80 dye injections in the mouse TEC lines.

TEC/TEC gap junctions. In this respect, immunocytochemistry on thymus frozen sections revealed positive labeling on TEC (determined in double-labeling experiments with an anticytokeratin antibody).

From a functional point of view, we showed that when TEC were cultured in the presence of octanol, they consistently exhibited a partial decrease in thymulin production, an effect that could be reversed after washing the cultures with octanol-free medium.

ARE THERE COMMUNICATING JUNCTIONS BETWEEN MICROENVIRONMENTAL CELLS AND THYMOCYTES ?

We also investigated the possibility of transient communicating junctions between TEC and thymocytes. First, we showed that round, freshly-isolated lymphocyte-rich TNC could be specifically stained with the anti-connexin 43 antibody. In addition, injection of lucifer yellow in the epithelial component of spread TNCs revealed communication with intra-TNC thymocytes in 10% of TNC complexes .

Since we had evidenced TEC/thymocyte heterotypic gap junctions, we asked whether thymocytes could also make communicating junctions with other cells of the thymic microenvironment. We isolated phagocytic cells of the thymic reticulum (P-TR-C), according to the method originally described by Papiernik et al.[11]. Inter-P-TR-C communication was not detected by dye injection experiments on 100 cells. As reported by the same investigators, P-TR-C can rosette with thymocytes[12]. Nonetheless, after performing dye transfer in more than 75 P-TR-C (previously allowed to rosette with thymocytes), no adhered thymocyte was labeled (Fig. 1).

CONCLUDING REMARKS

The data discussed above strongly point to the existence of communicating junctions in the thymus. The homotypic TEC/TEC gap junctions suggest that the whole TEC network may be electrotonically coupled and thus behaving like a syncitium, a concept previously postulated by Kendall et al.[13.] Yet, it is also conceivable that such cell coupling is restricted to small TEC areas, yielding distinct microenvironments independently coupled.

Additionally, it is important to note that TEC also make heterotypic communications with thymocytes through gap junctions, as ascertained with the studies of thymic nurse cell complexes and the use of stimulated thymocytes laid down on the mouse TEC line. Given thymocyte migration within the thymic parenchyma during their differentiation process, TEC/thymocyte junctions should be rapidly disassembled. This hypothesis requires demonstration is compatible with the fact that only a minor percentage of TNC are internally coupled by gap junctions at a given moment. In fact, a similar system has already been described for the differentiation of gonocytes that form transient gap junctions with the sessile Sertoli cells [14].

In conclusion, we postulate that gap junctions may represent a novel pathway for intrathymic cellular interactions, involving not only TEC/TEC but also TEC/thymocyte direct communication.

ACKNOWLEDGMENTS

We thank Drs. D. Goodenough, B. Nicholson and G.I. Fishman for providing anti-connexin antibodies. This work was partially supported with grants from CNPq (Brazil), INSERM (France) and CEC (Belgium).

REFERENCES

1. J. Sprent, D. Lo, E.O. Gao, and Y. Ron. T cell selection in the thymus. *Immunol. Rev.* 101:173 (1988).
2. W. van Ewijk. T-cell differentiation is influenced by thymic microenvironments. *Ann. Rev. Immunol.* 9:591 (1991).

3. W. Savino, and M. Dardenne. Thymic hormone containing cells. VI. Immunohistologic evidence for the simultaneous presence of thymulin, thymopoietin and thymosin α1 in normal and pathologic human thymuses. *Eur. J. Immunol.* 14 : 4987 (1984).

4. P.T. Le, D.T. Tuck, C.A. Dinarello, B.F. Haynes, and K.H. Singer. Human thymic epithelial cells produce interleukin-1. *J. Immunol.* 138:2520 (1987).

5. P.T. Le, S. Lazorick, L.P. Whichard, Y.C. Yang, S.C. clarck, B.F. Haynes, and K.H. Singer. Human thymic epithelical cells produce IL-6, granulocyte-monocyte CSF and leukemia inhibitory factor. *J. Immunol.* 145:3310 (1990).

6. L.W. Vollger, D.T. Tuck, T.A. Springer, B.F. Haynes and K.H. Singer. Thymocyte binding to human thymic epithelial cells is inhibited by monoclonal antibodies to CD2 and LFA-3 antigens. *J. Immunol.* 138:358 (1989).

7. W. Savino, D.M.S. VIlla Verde, and J. Lannes Vieira. Extracellular matrix proteins in intrathymic T cell migration and differentiation? *Immunol. Today* 14:651 (1993).

8. M.V.L. Bennett, and D..A. Goodenough. Gap junctions, electronic coupling, and intercellular communication. *Neurosci. Res. Prog. Bull.* 165:373 (1978).

9. M.V.L. Bennett, and D.C. Spray. "Gap junctions". Cold Spring Harbor, N.Y.: Cold Spring Harbor Laboratory (1985).

10. H. Wekerle, U.P. Ketelsen, and M. Ernst. Thymic nurse cells lymphoepithelial cell complexes in murine thymuses:morphological and serological characterization. *J. Exp. Med.* 151: 925(1980).

11. M. Papiernik, B. Nabarra, W. Savino, C. Pontoux, and S. Barbey. Thymic reticulum in mice. II. Culture and characterization of non epithelial phagocytic cells of the thymic reticulum : their role in the syngeneic stimulation of thymic medullary lymphocytes. *Eur. J. Immunol.* 13:147 (1983).

12. S. El Rouby, F. Praz, L. Halbwachs-Mecarelli , and M. Papiernik. Thymic reticulum in mice.IV. The rosette formation between phagocytic cells of the thymic reticulum and cortical type thymocytes is mediated by complement receptor type three. *J. Immunol.* 134:326 (1985).

13. M.D. Kendall. The syncytial nature of epithelial cells in the thymic cortex. *J. Anat.* 147:95 (1986).

14. McGimley, D. Posalaky, Z. Porvazmik, and L. Russell. Gap junctions between sertoli and germ cells or not seminiterous tubules. *Tissue Cell* 11, 741 (1979).

AIDS AND LYMPHOPROLIFERATIVE DISEASES

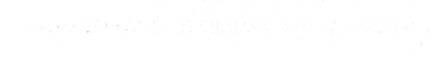

COMPLEMENT AND ANTIBODY ENHANCE BINDING AND UPTAKE OF HIV-1 BY BONE MARROW CELLS

Bart A. van de Wiel[1], Leendert J. Bakker[2], Loek de Graaf[2],
Roel A. de Weger[1], Jan Verhoef[2], Jan G. van den Tweel[1], and Piet Joling[1]

[1]Departments of Pathology and [2]Clinical Microbiology
University Hospital, Utrecht, The Netherlands

INTRODUCTION

Infection of bone marrow cells by HIV-1 might be a principle cause for the bone marrow myelodysplasia and peripheral blood cytopenias in HIV-1 infected patients[1]. Infection of immature cells in bone marrow may have long-lasting effects on the haematopoiesis[2]. Although the CD4 molecule is considered as the major receptor of HIV-1, also other factors may be decisive for binding and modulation of the retrovirus[3-5]. In this study we present data of the binding and the infection of bone marrow cells by HIV-1. Furthermore the role of anti-HIV-1 antibody and complement on binding of HIV-1 is evaluated.

MATERIALS AND METHODS

Bone marrow aspirates. Bone marrow cells were obtained through sternal punction of patients during thoracotomy. Samples were aspirated in RPMI-1640 medium supplemented with heparin. To obtain a mononuclear cell fraction, cells were separated on Ficoll (Pharmacia, Uppsala, Sweden).

Human Immunodeficiency Virus. HIV-1 strain HTLV-IIIB was obtained from the culture supernatant of infected SUP-T1 cells. For in vitro experiments high titered culture supernatants ($TCID_{50}$ 3×10^6/ml) or purified virus conjugated to fluorescein isothiocyanate (FITC) was used as described by Bakker et al[5].

Sera and MAb. Sera from control individuals, negative for anti-HIV-1 antibodies (detected by ELISA and Western blotting), were pooled and part was stored immediately after harvesting in aliquots at -70°C (fresh serum). Another part was heat-inactivated for 30 min at 56°C to inactivate complement activity. This pooled serum was designated as control serum. Sera from HIV-1 positive individuals containing anti-HIV-1 antibodies (detected by ELISA and Western blotting) were pooled and heat-inactivated. This pooled serum was designated as HIV-1 serum. Serum from a patient with C3-deficiency was obtained from the Department of Immunology, University Hospital for Children and Youth "Het Wilhelmina Kinderziekenhuis" (Utrecht, The Netherlands). This serum was designated as C3-deficient serum. Adding C3 to this serum completely restored complement activity. All sera were stored at -70°C until use. Monoclonal antibody (MAb) CD34 (IgG1; Becton Dickinson, San Jose, CA) is directed against a 105-120 kD glycoprotein (GP) on hematopoietic progenitor cells; CD14 (IgG2b; Becton Dickinson) is directed against a 55kD GP on monocytes/macrophages; Fibroblast (IgG1; Dako, Glostrup, Denmark) is directed against fibroblasts in normal and inflammatory tissues; STRO-1 (IgM) was a gift of Dr Torok-Storb (Seattle, WA, USA) and is directed against stromal cells[6].

Binding assay and analysis. A total of 5×10^5 isolated cells was resuspended in 50 μl FITC-conjugated HIV-1 (HIV-1/FITC) in PBS. The incubation mixture was supplemented with 20% (v/v) HIV-1 serum or with 20% (v/v) fresh or heated control serum. Incubation was done at 37°C for 30 min. Thereafter the cells were washed twice in PBS at 4°C and fixed in 1% paraformaldehyde. Flow cytometric analysis was performed on the cells using a FACStar (Becton Dickinson, San Jose, CA) as described by Joling et al[7]. Cells were separated on the basis of forward and side scatter properties into 4 different subpopulations. Part of the cells was processed for conventional transmission electron microscopy and investigated for the presence of virions.

PCR analysis. Cells were analyzed for the presence of HIV-1 and ß-globine DNA using a nested PCR assay as described by Nottet et al[8].

RESULTS AND DISCUSSION

The mononuclear cell fraction of bone marrow aspirate was isolated and in vitro infected with HIV-1 (strain HTLV-IIIB). Both after 14 and 21 days, infection was clearly demonstrable by the detection of viral HIV-1 DNA in the cells and HIV-1 *gag* p24 in the culture supernatants. Conventional transmission electron microscopy revealed HIV-1-like virus particles (80 to 120 nm in diameter), showing the typical electron-dense conical shaped cores, in association with plasma membrane invaginations of plasma cells and mononuclear phagocytes[9]. Occasionally budding figures were observed in granulocyte-like cells. After 21 days a low number of cells contained virus. These results indicate that a low but definite number of bone marrow cells can be infected by HIV-1 and produce virus.

In order to determine the amount of HIV-1 infected cells, the total fraction of bone marrow cells was incubated with HIV-1/FITC and analyzed on a FACScan. Under these conditions only a small fraction of the bone marrow cells (2-6%) was HIV-1 positive, which is in accordance with the electron microscopical results. Since bone marrow cells are highly heterogeneous, the cells were separated on the basis of different scatter properties into 4 different populations. These populations were named after the mature cell types with comparable scatter profiles: lymphoid, monocyte-like, granulocyte-like and blastoid cells. Subsequently, binding of HIV-1/FITC to each population was studied (Figure 1). In the presence of medium alone binding was relatively low in the lymphoid cells whereas higher frequencies were found in the monocyte-like and the blastoid cells.

Although HIV-1 infection of various cell types is mediated via the CD4 molecule[10], several studies have suggested that infectivity may also occur through a anti-HIV-1 antibody or a complement mediated mechanism[3-5] by binding to Fc- or complement receptors. This was evaluated by incubating the cells in the presence of culture medium supplemented with different serum sources. Heat-inactivated control serum did not alter binding of HIV-1/FITC to bone marrow cells (Figure 1).

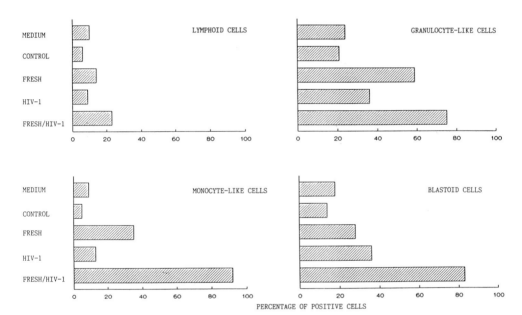

Figure 1.   Binding of HIV-1 to subpopulations of bone marrow cells. Bone marrow cells were incubated with HIV-1/FITC in the presence of culture medium alone or supplemented with heat-inactivated control or fresh serum, HIV-1 serum or a combination of fresh and HIV-1 serum. Binding was assessed by FACScan analysis and expressed as percentage of positive cells within each subpopulation.

However, a significant increase in the numbers of HIV-1 positive cells in the bone marrow subpopulations occured when cells were incubated in the presence of fresh serum, particularly in the monocyte-like (59%) and in the granulocyte-like (35%) population. Incubation with HIV-1 serum showed a minor effect on binding of HIV-1/FITC in the monocyte-like and in the granulocyte-like population. In contrast, the effect of HIV-1 serum surpassed the effect of fresh serum in the blastoid cell population. The combination of fresh serum and HIV-1 serum resulted in summation of the individual serum effects in the monocyte-like population, whereas a clearly enhancing effect was seen in the granulocyte-like and blastoid population. These data are in agreement with results reported for monocytes and follicular dendritic cells, where an enhancing effect of anti-HIV-1 antibody with fresh serum was shown[7,8].

These data point to a possible role of complement (in fresh serum) in binding of HIV-1 to bone marrow cells. This aspect could be studied using serum lacking complement component C3. Control experiments using fresh serum gave substantial fluorescence signal compared to control values of heat-inactivated serum (Figure 2).

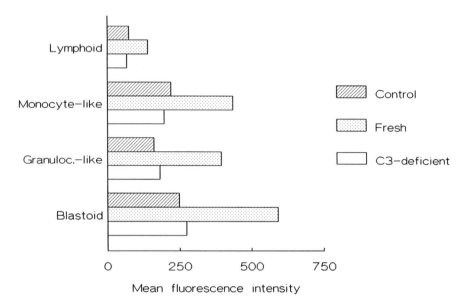

Figure 2.   The role of complement component C3 of binding on HIV-1/FITC to bone marrow cells. The cells were incubated with HIV-1/FITC in the presence of heat-inactivated control serum, fresh serum or C3-deficient serum. Binding was assessed by FACScan analysis and expressed as arbitrary units of fluorescence (mean value).

Using C3-deficient serum, the mean fluorescence intensity returned to control values indicating that complement component C3 is the factor in fresh serum mediating the HIV-1/FITC binding to bone marrow cells. The role of complement in HIV-1 infection has recently been supported by the demonstration of the capacity of HIV-1 *env* gp41 to activate the classical pathway of complement by the binding and activation of complement component C1[11]. Activation leads to deposition of C3b on the virus and on infected cells and subsequent binding of opsonized virus to complement receptors could lead to HIV-1 infection of target cells[4,5]. Under serum-free conditions binding of HIV-1/FITC to bone marrow cells is low. In vivo, special circumstances like inflammation can disrupt the bone marrow/blood barrier, resulting in the introduction of additional serum factors. In this situation increased numbers of bone marrow cells can be infected by HIV-1.

The expression of CD4, the major receptor for HIV-1, on HIV-1 positive cells was measured using two-colour fluorescence analysis. In the total fraction of bone marrow cells CD4+/ HIV-1/FITC+ cells were detected, suggesting that the binding of the MAb CD4 did not interfere with HIV-1/FITC labelling, though both mAb CD4 and HIV-1 are regarded to bind to the same molecule. In the monocyte-like population CD4+/ HIV-1/FITC+ cells are present in low numbers, increasing up to 28% in the presence of fresh serum. However, CD4$^-$/ HIV-1/FITC$^+$ cells were also present in the same population up to 17%, in the presence of fresh serum. Similar results were found with the granulocyte-like population. Low numbers of both phenotypes were found in the lymphoid and the blastoid population. This suggests the existence of a CD4 independent pathway for HIV-1 infection in bone marrow cells. Preliminary results of the expression of other cell markers showed that quantities of HIV-1/FITC positive bone marrow cells express CD34, CD14 or STRO-1, whereas the fibroblast marker was almost absent, as measured by two-colour fluorescence analysis. These results indicate HIV-1 infection of bone marrow progenitor cells and cells of the monocyte/macrophage lineage, which is in accordance with earlier findings[12-13]. The possible infection of stromal cells, suggested by the STRO-1 positivity of HIV-1/FITC positive cells, is a novel finding since thus far HIV-1 infection only has been demonstrated in stromal cell lines[14].

REFERENCES

1.   J.L. Spivak, B.S. Bender, and T.C. Quinn, Hematologic abnormalities in the acquired immune deficiency syndrome, *Am. J. Med.* 77:224 (1984).
2.   C.C. Stella, A. Ganser, and D. Hoelzer, Defective in vitro growth of the hemopoietic progenitor cells in the acquired immunodeficiency syndrome, *J. Clin. Invest.* 80:286 (1987).
3.   A. Takeda, C.U. Tuazon, and F.A. Ennis, Antibody-enhanced infection by HIV-1 via Fc receptor-mediated entry, *Science* 242:580 (1988).
4.   V. Boyer, C. Desgranges, M.-A. Trabaud, E. Fischer, and M.D. Kazatchkine, Complement mediates human immunodeficiency virus type 1 infection of a human T cell line in a CD4- and antibody-independent fashion, *J. Exp. Med.* 173:1151 (1991).
5.   L.J. Bakker, H.S.L.M. Nottet, N.M. de Vos, L. de Graaf, J.A.G. Van Strijp, M.R. Visser, and J. Verhoef, Antibodies and complement enhance binding and uptake of human immunodeficiency virus type 1 by human monocytes, *AIDS* 6:35 (1992).
6.   P. Simmons, and B. Torok-Storb, Identification of stromal cell precursors in human bone marrow by a novel monoclonal antibody, STRO-1, *Blood* 78:55-62 (1991).
7.   P. Joling, L.J. Bakker, J.A.G. van Strijp, T. Meerlo, M.E.M. Dekker, J. Goudsmit, J. Verhoef, and H.-J. Schuurman, Binding of human immunodeficiency virus type 1 to follicular dendritic cells in vitro is complement dependent, *J. Immunol.* 150:1065 (1993).
8.   H.S.L.M. Nottet, I. Janse, N.M. de Vos, L.J. Bakker, M.R. Visser, and J. Verhoef, Antibody mediated enhancement of HIV-1 infection of an EBV transformed B cell line is CD4 dependent, *Eur. J. Clin. Invest.* 22:670 (1992).
9.   T. Meerloo, H.K. Parmentier, A.D.M.E. Osterhaus, J. Goudsmit, and H.-J. Schuurman, Modulation of cell surface molecules during HIV-1 infection of H9 cells, *AIDS* 6:1106 (1992).
10.   A.G. Dalgleish, P.C.L. Beverly, P.R. Clapham, D.H. Crawford, M.F. Greaves, and R.A. Weiss, The CD4 (T4) antigen is an essential component of the receptor for the AIDS retrovirus, *Nature* 312:763 (1984).
11.   C.F. Ebenbichler, N.M. Thielens, R. Vornhagen, P. Marschang, G.J. Arlaud, and M.P. Dierich, Human immunodeficiency virus type 1 activates the classical pathway of complement by direct C1 binding through specific sites in the transmembrane glycoprotein gp41, *J. Exp. Med.* 174:1417 (1991).
12.   T.M. Folks, S.W. Kessler, J.M. Orenstein, J.S. Justement, E.S. Jaffe, and A.S. Fauci, Infection and replication of HIV-1 in purified progenitor cells of normal human bone marrow, *Science* 242:919 (1988).
13.   S. Gartner, P. Markovits, D.M. Markovits, M.H. Kaplan, R.C. Gallo, and M. Popovic, The role of mononuclear phagocytes in HTLV-III/LAV infection, Science 233:215 (1986).
14.   H.N. Sternberg, J. Anderson, C.S. Crumpacker, and P.A. Chates, HIV infection of the BS-1 human stroma cell line: effect on murine hematopoiesis, *Virology* 193:524 (1993).

FOLLICULAR DENDRITIC CELLS (FDC) ARE NOT PRODUCTIVELY INFECTED WITH HIV-1 IN VIVO

Jörn Schmitz[1,2], Jan van Lunzen[2], Klara Tenner-Racz[3,4] Gudrun Großschupff[3], Paul Racz[4], Herbert Schmitz[1], Manfred Dietrich[2], and Frank Hufert[5]

From the Departments of Virology[1] and Pathology[4] and the Clinical Medicine Section[2], Bernhard Nocht Institute, Hamburg, Germany; the Department of Hematology, Allgemeines Krankenhaus St. Georg[4], Hamburg, Germany; and the Institute for Medical Microbiology and Hygiene[5], Freiburg, Germany

INTRODUCTION

During HIV-1 infection a progredient destruction of FDC is generally observed[1]. By electron microscopy, immunohistochemistry and in situ hybridization high amounts of HIV-1 particles and HIV-1 antigen can be detected on the network of FDC, even in the early phase of the infection. For long periods of time, HIV-1 particles persist in the germinal centers. A part of these particles may be still infectious and T helper cells gain infection, when they invade the germinal centers[2]. Intracellular virus particles in FDC or budding from FDC have been observed in rare occasions[3,4], but others could not confirm a productive infection of FDC by electron microscope[5]. The massive staining of the FDC network for HIV-RNA in in situ hybridization has been interpreted as a productive infection of FDC[6]. Yet, a clear distinction between trapped antigen-antibody complexes and a possible production of HIV-1 by FDC is difficult. We investigated whether or not the destruction of FDC is due to HIV-1 infection in vivo. FDC were isolated by magnetic activated cell sorting (MACS) or fluorescence activated cell sorting (FACS) from lymph nodes of five HIV-1 infected patients. In the MACS enriched cellfraction HIV-1 RNA and HIV-1 particles were detected by in situ hybridization and electron microscopy. The proviral load was detected in FACS purified FDC.

MATERIALS AND METHODS

Surgical biopsy of enlarged lymph nodes from five HIV-1 infected patients (CDC stage II/III) were taken after written informed consent for diagnostic purposes. The duration of the infection after diagnosis of HIV-1 ranged between a few months (shortly after seroconversion) up to nine years. Rountine histopathology showed that malignant disorders or opportunistic infections could be excluded in causing the lymphadenopathy.

Isolation of FDC was performed as described elsewhere[7]. Briefly, the lymphatic tissue was cut into small pieces and digested by collagenase class IV (450 U/ml; Worthington, Freehold, NJ) at 37° C for 60 minutes. Subsequently, the digested cell suspension was passed through a 120 μm nylon mesh and the cell suspension was layered onto a discontinuous density gradient and centrifuged at 8,500 x g for 1 h. The interphase was collected and the cell suspension (containing 1.0 - 3.0 % FDC) were split for further enrichment of FDC either by MACS or FACS.

MACS-enrichment of FDC was performed as described previously[8]. Briefly, the cell suspension was stained with Ki-M4, previously couppled to biotin. Subsequently, the cell suspension was incubated with strepavidin-conjugated microbeads (Miltenyi Biotec, Bergisch-Gladbach, Germany). The cellfraction was filled on a steelwool column (type B1; Miltenyi Biotec), adjusted to the MACS (Miltenyi Biotec). Unlabeled cell were rinsed out. Finally, the column was removed from the magnetic field and the attached cells were eluted. The cells were resuspended in plasma, clotted with Thromboplastin-IS (Baxter; Dade Division, Miami, USA) and fixed either by 4% glutaraldehyde for electron microscopy or 1.3 M formaldehyde for in situ hybridization. For electron microscopy ultrathin sections were investigated using a Philips 201 electron microscope operating at 80 kV. In situ hybridization was done on 5 μm sections using ^{35}S-labeled antisense RNA probes of HIV-1.

For detection of proviral load FDC were highly enriched by FACS. Subsequently, staining FDC with Ki-M4 and anti mouse IgG-FITC the cells with a higher forward scatter than lymphocytes and a positive reaction with Ki-M4 were excepted for sorting of FDC. The purity of all enriched cell fractions was confirmed by immunofluorescence of the cells sorted directly onto glass slides and post-sort reanalysis on FACS.

The proviral DNA load of the obtained cell fractions were estimated in limiting dilution assays by nested polymerase chain reaction (PCR). The cell samples contained 1.0×10^2 to 1.0×10^5 FDC and were prepared in triplicate. For control non-infected H9 cells, and 1.0×10^1 to 1.0×10^3 molecules of the HIV-1 plasmid pLAI were used. The 5'V3 NOT and 3'V3 NOT primers were used for the first PCR and PCR-1 and PCR-2 primers for the second PCR. The amplifications were applied on Perkin Elmer DNA amplification system 9600 (Perkin-Elmer-Cetus, Norwall, Conn., USA). The specific amplified DNA fragment was detected using a 2% agarose gel stained with ethidiumbromid.

RESULTS

In electron microscopy of MACS-enriched FDC (a mean of 25%) appeared as large rounded cells with one or two nuclei containing loose chromatin. Even after mechanical and enzymatical disruption the cells showed the characterizing long cytoplasmatic extensions. Sometimes FDC envoled lymphocytes forming round clusters. A massive concentration of HIV particles could regularly be detected on or between the cytoplasmatic extensions (Fig. 1). Yet, intracytoplasmic virus particles or budding were not present. In in situ hybridization of MACS-enriched FDC we could detect HIV-RNA on the surface of FDC but not in the cytoplasm. In rare occasions, cells with lymphocyte morphology showed strong hybridization signals. The nested polymerase chain reaction of FACS purified FDC (purity over 93%) showed no positive reaction, except of on single cell sample with 10^5 cells.

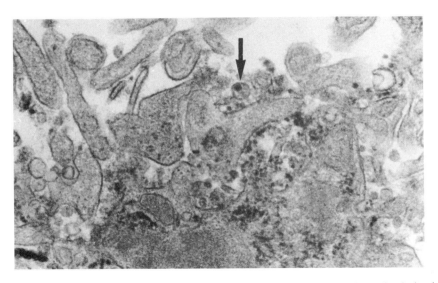

Figure 1. Extracellular HIV-1 particle (arrow) between the cytoplasmatic extensions of an isolated FDC obtained from a lymph node of an HIV-1 infected patient (x 30,000).

DISCUSSION

During HIV-1 infection an explosive hyperplasia of the germinal centers is generally followed by a continous disruption of the network of FDC[1]. The results described here show that the destruction of FDC is most likely not caused by an infection of FDC by HIV-1.

By applying in situ hybridization on isolated FDC we have found silver grains be associated with the cell surface of FDC, but not with the cell bodies. In contrast to Spiegel and coworkers[6] we feel that the diffusely distributed autoradiographic signal is mainly due to extracellular HIV RNA. Electron microscopy of the isolated FDC confirmed these results. Even after the isolation procedure retained virus particles could be demonstrated on the surface of FDC, but intracellular virusparticles or budding was not seen.

Since the PCR allows a clear detection of an infection with HIV-1 and thus overcomes the examination of the precise localisation of the HIV-antigen, we applied PCR on highly enriched FDC fractions in limiting dilution assays. With only one exception we could not find a positive signal in FDC. Similar results have been reported recently by Embretson and her coworkers[9], who could not detect HIV-DNA in FDC by in situ PCR.

Therefore infection of FDC seems to be exceptional. Further studies are needed to elucidate the exact pathomechanisms of FDC destruction during HIV-infection.

REFERENCES

1. P. Racz, K. Tenner-Racz, and H. Schmidt, Follicular dendritic cells in HIV-induced lymphadenopathy and AIDS. *Acta Path. Microbiol. Scand.* 97(Suppl. 8):16 (1989).

2. C.H. Fox, K. Tenner-Racz, P. Racz, A. Firpo, P.A. Pizzo, and A.S. Fauci, Lymphoid germinal centers are reservoirs of human immunodeficiency virus type 1 RNA. *J. Infect. Dis.* 164:1051 (1991).

3. K. Tenner-Racz, P. Racz, S. Gartner, J. Ramsauer, M. Dietrich, J.-C. Gluckman, and M. Popovic, Ultrastructural analysis of germinal centers in lymph nodes of patients with HIV-1 induced persistent generalized lymphadenopathy: evidence for persistence of infection. *Prog. AIDS Pathol.* 1:29 (1989).

4. J.A. Armstrong and R. Horne, Follicular dendritic cells and virus-like particles in AIDS-related lymphadenopathy. *Lancet* 2:370 (1984).

5. J. Diebold, C.L. Marche, J. Audouin, J.P. Aubert, A. Le Tourneau, C.L. Bouton, M. Reynes, J. Wizniak, F. Capron, and V. Tricottet, Lymph node modification in patients with the acquired immunodeficiency syndrome (AIDS) or with AIDS-related complex (ARC). A histological, immunohistological and ultrastructural study of 45 cases. *Pathol. Res. Pract.* 180:590 (1985).

6. H. Spiegel, H. Herbst, G. Niedobitek, H.D. Foss, and H. Stein, Follicular dendritic cells are a major reservoir for human immunodeficiency virus type 1 in lymphoid tissues facilitating infection of CD4+ T-helper cells. *Am. J. Pathol.* 140:15 (1992).

7. C.T. Schnizlein, M.H. Kosco, A.K. Szakal, and J.G. Tew, Follicular dendritic cells in suspension: Identification, enrichment, and initial characterization indicating immune complex trapping and lack of adherence and phagocytic activity. *J. Immunol.* 134:1360 (1985).

8. J. Schmitz, S. Petrasch, J. van Lunzen, P. Racz, H.D. Kleine, F. Hufert, P. Kern, H. Schmitz, and K. Tenner-Racz. Optimizing follicular dendritic cell isolation by discontinuous gradient centrifugation and use of the magnetic cell sorter (MACS). *J. Immunol. Methods* 159:189 (1993).

9. J. Embretson, M. Zupancic, J.L. Ribas, A. Burke, P. Racz, K. Tenner-Racz, and A.T. Haase, Massive covert infection of helper T lymphocytes and macrophages by HIV during the incubation period of AIDS. *Nature* 362:359 (1993).

ACKNOWLEDGMENT

Sponsorship: This work was supported in part by the grants from the Bundesministerium für Forschung und Technologie, Germany (FKZ BGA III-006-89/FVP 6, project A01 and C03), the Körber Foundation, Hamburg, Germany and the donation from Mrs G. Bruhn, Hamburg, Germany.

LYMPH NODE PATHOLOGY IN EXPERIMENTAL FIV INFECTION

John J. Callanan,[1] Paul Racz, [2] Hal Thompson[1]
and Oswald Jarrett[1]

[1]Department of Veterinary Pathology
University of Glasgow
Bearsden, Glasgow
Scotland
[2]Department of Pathology and Korber Laboratory
Bernhard-Nocht Institute for Tropical Medicine
Hamburg
Germany

INTRODUCTION

Feline immunodeficiency virus (FIV) was first isolated in 1986 from a colony of cats in California exhibiting multiple, and often chronic, infections (Pedersen et al, 1987). The virus was characterised as a T-lymphotropic lentivirus morphologically similar but antigenically distinct from human immunodeficiency virus (HIV), the cause of acquired immunodeficiency syndrome (AIDS) in man (Barré-Sinoussi et al, 1983; Gallo et al, 1984). Subsequently the virus was isolated throughout the world (Harbour et al, 1988; Ishida et al, 1988) and analysis of stored serum samples indicated that FIV infection has been present since at least the 1960s in cat populations (Gruffydd-Jones et al, 1988; Shelton et al, 1990). It is likely that biting is the most common means of transmission of the virus (Yamamoto et al, 1989). Infection is persistent and can be detected by the demonstration of infectious virus in activated T cells from peripheral blood (Pedersen et al, 1987), by amplification of FIV nucleic acid sequences in blood or other cells by the polymerase chain reaction (PCR) (Dandekar et al, 1992) or by the demonstration of anti-FIV antibodies in the serum or plasma (Pedersen et al, 1987; Hosie & Jarrett, 1990).
FIV infections have been associated with gingivitis/stomatitis, respiratory tract infections, enteritis, dermatitis, weight loss, pyrexia, lymphadenopathy, opportunistic infections (Pedersen et al, 1987; Ishida et al, 1988; Gruffydd-Jones et al, 1988; Hosie et al, 1989; Yamamoto et al, 1989), immune dysfunctions (Novotney et al, 1990; Sieblink et al, 1990; Hoffman-Fezer et al, 1992; Ishida et al, 1992), haematological alterations (Yamamoto et al,

1989; Shelton et al, 1990; Sparkes et al, 1993), pathology of the central nervous system and eyes (Dow et al, 1990; Hurtel et al, 1992; English et al, 1990; Hopper et al, 1989) and neoplasia (Alexander et al, 1989; Shelton et al, 1990).

Experimental infection of kittens and young adult cats with FIV causes a syndrome characterised by generalised lymph node enlargement. Coexisting with this generalised lympadenopathy are episodes of neutropenia, lymphopenia, pyrexia, dullness and anorexia (Pedersen et al, 1987; Yamamoto et al, 1988; Callanan et al, 1992; Moraillon et al, 1992; Mandell et al, 1992). The purpose of the present study was to define the histopathological changes in the lymph nodes of FIV infected cats during the first year of infection and to compare these changes with those observed in the lymph nodes of HIV-infected persons. Findings from this study have been described in greater detail elsewhere (Callanan et al, 1993).

MATERIALS AND METHODS

Ten 11-14 month old specific pathogen free cats were infected intraperitoneally with 2000 infectious units of FIV/GL-8. Three uninfected and non-immunised age-matched cats provided a reference of normal lymphoid tissue. In order to compare the follicular hyperplasia of FIV infection to that due to non-infectious agents, 5 age-matched controls which were immunised with ovalbumin in AL(OH)$_3$ (T-dependent antigen), DNP-Ficoll (T-independent antigen) and a killed feline respiratory virus vaccine (Feliniffa, Rhone Merieux) were used.

Cats were selectively sacrificed in groups of three (2 infected and 1 immunised control) at 4, 8, 16, 32 and 52 weeks after infection and were submitted to a detailed post mortem examination. However one infected cat became ill and required euthanasia at 6 weeks rather than the intended 16 weeks after infection.

Lymph nodes were fixed in formalin, post-fixed in mercuric chloride, paraffin embedded, sectioned and stained with Giemsa and haemotoxylin and eosin. Cryostat sections were prepared from popliteal and retropharyngeal lymph nodes. These sections were fixed in acetone at room temperature for 10 minutes. Monoclonal antibodies to feline CD4 (VPG34) and CD8 (VPG 9) (Willett et al, 1991) and to the follicular dendritic cell (FDC) network (anti-human CD21: Scottish Antibody Production Unit) were used employing an avidin-biotin technique (Vectastain ABC Kit, Vector Labs, Peterborough, UK).

RESULTS

After infection with FIV all cats in this study developed a generalised lymph node enlargement which commenced 3-6 weeks after infection and persisted in some cases up to one year. The architecture and cell content of the feline lymph node was similar to that of man and many other species (Racz et al, 1986) and the alterations in lymph node morphology were identified in the follicular, extrafollicular and sinus regions (Figure 1).

Follicles

The feline secondary follicle contains a mantle zone and a germinal centre composed of centrocytes, centroblasts, immunoblasts, follicular dendritic cells, macrophages, small numbers of CD4[+] lymphocytes and occasional CD8[+] lymphocytes. An increase in the number and size of the follicles was the earliest change observed in FIV infection. There was attenuation of the mantle zone and zonation of the germinal centre. There was a generalised increase in cellularity within the germinal centres with a significant increase in the numbers of CD8[+] and CD4[+] lymphocytes. Immunoblasts were also significantly increased in number and appeared to migrate to the extrafollicular parenchyma. With

Morphological Changes in Lymph Nodes of Cats with Experimental FIV Infection

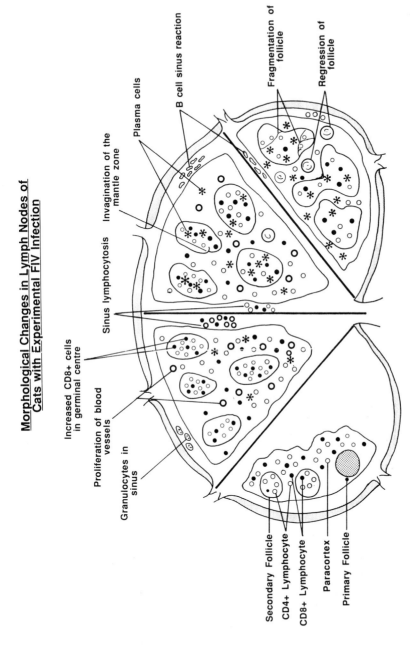

Figure 1. Sequential pathological findings in the lymph nodes of FIV experimentally infected cats (adapted from Racz et al, 1986)

Increased CD8+ cells in germinal centre

Proliferation of blood vessels

Granulocytes in sinus

Sinus lymphocytosis

Invagination of the mantle zone

Plasma cells

B cell sinus reaction

Fragmentation of follicle

Regression of follicle

Secondary Follicle

CD4+ Lymphocyte

CD8+ Lymphocyte

Paracortex

Primary Follicle

Normal ◄——► Progression of Infection

progression of infection the number of CD8$^+$ lymphocytes in the germinal centres remained high but the CD4$^+$ numbers returned to normal levels. During the first year of infection the FDC network remained intact and there was a gradual increase in the concentration of intrafollicular plasma cells.

As the germinal centres continued to increase in size they became irregular in shape and there was often follicular fusion. In these later stages of infection there was also fragmentation, regression and depletion of individual follicles.

Extrafollicular Lymphoid Tissue

After infection there was an initial expansion of paracortical tissue and of medullary cords with an increase in the numbers of mitotic cells and immunoblasts and a prominent high endothelial venule network. Later there was also an increase in centrocytic-like cells especially surrounding the follicles. Throughout infection there was a gradual increase in the number of plasma cells. With progression of infection the paracortex decreased in size and was eventually compressed by the florid follicular hyperplasia. No major alteration in the CD4:CD8 ratio was seen.

Sinus Reactions

Throughout infection there was enhanced cellularity in the sinuses which contained lymphocytes, immunoblasts, macrophages, mast cells and plasma cells. In both the early and later stages of this study polymorphonuclear leucocytes were also found and a prominent sinus lymphocytosis was identified. With progression of infection sinus B-cell reactions were frequently observed.

Acute Illness

One cat developed an acute illness at 5 weeks after infection characterised by pyrexia, dullness and profound leucopenia. In this animal the lymph nodes contained many follicles which were depleted. These follicles consisted mainly of large cells with pale cytoplasm and a loose chromatin structure. They were arranged in a whorl pattern and many cells resembled FDCs and stained positive with anti-CD21 monoclonal antibodies. Other follicles showed necrosis or regressive changes. There was also an increase in the plasma cell content within the extrafollicular tissue and the pathology resembled that seen in Castleman's disease in man.

DISCUSSION AND CONCLUSIONS

The findings within lymphoid tissues in the first year of experimental infection closely resemble those identified in HIV lymphadenitis (Dieblod et al, 1985; Racz et al, 1986; Ost et al, 1989). The initial lymphadenopathy observed after experimental FIV infection is due to moderate or marked follicular hyperplasia accompanied by paracortical activation and expansion. This is augmented from two months after infection by a strong humoral response with the appearance of numerous plasma cells in the follicles and extrafollicular parenchyma. From two months after infection there is gradual follicular enlargement with the formation of irregular and fused follicles. At eight to twelve months after infection the first evidence of follicular exhaustion and involution is apparent with the appearance of hyalinised follicles.

In addition, in this period characteristic features of HIV lymphadenitis are noted: mantle zone invaginations, increased follicular CD8[+] cells, sinus lymphocytosis and sinus B-cell reactions.

The maintenance of active germinal centres requires the constant presentation of antigen in the form of immune complex deposition on the FDCs (vanRooijen, 1990). In HIV infection, antigen-antibody complexes are present on the surface of the FDC (Tenner-Racz et al, 1985). Whether the FDC is itself infected with with HIV remains controversial (Speigel et al, 1992; Stahmer et al, 1991). Recent investigations by two groups showed that HIV is active in the lymphoid tissue even throughout periods of clinical latency and at times when there are very few cells in the blood carrying proviral DNA (Embretson et al, 1993; Pontaleo et al, 1993). By both *in situ* hybridisation or PCR combined with *in situ* hybridisation it was demonstrated that there is mechanical filtering and trapping of virus by FDCs which probably facilitates the infection of CD4[+] cells sequestered in the lymph node. With progression of HIV infection there is gradual destruction of the FDC network probably mediated by several mechanisms but certainly associated with an increased number of CD8[+] lymphocytes within the germinal centres. While it is likely that FIV antigen-antibody complexes on FDCs are responsible for the persistent follicular hyperplasia seen in this study, it is not yet known if the FDC in the cat harbours virus or what the fate of the FDC network will be. Although an increase in CD8[+] cells was identified within the germinal centre, in the first year of infection the FDC framework remained intact indicating that the production of B memory cells and plasma cells was not disturbed and the ability of the animals to respond to new antigens was not hindered. However in studies on lymph node morphology in cats in the end stages of natural infection the FDC network is damaged (Rideout et al, 1992). Much of the antibody produced by these cells is specific for the core and envelope proteins of HIV (Laman et al, 1991). Whether this is also the case with FIV is not yet known.

In the first year of FIV infection lymphadenitis strongly resembles the lymphadenopathies observed during HIV infection with strong similarities to the persistent lymphadenopathy stage of infection. A greater understanding of the disease mechanisms requires the detection of virus by immunohistochemical and *in situ* hybridisation techniques.

Acknowledgements

The authors acknowledge the advice of Dr K. Tenner-Racz and assistance of Mr C. Patterson, Mr B O'Neil, Mr I. McMillan, Mr R Irvine, Mr J. Murphy and Ms B Guhlk. This study was funded by the Wellcome Trust. P.R. is supported by BMFT (Bundesministerium fur Forschung und Technologie, SKZ 111-006-89, Bonn) and Korber Foundation, Hamburg. Collaboration between laboratories was supported by the European Commission Concerted Action on Feline AIDS.

REFERENCES

Alexander, R., Robinson, W.F., Mills, J.N., Sherry, C.R., Sherard, E., Paterson, A.J., Shaw, S.E., Clark, W.T. and Hollingsworth, T., 1989, Isolation of feline immunodeficiency virus from three cats with lymphoma, *Aus Vet Pract* 19:93.

Barré-Sinoussi, F., Chermann, J.C., Rey, F., Nugeyre, M.T., Charmaret, S., Gruest, J., Dauguet, C., Axler-Blin, C., Vezinet-Brun, F., Rouzioux, C., Rozenbaum, W. and Montagnier, L., 1983, Isolation of a T-lymphotropic retrovirus from a patient at risk for acquired immune deficiency syndrome (AIDS), *Science* 220:868.

Callanan, J.J., Thompson H., Toth, S.R., O'Neil, B., Lawrence, C.E., Willett, B. and Jarrett, O., 1992, Clinical and pathological findings in feline immunodeficiency virus experimental infection, *Vet Immunol Immunopath* 35:3

Callanan, J.J., Racz, P., Thompson H. and Jarrett O., 1993, Morphological characterisation of the lymph node changes in feline immunodeficiency virus infection as an animal model of AIDS, in: " *Animal Models of HIV and Other Retroviral Infections*" P. Racz, N.L. Letvin, J.C. Gluckman, eds, Karger, Basel.

Dandekar, S., Beebe, A.M., Barlough, J., Phillips, T., Elder, J., Torten, M. and Pedersen, N., 1992, Detection of feline immunodeficiency virus (FIV) nucleic acids in FIV-seronegative cats, *J Virol* 66:4040.

Diebold, J., Marche, C.L., Audouin, J., Aubert, J.P., LeToourneau, A., Bouton, C.L., Reynes, M., Wizniak, J., Capron, F. and Tricottet, V., 1985, Lymph node modification in patients with the acquired immunodeficiency syndrome (AIDS) or with AIDS related complex (ARC), *Pathol Res* 161:590.

Dow, S.W., Poss, M.L. and Hoover E.A., 1990, Feline immunodeficiency virus: a neurotropic lentivirus, *J AIDS* 3:658.

Embretson, J., Zupancic, M., Ribas, J.L., Burke, A., Racz, P., Tenner-Racz, K. and Hasse, A.T., 1993, massive covert infection of helper T lymphocytes and macrophages by HIV during the incubation period of AIDS, *Nature* 362:359.

English, R.V., Davidson, M.G., Nasisse, M.P., Jamieson, V.E. and Lappin, M.R., 1990, Intraocular disease associated with feline immunodeficiency virus infection in cats, *J Amer Vet Med Assoc* 196:1116.

Gallo, R.C., Salahuddin, S.Z., Popovic, M., Sherer, G., Kaplan, M., Haynes, B.F., Parker, T.J., Redfield, R., Oleske, J., Safai, B., White, G., Foster, P. and Markham, P.D., 1984, Frequent detection and isolation of cytopathic retroviruses (HTLV-III) from patients with AIDS and at risk for AIDS, *Science* 224:500.

Gruffydd-Jones, T.J., Hopper, C.D., Harbour, D.A., and Lutz, H., 1988, Serological evidence of feline immunodeficiency virus infection in UK cats from 1975-76, *Vet Rec* 123:569.

Harbour, D.A., Williams, P.D., Gruffydd-Jones, T.J., Burbridge, J. and Pearson, G.R., 1988, Isolation of a T-lymphotropic lentivirus from a persistently leucopenic domestic cat, *Vet Rec* 122:84.

Hoffmann-Fezer, G., Thum, J., Ackley, C., Herbold, M., Mysliwietz, J., Thefeld, S., Hartmann, K. and Kraft, W., 1992, Decline in CD4+ cell numbers in cats with naturally acquired feline immunodeficiency virus infection, *J Virol* 66:1484.

Hopper, C.D., Sparkes, A.H., Gruffydd-Jones, T.J., Crispin, S.M., Muir, P., Harbour, D.A. and Stokes, C.R., 1989, Clinical and laboratory findings in cats infected with feline immunodeficieny virus, *Vet Rec* 125:341.

Hosie, M.J., Robertson, C. and Jarrett, O., 1989, Prevalence of feline leukaemia virus and antibodies to feline immunodeficiency virus in cats in the United Kingdom, *Vet Rec* 128:293.

Hosie, M.J. and Jarrett, O., 1990, Serological responses of cats to feline immunodeficiency virus, *AIDS* 4:215.

Hurtrel, M., Ganiere, J-P., Gueifi J-F., Chakrabarti, L., Maire, M-A., Gray, F., Montagnier, L. and Hurtrel, B., 1992, Comparsion of early and late feline immunodeficiency virus encephalopathies, *AIDS* 6:399.

Ishida, T., Washizu, T., Toriyabe, K. and Motoyoshi, S., 1988, Detection of feline T-lymphotropic lentivirus (FTLV) infection in Japanese domestic cats, *Jpn J Vet Sci* 50:39.

Ishida, T., Taniguchi, A., Matsumura, S., Washizu, T. and Tomoda, I., 1992, Longterm clinical observations on feline immunodeficiency virus infected asymptomatic carriers, *Vet Immunol Immunopath* 35:15.

Laman, J.D., Racz, P., Tenner-Racz, K., Klasmeier, M., Fasbender, M.J., Neelen, C., Zegers, N.D., Dietrich, M., Boersma, W.J.A. and Claassen, E., 1991, Immunocytochemical determination of antigenand epitope specificity of HIV-1 specific B cells in lymph node biopsies from HIV-1 infected individuals, *AIDS* 5:255.

Mandell, C.P., Sparger, E.E., Pedersen, N.C. and Jain, N.C., 1992, Long-term haematological changes in cats experimentally infected with feline immunodeficiency virus (FIV), *Comp Haem Int* 2:8.

Moraillon A., Barre-Sinoussi, F., Parodi, A., Moraillon, R. and Dauguet, D., 1992, In vitro properties and experimental pathogenic effects of three strains of feline immunodeficiency viruses (FIV) isolated from cats with terminal disease, *Vet Microbiol* 31:41.

Novotney, C., English, R., Housman, J., Davidson, M.G., Nasisse, M.P., Chian-Ren, J., Davis, W.C. and Tompkins, M.B., 1990, Lymphocyte population changes in cats naturally infected with feline immunodeficiency virus, *AIDS* 4:1213.

Ost, A., Baroni, C.D., Biberfeld, P., Diebold, J., Moragas, A., Noel, H., Pallesen, G., Racz, P., Schipper, M., Tenner-Racz, K. and van den Tweel, J.G., 1989, Lymphadenopathy in HIV infection: histological classification and staging, *APMIS* suppl 8:7.

Pedersen, N.C., Ho, E.W., Brown, M.L. and Yamamoto, J.K., 1987, Isolation of a T-lymphotropic virus from domestic cats with an immunodeficiency-like syndrome, *Science* 235:790.

Pantaleo, G., Graziosi, C., Demarest, J.F., Butini, L., Montroni, M., Fox, C.H., Orenstein, J.M., Kotler, D.P. and Fauci, A.S. (1993) HIV infection is active and progressive in lymphoid tissue during the clinically latent stage of disease, *Nature* 362:355.

Racz, P., Tenner-Racz, K., Kahl, C., Feller, A.C., Kern, P. and Dietrich, M, 1986, The spectrum of morphological changes of lymph nodes from patients with AIDS or AIDS-related complexes, *Prog Allergy* 37:81.

Rideout B.A., Lowensteine, L.J., Hutson, C.A., Moore, P.F. and Pedersen, N.C., 1992, Characterization of morphologic changes and lymphocyte subset distribution in lymph nodes from cats with naturally acquired feline immunodeficiency virus infection, *Vet Pathol* 29:391.

Shelton, G.H., Grant, C.K., Cotter, S.M., Gardner, M.B., Hardy, W.D. and DiGiacomo, R.F., 1990, Feline immunodeficiency virus and feline leukemia virus infections and their relationships to lymphoid malignancies in cats: a retrospective study (1986-1988), *J AIDS* 3:623.

Sieblink, K.H.J., Chu, I-H., Rimmelzwaan, G.F., Weijer, K., Van Herwijnen, R., Knell, P., Egberink, H.F., Bosch, M.L. and Osterhaus, A.D.M.E., 1990, Feline immunodeficiency virus (FIV) infection in the cat as a model for HIV infection in man: FIV-induced impairment of immune function, *AIDS Res Hum Retroviruses* 6:1373.

Sparkes, A.H., Hopper, C.D., Millard, W.G., Gruffydd-Jones, T.J. and Harbour, D.A., 1993, Feline immunodeficiency virus infection: clinicopathologic findings in 90 naturally occurring cases, *J. Vet Int Med* 7:85.

Spiegel, H., Herbst, H., Niedobitek, G., Foss, H-D. and Stein, H., 1992, Follicular dendritic cells are a major resevoir for human immunodeficiency virus type 1 in lymphoid tissues facilitating infection of CD4+ helper cells, *Am J Pathol* 140:15.

Stahmer, I., Zimmer, J.P., Ernst, M., Fenner, T., Finnern, R., Schmitz, H., Flad, H.D. and Gerdes, J., 1991, isolation of normal human follicular dendritic cells and CD4-independent in vitro infection by human immunodeficiency virus (HIV-1), *Eur J Immunol* 21:1873.

Tenner-Racz, K., Racz, P., Diettrich, M. and Kern, P., 1985, Altered follicular dendritic cells and virus-like particles in AIDS and AIDS-related lymphadenopathy, *Lancet* i:105.

van Rooijen, N., 1990, Antigen processing and presentation in vivo; the microenvironment as a crucial factor, *Immunol Today* 11:426.

Willett, B.J., Hosie, M.J., Dunsford, T.H., Neil, J.C. and Jarrett, O., 1991, Productive infection of T-helper lymphocytes with feline immunodeficiency virus is accompanied by reduced expression of CD4, *AIDS* 5:1469.

Yamamoto, J.K., Sparger, E., Ho, E.W., Anderson, P.R., O'Connor, T.P., Mandell, C.P., Lowensteine, L., Munn, R. and Pedersen, N.C., 1988, The pathogenesis of experimentally induced feline immunodeficiency virus infection, *Am J Vet Res* 49:1246.

Yamamoto, J.K., Hansen, H., Ho, E.W., Morishita, T.Y., Okuda, T., Sawa, T.R., Nakamura, R.M. and Pedersen N.C., 1989, Epidemiologic and clinical aspects of feline immunodeficiency virus infection in cats from the continental United States and Canada and possible mode of transmission, *J Amer Vet Med Assoc* 194:213.

LYMPHOCYTE LIFESPAN IN MURINE RETROVIRUS-INDUCED IMMUNODEFICIENCY

Michel Moutschen, Sonia Colombi, Manuel Deprez,
Roland Greimers, France Van Wijk, Christophe Hotermans,
and Jacques Boniver

Department of Pathology
CHU Sart-Tilman
4000 Liège, Belgium

INTRODUCTION

Infection of mice with the Duplan-Latarjet strain of RadLV, also called RadLV-Rs, induces a syndrome characterised by polyclonal proliferation of B- and CD4[+] T-cells and the simultaneous appearance of an *in vitro* refractoriness to mitogen stimulation involving both lymphocyte subsets. This syndrome, initially observed by Mistry and Duplan[1] and described later as MAIDS (for Murine Acquired Immunodeficiency Syndrome) by Mosier and Morse[2], is due to the infection of B-cells by a defective virus present in the RadLV-Rs viral mixture[3]. MAIDS is clearly not a perfect model of human AIDS, since there is neither infection of CD4[+] T-cells nor CD4[+] T-cell lymphopaenia in the murine infection. Nevertheless, since CD4[+] T-cell modifications in MAIDS are functional (i.e. not due to direct cytopathic effects of the virus on the CD4 subset), MAIDS could be a valuable model to study the immunodeficiency associated with certain states of antigenic activation such as chronic graft-versus-host disease, autoimmune diseases, and perhaps some aspects of the early stages of HIV infection when the frequency of infected CD4[+] T-cells is still low, at least in the peripheral blood.

Cell lifespan could be a critical parameter to understand the functional effects of sustained polyclonal activation on the homeostasis of the immune system and on its ability to provide secondary responses (i.e. to TCR stimulation *in vitro*). The growing numbers of B-cells and CD4[+] T-cells in MAIDS indicate a dysregulation of homeostatic mechanisms which control lymphocyte numbers. Although increased proliferative activity takes place within the lymphoid organs of infected animals, it is presently unknown if the cell lifespan within these subsets is unchanged, increased (and therefore participating in the accumulation of lymphocytes in the LN) or reduced (as a homeostatic mechanism compensating for proliferation). As a approach to define the cell lifespan in MAIDS, we

In Vivo Immunology, Edited by E. Heinen *et al.*
Plenum Press, New York, 1994

studied the persistence after arrest of cell production by hydroxyurea (HU) adminsistration. HU eliminates cycling cells in a few hours, therefore cell depletion observed at later time points does not reflect direct cytotoxic effects of the drug but rather the lack of replenishment from the cycling pool eliminated earlier [4,5]. Our results show that the frequency of short-lived cells increases in the infected animals especially within B-cells and CD4[+] T-cells with a primed/memory phenotype.

MATERIALS AND METHODS

Mice , Cell Suspensions and Viral extract

Male C57Bl/Ka (H-2b) mice were bred in our facility. Mice were injected twice i.p. at the age of 4 and 5 weeks with 0.25 ml RadLV Duplan MuLV stock solution. Aged-matched control mice were injected twice with 0.25 ml saline. Extract was prepared from the lymph nodes of three mice injected two months previously with RadLV-Rs extract 64. RadLV-Rs extract 64 was kindly provided by E. Legrand (INSERM 117 Bordeaux, France) and was described previously[1]. The cell-free supernatant constituted the extract. The virus preparation contained 1.0×10^3 PFU of ecotropic virus /ml.

Antibodies and Flow cytometry

The mAb used were fluorescein isothiocyanate (FITC) conjugated anti-Thy-1.2 (30-H12), phycoerythrin (R-PE) labelled anti-CD4/L3T4 (GK1.5) (Becton Dickinson, Erembodegem, Belgium), biotinylated anti-mouse CD44 (IM7) and FITC-labelled anti-B220 (6B2). Streptavidin-PE (Dako) and streptavidin-Red[613] [®] (Gibco BRL) were used as a second step reagent to reveal biotinylated antibodies. Single cell suspensions were stained with optimal amounts of mAb on ice for 20 minutes in PBS with 2% BSA and 0.1% sodium azide. Cells were washed twice and counterstained with streptavidin-PE or streptavidin-Red[613]. After additional washes, cells were analysed on a FACStar Plus[®] (Becton Dickinson). Data were collected and processed using the LYSIS II software (Becton Dickinson).

Hydroxyurea treatment

HU (Sigma) was dissolved in phosphate-buffered saline (PBS) and administered i.p. at 1 mg/g body weight in two separate injections with a 7-h interval according to the protocol of Rocha *et al.* [4] Control animals received two i.p. injection of PBS with a 7-h interval. Mice were sacrificed at various times after HU administration. LN were dissected and weighted. Cell suspensions were prepared from the pooled LN from three mice in each group.

RESULTS

Major Cell Depletion is Observed in the LN of Infected Mice 24 h after HU Administration

HU administration had no early effects (1h after the second i.p. injection) on the total number of mononucleated cells in the lymph nodes of normal and infected mice. 24 hours after the second injection, no variation was visible in the LN from control mice, however a major cell depletion (around 50%) was observed in the LN of mice infected with RadLV-Rs (figure 1).

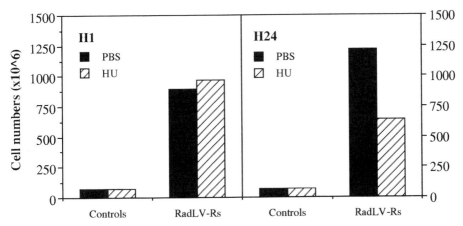

Figure 1. Effects of HU on LN cell numbers in MAIDS (Wk 7 postinfection).

Increased Susceptibility of CD4 T-cells with a Memory Phenotype to HU Treatment

Phenotypic analysis of T-cell subsets in HU-treated mice vs PBS-injected controls revealed the differential susceptibility of each subset to cell depletion. In non-infected mice, CD8[+] T-cells displayed a higher susceptibility than CD4[+] T-cells (figure 2). Infected mice (wk 7 postinfection) showed a higher depletion rate within both subsets, with slightly higher values for CD4[+] cells.

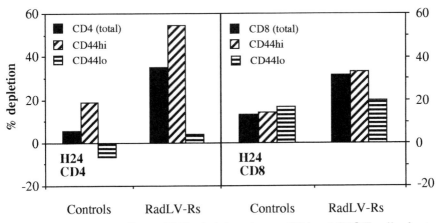

Figure 2. Differential effects of HU administration on CD4 and CD8 T-cell subsets.

Compared to non-infected mice, the increase of the frequency of short-lived cells was therefore more important for CD4+ cells (6-fold increase) than for CD8+ cells (2-fold increase). The depletion of CD4+ cells mostly reflected the loss of cells with a memory/primed CD44hi phenotype in non-infected as well as in RadLV-Rs infected mice. The sensibility of the naive CD44lo CD4 subset to HU administration was not influenced by RadLV-Rs infection whereas the depletion rate of CD4 cells with a memory phenotype was dramatically higher in the infected mice, reaching 58% (figure 2). RadLV-Rs infection was also associated with the appearance of an abnormal CD4+ subset lacking Thy-1 expression. Although the CD4+ Thy-1- subset showed a slightly higher depletion at 24 h, both subsets reached similar values 72 h after HU administration (not shown).

Increased Susceptibility of B-cells (especially B220lo) to HU Treatment

The frequency of short-lived cells was higher in B-cells than in T-cells for control as well as infected animals. As for T-cells, RadLV-Rs infection was associated with an important increase of the depletion rate of B-cells (4-fold increase) (figure 3).

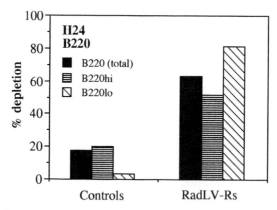

Figure 3. Effects of HU on B-cell numbers (Wk 7 postinfection).

An abnormal B-cell subset with a low membrane expression of B220 (B220lo) appeared in the LN of the infected mice. Interestingly, this subset showed an even higher sensibility to HU treatment with around 80% depletion at 24h (figure 3).

DISCUSSION

Infection of mice with the RadLV-Rs virus was associated with an increased frequency of short-lived lymphocytes in the LN. This increase was more important for CD4 cells with a memory phenotype and for B-cells. Some effects were also observed on CD8+ T-cells. It could be argued against such an interpretation that cell depletion induced by HU at 24h might still be due to direct killing of cycling cells rather than to secondary effects due to early depletion of the cycling pool. It would therefore be logical to observe higher depletion rates in RadLV-Rs infected animals where the proportion of proliferating cells is increased. Although some direct killing could participate in the depletion observed at 24h, we believe that this mechanism cannot explain the high depletion rates observed in the infected animals since (1) minor depletion (less than 15%) is observed at 1h after the second i.p. injection (i.e. 8 h after the first injection) and (2) the proportion of cycling CD4 cells in RadLV-Rs infected mice remains under 10% and cannot explain the high depletion rates observed in these animals. Furthermore, non specific toxic effects of the drug are also unlikely since some subsets (i.e. CD4$^+$ cells with a naive CD44^{lo} phenotype) are not influenced by HU treatment.

The increased frequency of short-lived CD4$^+$ T-cells in the LN of mice with MAIDS could explain why CD4$^+$ T-cells fail to proliferate in vitro. It remains to determine which mechanisms are responsible for this shorter lifespan. It is tempting to speculate that after transient proliferation in response to retrovirus-dependent activation signals, CD4$^+$ T-cells rapidly undergo programmed cell death *in vivo*, although we did not detect DNA hypoploidy in unstimulated cell suspensions from the LN of infected mice. The resistance of CD4$^+$ T-cells with a naive phenotype to HU treatment in the infected animals suggests that the major expansion of the CD4 memory pool in these animals results more from proliferation of CD44^{hi} cells than from phenotypic conversion from the naive pool.

The validity of MAIDS as a model for HIV infection has been questioned. The present data illustrate that despite the absence of CD4$^+$ T-cell lymphopaenia, CD4$^+$ T-cell lifespan is strikingly reduced in MAIDS. They advocate for further examination of the functional effects of retrovirus-related abnormal activation signals on the homeostasy of T-cell numbers in HIV infection.

ACKNOWLEDGEMENTS

MM is supported by a grant from the FNRS and Télévie. SC is supported by a grant from the IRSIA. This work is supported in part by the FRSM and the Centre Anticancéreux près l'Université de Liège. The authors wish to thank Gaby Zeimers and Elizabeth Franzen-Detrooz for expert technical assistance and Dr E. Legrand for having provided the virus.

REFERENCES

1. Mistry PB, Duplan JF. Propriétés biologiques d'un virus isolé d'une radioleucémie C57BL. *Bull Cancer* (Paris) 1973, 60:287-300.

2. Mosier DE, Yetter RA and Morse III HC. Retroviral induction of acute lymphoproliferative disease and profound immunosuppression in adult C57BL/6 mice. *J Exp Med* 1985, 161:766-784.

3. Aziz DC, Hanna Z, Jolicoeur P. Severe immunodeficiency disease induced by a defective murine leukaemia virus. *Nature* 1989, 338:505-508.

4. Rocha BB, Freitas AA, Coutinho AA. Population dynamics of T lymphocytes, renewal rate and expansion in the peripheral lymphoid organs. *J Immunol* 1983, 131:2158-2164.

5. Freitas AA, Rocha BB. Lymphocyte lifespans : homeostasis, selection and competition. *Immunol Today* 1993, 14:25-29.

ANALYSIS OF HIV INFECTIONS IN HUMAN MACROPHAGE-LIKE CELL LINES

Lea Brys[1], Ann Van Gyseghem[1], Steven Verhaegen[1], Erik Saman[2], and Patrick De Baetselier[1]

[1]Instituut voor Moleculaire Biologie
 Vrije Universiteit Brussel, Brussel
[2]Innogenetics, Gent

INTRODUCTION

The macrophage tropism of early HIV isolates[1] suggests that monocyte-derived cells may be a more general target for various HIV quasi-species. The question is thus raised whether cells of the mononuclear phagocyte lineage may be the first cells in the body to be infected with HIV. At least three forms of HIV replication have been documented to occur in monocytes[2] : (i) latent infections with viral DNA but no viral RNA, (ii) low permissive infections with numerous virions accumulated within intracellular vacuoles and (iii) highly replicative infections resulting in cytopathicity and formation of multinucleated giant cells. Both latently infected macrophages and low level infected macrophages may constitute a large intracellular reservoir for HIV in the body. In fact, according to a recent study[3] extraordinary large numbers of latently infected CD4[+] lymphocytes and macrophages can be detected throughout the lymphatic system from early to late stages of infection.

The predominant mechanism of virus entry for infection of macrophages is CD4-dependent. This does not preclude other CD4-independant routes of infection. Indeed, HIV may enter macrophages through phagocytosis, FcR- and C3R-mediated endocytosis or interaction with mannose-specific receptors. Interestingly, HIV isolates that do not replicate in monocytes (i.e. T-cell-tropic HIV) will infect these cells after treatment with enhancing anti-HIV antibodies and such antibody-mediated enhancement is not inhibited by anti-CD4[4]. Hence, formation of immune complexes (virus plus immunoglobulin and/or complement) can contribute not only to the attachment of HIV to follicular dendritic cells but also to sequestration of HIV in monocytes/macrophages. This may result in a state of clinical latency during which HIV accumulates in the lymphoid organs (trapped on FDC's and sequestered in macrophages) without signs of viral burden and viral replication in the peripheral blood[3,5]. The capacity of the macrophage to function as a persistent reservoir for HIV may assign a cardinal role to this cell type in the pathogenesis of HIV disease. In this report we will provide evidence that the level of CD4 determines the level of HIV

In Vivo Immunology, Edited by E. Heinen *et al.*
Plenum Press, New York, 1994

replication in macrophage-like cell lines and that established low replicative infections represent a reservoir for continuous release of infectious viruses.

RESULTS

Infection of human macrophage cell lines (i.e. THP1 and U937) with the HTLV IIIB strain of HIV-1 results in productively infected cells. Virus production does not lead to cytopathic effects and consequently permanent HTLV IIIB producing cell lines can be easely obtained. Hereby it is worthwhile to mention that a marked cytopathic effect and cell death is only observed when these cell lines are contamined with mycoplasma.

Both U937 and THP-1 express the CD4 molecule and viral entry in these cell lines might occur via this primary receptor for HIV. In order to analyse the possible contribution of CD4 to the productive infection of HTLV IIIB in the U937 and THP-1 cell lines, attempts were made to generate CD4⁻ cell mutants. To this end, U937 and THP-1 were treated with the mutagen ethyl-methyl sulfonate and subsequently selected for the absence of CD4 via panning on anti-CD4 coated petri dishes. The negatively selected populations were cloned and different clones were analysed for the expression of CD4 and their susceptibility to productive infections with HTLV IIIB.

CD4 expression in the different clones was evaluated by membrane immunofluorescence and Northern-blotting analysis. The results compiled in Table 1 demonstrate that certain mutant cell lines score completely negative for the membrane expression of CD4 while other clones manifest a reduced yet significant expression of CD4 (i.e. U-16, THP-30; Table 1). The lack of CD4, as detected by immunofluorescent staining was confirmed by Northern blotting analysis which revealed a complete absence of mRNA species for CD4 (data not shown).

Table 1. Membrane CD4 expression on CD4⁻ selected U937 and THP-1 variants.

Cell line (origin)[1]		Membrane fluorescence[2]		
		CD4 (MT 310)	CD4 (LEU3)	CD4 (OKT4A)
Parental:	U-937	+	+	+
CD4⁻ selected :	U-13	-	-	-
	U-14	-	-	-
	U-15	-	-	-
	U-16	±	±	±
Parental :	THP-1	+	+	+
CD4⁻ selected :	THP-29	-	-	-
	THP-30	±	±	±
	THP-36	-	-	-
	THP-38	-	-	-

[1] CD4⁻ selected : cloned cell lines obtained from the parental U-937 and THP-1 following mutagenization with EMS and negative selection for CD4 epxression.

[2] Score for CD4 membrane fluorescence : + from 80 to 100% positive cells, ± from 10 to 30% positive cells, -no fluorescent cells (% fluorescent cells scored on a FACstar⁺). MT310, LEU3 and OKT4A are different anti-CD4 monoclonal antibodies.

The different clones were infected with HTLV IIIB and virus production was followed via an antigen capture test. The results (Fig. 1) demonstrate a lack of production of viral components by the cell lines that were completely negative for the membrane expression of CD4 (Table 1). Mutant cell lines with a reduced expression of CD4 were productively infected, yet virus production was significantly delayed as compared to the parental cell lines (Fig. 1). Collectively these results indicate that CD4 serves as the receptor for viral entry into these macrophage-like cell lines.

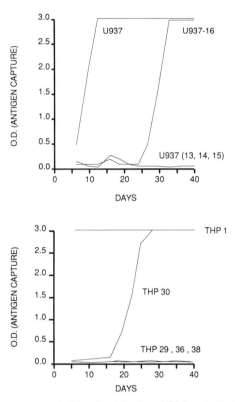

Figure 1. Detection of viral components following infection of CD4$^-$ mutant cell lines with HTLV IIIB.

The absence of productive HIV infection in the CD4$^-$ mutant cell lines does not exclude the possibility that these cells are latently infected. To test this possibility CD4$^-$ cell lines were selected for additional infection experiments and presence of viral components was assessed by following means : (i) direct detection of viral antigens in the culture supernates via an antigen capture ELISA, (ii) indirect detection of viral antigens in the supernates of co-cultures with a CD4$^+$ T cell line (MT4), (iii) PCR with combined LTR, GAG and POL primers, (iv) membrane expression of P24 antigens by immunofluorescent staining, (v) reverse transcriptase (RT) activity. The results, compiled in Table 2, compare the pattern of virus production in the parental THP-1 cell line and the thereof derived CD4$^-$ mutant cell line THP-36.

According to these results the THP-36 cell line is productively infectable with HTLV IIIB since presence of infectious viral particles can be evidenced upon coculture with the CD4$^+$ acceptor cell line MT4. Yet this represents an extremely low amount of virus that is not detectable with other detection systems till day 40 post infection. However, virus production increases with time and becomes detectable at day 60-70 post-infection by direct antigen capture and PCR. Still, at this time point we were unable to detect membrane-associated P24 antigens and reverse transcriptase activity remained very low (3% of the activity measured in the parental cell line). Similar results were obtained with other CD4⁻ mutant cell lines indicating that these cell lines can be infected in a CD4-independent fashion.

To exclude completely the involvement of CD4 in the HIV-1 infection of these mutant cell lines infections were performed in the presence of anti-CD4 antibodies. Suprisingly, pretreatment of the CD4⁻ mutant cell lines with anti-CD4 antibodies abolished completely the productive HTLV IIIB infection in these cell lines (examplified for the THP-36 cell line, Table 2). Hence, despite non-detectable levels of CD4 expression (Table 1) in the mutant cell lines, CD4 appears to be implicated in the productive infection with HTLV III B. These results suggest that the putative CD4⁻ mutant cell lines harbour enough CD4 molecules to sustain a low yet detectable productive HIV-1 infection. Therefore the possible presence of minor amounts of CD4 mRNA species was evaluated by a coupled reverse transcriptase/PCR. These experiments revealed indeed that the putative CD4⁻ mutant cell lines contain extremely low yet detectable levels of CD4 mRNA molecules (data not shown).

Table 2. Detection of viral components in HTLV IIIB infected $CD4^+$ and $CD4^-$ macrophage cell lines.

Cell line[1]	Detection[2] system	Presence of viral components (days after infection)						
		10	20	30	40	50	60	70
THP-1	Ag capture (direct)	+++	+++	+++	+++	+++	+++	+++
	Ag capture (coculture)	+++	+++	+++	+++	+++	+++	+++
	PCR	+++	+++	+++	+++	+++	+++	+++
	P24/IFA	+++	+++	+++	+++	+++	+++	+++
	RT	+++	+++	+++	+++	+++	+++	+++
THP-36	Ag capture (direct)	-	-	-	±	+	++	+++
	Ag capture (coculture)	+++	+++	+++	+++	+++	+++	+++
	PCR	-	-	-	-	-	+	+++
	P24/IFA	-	-	-	-	-	-	-
	RT	-	-	-	-	-	-	-
THP-36	Ag capture (direct)	-	-	-	-	-	-	-
(anti-CD4)	Ag capture (coculture)	+++	+++	+++	+++	-	-	-
	PCR	-	-	-	-	-	-	-
	P24/IFA	-	-	-	-	-	-	-
	RT	-	-	-	-	-	-	-

[1] THP-1 ($CD4^+$) and THP-36 ($CD4^-$) were infected with 510^2 TCD50 HTLV IIIB.
In one experiment the THP-36 cell line was pretreated with anti-CD4.

[2] Ag capture (direct) = detection of viral antigens in culture supernates by the Innotest HIV antigen capture assay. Ag capture (coculture) = detection of viral antigens in supernates of co-cultures with $CD4^+$ indicator cells by the Innotest HIV antigen capture assay. PCR = polymerase chain amplification with LTR, GAG and ENV primers. IFA = immunofluorescence assay for P24 antigens. RT = reverse transcriptase.

DISCUSSION

The herein desribed results demonstrate that the level of CD4, expressed on macrophage-like cell lines, determines the form of HIV replication : (i) high levels of CD4 lead to highly replicative infections, (ii) reduced levels of CD4 (70 to 90% reduction) result in a delayed but still high replicative infection and (iii) virtual absence of CD4 leads to low permissive infections. Though our research strategy aimed at demonstrating CD4-independant ways of HIV infection in macrophage-like cell lines, we could not substantiate unequivocally the existance of CD4-independant mechanisms of HIV entry. Indeed, despite undetectable levels of CD4 expression, the CD4 molecule was found to be implicated in the low permissive infection of the putative CD4$^-$ macrophage-like cell lines by HTLV IIIB and furthermore PCR corroborated the presence of intracellular CD4 message. Yet it should be hereby emphasized that 70 PCR cycles were required to detect CD4 mRNA species indicating an extremely low level of such molecules that could be attributed to transcriptional leakage. This observation may be important in view of different reports, claiming the productive infection of phenotypically and/or genotypically CD4$^-$ human cell lines (i.e. glial cells, colorectal cells, fibroblastoid cells a.o.), via alternative pathways for viral entry. The low permissive infection observed with the mutant cell lines may reflect the pattern of HIV replication in monocytes/macrophages in vivo[2]. In fact, in the early stage of infection progeny virion production was only detectable via coculture with CD4$^+$ T cell lines. After 40 days low permissive infection became replicative yet even at this stage the level of progeny virion production was extremely low as compared to the infected parental cell lines. Hence, the infected mutant cell lines represent a reservoir for low levels of continued infection and a similar situation might occur during HIV infections in vivo.

ACKNOWLEDGEMENTS

This work was supported by the N.F.W.O. project n° 3.3032.91.

REFERENCES

1. S. Schwartz, B.K. Kelber, E.V. Fenyö, and G.N. Pavlakis, Rapidly and slowly replicating human immunodeficiency virus type 1 isolates can be distinguised according to target-cell tropism in T-cell and monocyte cell lines, *Proc. Natl. Acad. Sci.*, 86:7200 (1989).

2. H.E. Gendelman, J.M. Orenstein, L.M. Baca, B. Weiser, H. Burger, D.C. Kalter, and M.S. Meltzer, The macrophage in the persistence and pathogenesis of HIV infections, *AIDS*, 3:475 (1989).

3. J. Embretson, M. Zupancic, J.L. Ribas, A. Burke, P. Racz, K. Tenner-Racz, and A.T. Haase, Massive covert infection of helper T lymphocytes and macrophages by HIV during the incubation period of AIDS, *Nature*, 362:359 (1993).

4. J. Homsy, M. Meyer, M.Tateno, S. Clarkson, and J.A. Levy, The Fc and not CD4 receptor mediates antibody enhancement of HIV infection in human cells, *Science*, 244:1357 (1989).

5. G. Pantaleo, C. Graziosi, J.F. Demarest, L. Butini, M. Montroni, C.H. Fox, J.M. Orenstein, D.P. Kotler, and A.S. Fauci, HIV infection is active and progressive in lymphoid tissue during the clinically latent stage of disease, *Nature*, 362:355 (1993).

THE PIVOTAL ROLE OF THE IMMUNOGLOBULIN RECEPTOR OF TUMOR CELLS FROM B
CELL LYMPHOMAS OF MUCOSA ASSOCIATED LYMPHOID TISSUE (MALT)

Axel Greiner, Alexander Marx, Bernd Schmaußer and
Hans Konrad Müller-Hermelink

Pathologisches Institut der Universität Würzburg
Josef-Schneider-Straße 2
97080 Würzburg
Deutschland

Introduction

B-cell lymphomas of mucosa-associated lymphoid tissue (MALT) occur commonly in sites that are normally devoid of lymphoid tissue (Isaacson,
1987). The low grade MALT-type lymphomas do not share the cytogenetic
alterations that characterize comparable low grade nodal lymphomas and
tend to remain localized (Isaacson, 1992). It has been postulated that
the acquired lymphoid tissue accumulates in response to infection with
Helicobacter pylori (H.p.)(Wotherspoon, 1991). This led to the hypothesis that the lymphomatous gastric lesion may progress into malignancy
and that specific antigen- Ig-receptor-interaction may affect the
pathogenesis of the tumor (Hussell, 1993 a). Therefore, the tumor
immunoglobulins harbour important clues for the possible role in B cell
proliferation and the nature of the preceding immune response.

Materials and Methods

MALT-type lymphoma immunoglobulins were produced by fusing lymphoma
cells with the heteromyeloma HAB-1 or NS0. HumAb were selected by
corresponding to the lymphoma immunoglobulin with respect to the isotype, the reacting pattern and the isoelectric point in isoelectric
focussing (IEF) tests. Tissue samples were collected from the frozen-
tissue bank of the Institute of Pathology of the University of Würzburg,
bacterial lysates obtained from the Department of Microbiology. Monoclo-

In Vivo Immunology, Edited by E. Heinen *et al.*
Plenum Press, New York, 1994

nal anti-idiotypic antibodies were selected by exhibiting specificity in immunohistochemistry, Western blot and competetive ELISA for the tumor immunoglobulin and not for controls. Proliferation was measured as the 24h ^{3}H-thymidin uptake by purified B-cells from lymphoma and buffy-coat after stimulation for 72h.

Results

1) Specificity of the lymphoma immunoglobulins

No reactivity was found with Helicobacter pylori (data not shown). In contrast there was a specificity for different normal tissue components (Tab. 1). Some of the idotypes of different MALT-type lymphomas exhibited comparable patterns.

Tab. 1 Specificity of MALT-type lymphoma

1	IgM/κ	ANA, vascular tissue
2	IgM/κ	—
3	IgM/κ	ANA, neuronal tissue, connective tissue, striate muscle, vascular tissue, glandular tissue
4	IgM	—
5	IgM/κ	connective tissue, vascular tissue
6	IgM/λ	ANA, striate muscle, vascular tissue
7	IgG/κ	—
8	IgM/λ	—
9	IgM/κ	—
10	IgA/λ	neuronal tissue, ANA, striate muscle, IgA, IgM
11	IgM/λ	glandular tissue, vascular tissue

2) MALT- lymphoma idiotype occured in Gastritis

Immunoperoxidase staining demonstrated a strong reactivity of α-Id 27/165 only with the tumor (Fig.1) but not with normal nodal lymphoid tissue at identical antibody concentrations. The α-Id did not crossreact with 20 other MALT-type lymphomas nor with 26 nodal lymphomas or tissue samples from normal and non-H.p. associated chronic inflamed gastric antral and corpus mucosa. In 19 out of 20 tissue samples from patients with H.p.-associated chronic gastritis there was a strong binding of the anti-Id 27/165 to polyclonal B lymphocytes and plasma cells of the gastric mucosa (Fig. 2; Tab.2).

Tab.2 Immunoreactivity of anti-Id 27/165

Tissue	n	positive n	Immunoreactivity
Gastritis with H.p.	20	19	+++ <> -
Gastritis without H.p.	14	1	+/- <> -
Normal gastric mucosa	11	0	- <> -
Normal lymph node	5	0	- <> -
MALT-type lymphoma	20	0	- <> -
Nodal lymphoma	26	0	- <> -

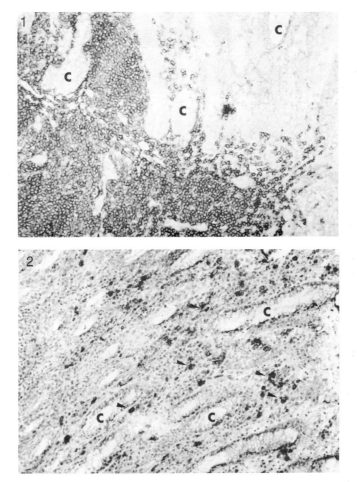

Fig.1 Staining with anti-Id 27/165 of tumor tissue (cryostat section, X 100) (c=crypt).
Fig.2 Staining of lymphocytes (arrow) with αId of chronic inflamed gastric mucosa associated with H.p. (cryostat section, X 100)(c=crypt).

3) 27/165 anti-idiotypic antibody has growth effect

A specific growth promotion effect on the lymphoma cells with the anti-idiotype antibody in combination with SAC was noted in comparison to the control. The effect was more pronounced than the effect with cytokine or mitogen stimulation alone (Fig. 3).

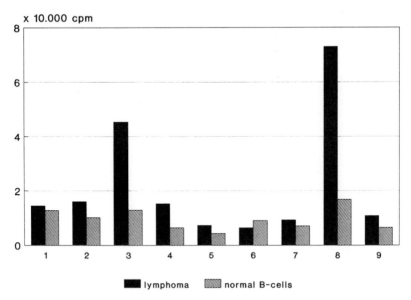

proliferation assay

Fig. 3 1= culture medium; 2= 1+PHA; 3= 1+SAC; 4= 1+EBV; 5= 1+Ionomycin 6= 1+100 IE IL-2; 7= 1+ 100 IE IL-6; 8= 3+ anti-Id; 9= 7+ anti-Id. 1μCi ^{3}H-Thymidin/well; data measured in triplets.

Discussion

The present investigation defining the target of lymphoma immunoglobulin specificity suggests an autoimmune rather than an anti-bacterial immune reactivity.

However, H.p. gastritis maintaining the proliferation of the lymphoma cells may be an event preceding the development of at least some low grade MALT-type lymphomas with autoantibody immunoreactivity (Greiner, submitted). This suggest a major role for antigen-driven lymphomagenesis in the process of monoclonal expansion as demontrated for follicular lymphoma recently (Zelenetz, 1992).

As shown in recent studies (Müller-Hermelink, 1992; Hussell, 1993 b) cross-linking of tumor-Ig using anti-idiotypic antibodies, mimick binding of antigen by the tumor cells, is likely to affect the progression of low grade MALT-type lymphomas. This is in contrast to other studies, which showed inhibition of proliferation using anti-idiotypic antibodies in different histiogenetic lymphomas like chronic lymphocytic leukaemia (CLL) or follicular lymphoma (Lowder, 1987; vanEndert, 1992). Induction of the proliferation response in low grade MALT-type lymphoma after cross-linking was induced by additional stimulation with a mitogen may indicate a dependency on additional signals. However, it is possible that the lymphoma cells are selected by binding to antigen presented on follicular dendritic cells or infiltrating T cells. Finally, this "activated" state could create prospicious conditions for further mutations and chromosomal translocations that may contribute to the progression into a high grade lymphoma.

Acknowledgments

The authors would like to thank M.Reichert and E.Schmitt for expert technical assistance. This work was supported by the "Deutsche Forschungsgemeinschaft" DFG Mu 579/3-1.

References

Greiner A, Marx A, Heesemann J, Leebmann J, Schmaußer B and Müller-Hermelink HK, Idiotype identity in a MALT-type lymphoma and B cells in Helicobacter pylori associated chronic gastritis, (submitted) (1993)

Hussell T, Isaacson PG, Crabtree JE, Dogan A, Spencer J, Immunoglobulin specificity of low grade B cell lymphoma of mucosa-associated tissue (MALT) type, Am J Path 142, 285-292 (1993 a)

Hussell T, Isaacson PG, Spencer J, Proliferation and differentation of tumor cells from B-cell lymphoma of Mucosa-associated lymphoid tissue in vitro, J Path 169, 221-227 (1993 b)

Isaacson PG, Spencer J, Malignant lymphoma of mucosa-associated lymphoid tissue, Histopathology 11, 445-462 (1987)

Isaacson PG, Extranodal lymphomas: the MALT concept, Verh Dtsch Ges Path 76, 14-23 (1992)

Lowder JN, Meeker TC, Campbell M, Garcia CF, Gralow J, Miller RA, Warnke R, Levy R, Studies on B lymphoid tumors treated with monoclonal anti-idiotype antibodies, Blood 69, 199-210 (1987)

Müller-Hermelink HK, Greiner A, Autoimmune diseases and malignant lymphoma, Verh Dtsch Ges Path 76, 96-109 (1992)

van Endert PM, Heilig B, Hämmerling GJ, Moldenhauer G, Monoclonal antibodies to idiotype inhibit in vitro growth of human B-cell lymphomas, Blood 79, 129-137 (1992)

Wotherspoon AC, Ortiz-Hidalgo C, Falzon M, Isaacson PG, Helicobacter pylori-associated gastritis and primary B cell gastric lymphoma, Lancet 338, 1175-1176 (1991)

Zelenetz AD, Chen TT, Levy R, Clonal Expansion in Follicular lymphoma occurs subsequent to antigenic selection, J Exp Med 176, 1137-1148 (1992)

TNF-α IS INVOLVED IN THE MECHANISM OF MURINE THYMIC LYMPHOMA PREVENTION BY BONE MARROW GRAFTING

Chantal Humblet, Johanne Deman, Anne-Michel Rongy, Roland Greimers, Jacques Boniver, Marie Paule Defresne

University of Liège
Department of Pathology,
CHU B35, B-4000 Liège, Belgium

INTRODUCTION

In C57 BL/Ka mice, whole body fractionated irradiation (4x1.75Gy at weekly intervals) induces thymic lymphomas in more than 90% of the animals after a latency period of 6-12 months (Kaplan 1967). During this latency period, potential neoplastic cells (or preleukemic cells (PLC)) are detected in the thymus: these cells require the thymic microenvironment for progression to lymphoma (Boniver et al.1981 ; Haran-Ghera 1978). Simultaneously to their appearance, several components of thymic lymphopoiesis are altered: the prothymocyte activity is drastically reduced in the bone marrow (Boniver et al.1981 ; Van Bekkum et al.1984); in the thymus, thymocyte subpopulations are modified (Rongy et al. 1990) and some properties of the thymic epithelium are altered (Defresne et al. 1986).

Interestingly, lymphoma development can be inhibited if a bone marrow graft is given early after the split dose irradiation (Kaplan et al.1953). This treatment does not inhibit the emergence of preleukemic cells nor the alterations of the thymic lymphopoiesis (Defresne et al. 1986). However, one to two months after the treatment, preleukemic cells disappear, the thymic microenvironment and T-cell subpopulations are restored (Defresne et al.1986 ; Rongy et al.1990 ; Sprecher et al.1989).

This marrow mediated thymic reconstitution might lead to the recovery of intrathymic paracrine secretion which would eliminate preleukemic cells directly or indirectly. Tumor necrosis factor alpha (TNF-α) is a good candidate for such effects. Indeed, it has been shown that some subsets of thymic cells can produce TNF-α (Deman et al.1992) which has some effects on thymic epithelial cells (Defresne et al.1990) and which is cytotoxic for neoplastic cells (Ruddle 1987 ; Beutler and Cerami 1987).

The present paper reports some selected data which indicate that exogenous TNF-α injected into irradiated mice mimick the effects of the bone marrow graft.

MATERIALS AND METHODS

Animals: C57BL/Ka mice originating from Stanford University (Stanford CA) were raised in our animal colony.

Irradiation: Five to six-week old mice were whole body irradiated with 4 doses of 1.75Gy applied at weekly intervals.

In Vivo Immunology, Edited by E. Heinen *et al.*
Plenum Press, New York, 1994

TNF-α treatment: Murine r-TNF-α (1,2 10^7 U/mg), produced by Genentech and kindly provided by Boehringer Ingelheim International was diluted in RPMI 1640 supplemented with 10% fetal calf serum. 200μl aliquots containing 2.5×10^4 U TNF-α were injected I.P. on day 1 after the last 1.75Gy irradiation. Three injections per week during 6 weeks were performed.

Detection of preleukemic cells: The preleukemic cells are detected by an in vivo assay described previously by Goffinet et al.(1983).

Analysis of thymocyte subpopulations: immunofluorescence staining was previously described by Rongy et al.(1990).

Thymic nurse cells Isolation: TNC were isolated by a slight modification (Houben-Defresne et al.1982) of the method originally described by Wekerle and Ketelsen (1980).

RESULTS

As shown in the table 1 and as previously published (Defresne et al.1986), a normal bone marrow graft inhibit the thymic lymphomas development in irradiated C57BL/Ka mice.

Treatment of irradiated mice with mu-TNF-α caused also a significant reduction in the incidence of lymphomas: the median incidence was 13% after injections of this cytokine whereas 90% of non treated animals develop tumors.

This inhibition of lymphoma development is related to the disappearance of preleukemic cells from the thymus. Whereas PLC were present in all the thymuses tested one month after the leukemogenic irradiation (data not shown), they disappeared thereafter from the majority of TNF-α injected mice: indeed, on day 60 after the irradiation, 100% of the thymuses of irradiated mice contained preleukemic cells whereas only 25% of the thymuses of TNF-α treated animals contained preleukemic cells (table 1).

Table 1. Effect of TNF-α treatment on the incidence of lymphomas and on the presence of preleukemic cells in mice which received a leukemogenic irradiation.

Mouse treatment		Incidence of lymphomas [1]	Proportion of irradiated thymuses containing preleukemic cells
4x1.75 Gy	Further treatment		
-	-	0%	0%
+	-	90%	100%
+	graft	5%	0%
+	muTNF-α	12%	25%

[1]:The presence of preleukemic cells was tested by an in vivo transplantation assay 60 days after the irradiation.

Simultaneously, thymocyte differentiation was restored. As previously described (Rongy et al.1990), there was a drastic decrease in CD4+CD8+ thymocytes and an increase in CD4-CD8- thymocytes in the irradiated mice. Treatment of these animals with rMuTNF-α did not prevent these alterations (data not shown), however they were reversible in the majority of the animals (Table 2).

The thymic nurse cells, which are elements of the thymic microenvironment involved in thymocyte differentiation, disappeared from the thymuses of irradiated mice, their number was completely restore by a bone marrow graft (Defresne and al.1986 ; table 2)

In mice which were injected with TNF-α, the number of TNCs increased to reach values intermediary between those seen in normal and in irradiated mice (table2).

Table 2. Effects of TNF-α treatment on thymocyte subpopulations and on thymic nurse cells in mice which received a leukemogenic irradiation.

Mouse treatment		Thymocyte differentiation [1]				number[1] of thymic nurse cells/thymus
4x1.75Gy	Further treatment	CD4- CD8-	CD4+ CD8+	CD4+ CD8-	CD4- CD8+	
-	-	3.1%	83%	8.9%	5%	17000
+	-	14.5%	46%	28.8%	10.7%	3000
+	BM graft	4.5%	84%	8.5%	3%	19000
+	muTNF-α	3.2%	82%	9.1%	5.7%	9000

([1]): thymocyte subpopulation and thymic nurse cells were analysed at day 60 after the irradiation.

DISCUSSION

We report here that repeated injections of rMuTNF-α prevent the development of thymic lymphomas in C57BL/Ka after a leukemogenic split dose irradiation. This effect is comparable with that obtained with a bone marrow graft.

Indeed, administration of rMuTNF-α induces the disapperance of preleukemic cells, restores thymocyte subpopulations and the thymic epithelium.

The observations on TNF-α inoculated mice raise many questions:
- what are the mechanisms leading to the partial restoration of thymic nurse cells and thymocyte differentiation?
- what are the mechanisms leading to the disappearance of preleukemic cells?
- does the bone marrow graft induce an intrathymic TNF-α production?

Concerning thymocyte differentiation, it has previously been show that TNF-α enhances the effects of other cytokines on the proliferation of thymocytes (Suda et al.1990); however to our knowledge, there is no evidence that it can directly induce phenotypic maturation of thymocytes. Another explanation would be that TNF-α restores the precursors compartment in the bone marrow: futher investigations are needed to test this hypothesis.

The increase in the number of the TNCs might be due either to thymocyte restoration, since TNC result from interactions between epithelial cells and immature thymocytes (Defresne et al.1986) or to a direct effect of TNF-α on the epithelial cells since TNF-α enhances in vitro the interactions between thymocyte precursors and thymic nurse cells derived epithelial cells (Defresne et al. 1990).

The mechanisms by which TNF-α induces the disappearance of PLC are still a matter of debate. As for the bone marrow graft, one can suggest that the restoration of thymic lymphopoiesis creates an environment incompatible with the progression of preneoplastic cells towards lymphoma growth. Alternatively, it could be suggested that TNF-α exerts a direct cytotoxic effect on PLC.

The last question is to know wether the bone marrow grafted cells induce an intrathymic TNF-α production. Preliminary results have shown that injections of rabbit anti-TNF-α antibodies into irradiated-marrow-grafted animals increase the incidence of lymphomas up to 40%. Moreover, it appeared that the number of cells containing TNF-α transcripts increases in the thymus of irradiated mice after a bone marrow graft. Thus, it seems that the effects of bone marrow graft are mediated by TNF-α.

TNF-α is probably not the only cytokine responsible for the inhibition of lymphoma development. Bone marrow graft probably restores intrathymically a cytokine cascade necessary for a normal T cell differentiation. Radiation induced lymphomas can also be prevented by IFN-γ (Boniver et al.1990) whereas administration of IL-4, a cytokine inhibiting the effects of IFN-γ upon thymocytes differentiation (Hodgkin et al.1990) abrogate the prophylactic effects of IFN-γ (C.Humblet et J.Plum in preparation).

Acknowledgments

This work was supported in part by the Fund for Medical Scientific Research (Belgium),Télévie, the Bekales Foundation, the Centre Anticancéreux près l'Université de Liège, the Research Fund of the Faculty of Médecine of Liège and Boehringer Ingelheim International.

REFERENCES

Beutler,B. and Cerami,A., 1987, Cachectin: more than a tumor necrosis factor.N.Engl.J.Med.316:379

Boniver,J.,Declève,A.,Lieberman,M.,Honsik,C.,Travis,M., and Kaplan,H.S., 1981,Marrow thymus interaction during radiation leukemogenesis in C57 BL/Ka mice. Cancer Res.41:390

Boniver,J.,Humblet,C. and Defresne,M.P., 1989, Tumor necrosis factor and interferon γ inhibit the development of radiation-induced thymic lymphomas in C57 BL/Ka mice.Leukemia 3:611

Defresne,M.P.,Greimers,R.,Lenaerts,P. and Boniver,J., 1986,Effects of bone marrow grafting on preleukemic cells and thymic nurse cells in C57 BL/Ka mice after a leukemogenic split dose irradiation.J.N.C.I.77:1079

Defresne,M.P.,Humblet,C.,Rongy,A.M.,Greimers,R. and Boniver,J., 1990, Effect of interferon γ and tumor necrosis factor-alpha on lymphoepithelial interactions within thymic nurse cells.Eur.J.Immunol.20:429

Deman,J.,Martin,M.T.,Humblet,C.,Delvenne,P.,Boniver,J. and Defresne,M.P, 1992, Analysis by in situ hybridization of cells expressing mRNA for TNFa in the developing thymus of mice.Developmental Immunology 2:103

Goffinet,G.,Defresne,M.P. and Boniver.J., 1983, Correlation of alkaline phosphatase activity to normal T cell differentiation and to radiation leukemia virus-induced preleukemic cells in the C57 BL mouse thymus.Cancer.Res.43:5416

Haran-Ghera,N., 1978,.Dependent and autonomous phases during leukemogenesis.Leukemia.2:11

Hodgkin, P.D., Cupp, J., Zlotnik, A., Howard,M., 1990, "IL-2, IL-6 and IFNγ have distinct effects on the IL-4 plus PMA-induced proliferation of thymocyte subpopulations", Cell Immunology. 126:57

Houben-Defresne,M.P.,Varlet,A.,Goffinet,G. and Boniver,J., 1982, Thymic nurse cells are the first site of virus replication after inoculation of the radiation leukemia virus. Leuk.Res.6:231

Kaplan,H.S., 1967,On the natural history of the murine leukemias.Cancer Res.27:1325.

Kaplan,H.S.,Brown,J. and Paull,J., 1953, Influence of bone marrow injection on involution and neoplasia of mouse thymus after systemic irradiation. J.N.C.I.14:303

Rongy,A.M.,Humblet,C.,Lelievre,P.,Greimers,R. and Boniver,J., 1990, Abnormal thymocyte subpopulations in split dose irradiated C57 BL/Ka mice before the onset of lymphomas. Effects of bone marrow grafting.Thymus.16:7

Ruddle,N.H., 1987,.Tumor necrosis factor and related cytokins.Immunol.Today.8:129

Sprecher,E.,Giloh,H.,Rahamin,E.,Yefenof,E. and Becker,Y., 1989,.Cytofluorometric analysis of thymic interdigitating cells from C57 BL/6 mice prior to and after leukemogenic x-irradiation. Leuk.Res.13:799

Suda, T., Murray, R., Fisher, M., Yokota, T., Zlotnik, A., 1990, TNFα and P40 induce day 15 murine fetal thymocyte proliferation in combination with IL-2, J. Immunol. 144:1783.

Suda, T., Murray, R., Guidos, C., Zlotnik, A., 1990, Growth-promoting activity of IL-1α, IL-6 and TNFα in combination with IL-2, IL-4 or IL-7 on murine thymocytes, J. Immunol. 144:3039.

Van Bekkum,D.W.,Boersma,W.J.A.,Eliason,J.F. and Knaan,S., 1984,.The role of prothymocytes in radiation-induced leukemogenesis in C57BL/Rij mice.Leuk.Res.8:461

Wekerle,H. and Ketelsen,U.P., 1980, Thymic nurse cells. Ia-bearing epithelium involved in T-lymphocyte differentiation?Nature.283:402

GERMINAL CENTRES

ANALYSIS OF GERMINAL CENTRES IN THE IMMUNE RESPONSE TO OXAZOLONE

Mike Ziegner and Claudia Berek

Deutsches RheumaForschungszentrum
Forschungslaboratorium Haus 10
13353 Berlin
Germany

INTRODUCTION

In a primary T-cell dependent immune response B-cell proliferation is observed in two areas of the spleen. In the first days after immunisation expansion of B-cell clones can be observed in the periarteriolar lymphocyte sheath. Here the development of plasma cells seems to take place. Then, around day 3 to day 4, antigen activated B-cells start to proliferate in the primary follicles. This leads to the formation of the germinal centre within which memory cells develop. The analysis of germinal centre B-cells at different timepoints after immunisation has shown that between days 10 and 14 somatic mutations rapidly accumulate in the variable regions of the antibody molecules (Berek et al., 1991). There is intraclonal diversification of the B-cell repertoire in the geminal centres (Jacob et al., 1991). We have now isolated DNA from single germinal centres of mice immunised with the hapten 2-phenyl-oxazolone (phOx). The data demonstrate that the affinity maturation of the primary immune response takes place in the germinal centres.

METHODS

BALB/c mice were immunized intraperitoneally with the antigen phOx coupled to chicken serum albumin. Two weeks later mice were killed and their spleens snap frozen. 50 μm histological sections were then prepared. In order to identify germinal centres tissue sections were stained with Peanut agglutinin-Biotin/Extravidin-Alkaline Phosphatase. Single germinal centres were isolated by hand using an inverted microscope. DNA was prepared and the VκOx1/Jκ5 rearrangements, characteristic for the immune response to phOx, amplified either by a one step or by nested PCR, cloned into M13 and sequenced.

RESULTS

Development of germinal centres 14 days after immunisation

The distribution of germinal centres over 12 tisssue sections (316 -327) is shown in Table 1. Altogether 18 different germinal centres (A to R) could be identified in a splenic fragment of 600 μm thickness. The relative size of each germinal centre in the whole fragment is indicated (Σ). Thus, in an animal immunised with phOx at day 14 about 4,5% of the splenic tissue is occupied by germinal centres. The area germinal centres cover in individual sections varies considerably. Furthermore, there are small germinal centres (B, D, E or J) which are seen only in a single section, whereas other ones (F, L, M and N) stretch over many 50μm sections. Germinal centre L may have developed from two independent follicles which merged in section 324.

Table 1. Distribution of germinal centres over a 600 μm splenic fragment

germinal centre	Σ	316	317	318	319	320	321	322	323	324	325	326	327
A	4,28	2,06	2,22										
B	0,31	0,31											
C	1,74	1,06	0,68										
D	1,06	1,06											
E	0,97	0,97											
F	4,21			1,04	1,26	0,77	0,73	0,40					
G	1,46				0,46	0,60	0,40						
H	2,30					0,90	0,78	0,62					
I	4,92					1,23	1,42	1,10	1,17				
J	0,77						0,77						
K	1,35						0,50	0,85					
L	8,85						0,51	0,86	1,51	1,41	0,80	1,69	2,07
M	3,53								0,62	1,07	0,98	0,42	0,46
N	8,19								0,43	1,98	2,92	2,20	0,66
O	1,17									0,85	0,32		
P	4,25										1,18	1,57	1,51
Q	3,64										0,51	1,50	1,62
R	2,27										0,76	0,83	0,68

Germinal centre area in relation to the total section size is indicated (values given in %)
VκOx1 positive fragments are boxed

Germinal centres expressing a VκOx1 L-chain

All fragments were analysed by PCR for the presence of a VκOx1/Jκ5 rearrangement. In good agreement with a previous analysis where in 30% of the germinal centers VκOx1 L-chains could be demonstrated (unpublished results) in this experiment 7 out of 18 analysed germinal centres gave a positive signal (indicated in table.1). One might have expected that succesive sections of the same germinal centre would be either all positive or all negative for VκOx1/Jκ5 rearrangements. However we found that only some, but not all sections of individual germinal centres were positive by PCR. This result may indicate that different parts of a single germinal centre may be occupied by different B-cell clones. Further work is nescessary to establish this point.

Clonal expansion without activation of the hypermutation mechanism

In the majority of these germinal centres L-chain sequences showed only few exchanges at a level no greater than expected by PCR. It seems that there is expansion of B-cell clones in germinal centres without accumulation of somatic mutations. This would result in a large clone size by the time the hypermutation mechanism becomes activated.

Only few somatic mutations will increase the affinity for the antigen. It has been estimated that approximately 25% of all mutations have a negative effect either on the structure of the antibody molecule or for the binding site (Weigert, 1986). Thus, with a random mutation mechanism many changes will give rise to low affinity variants. Activation of the hypermutation mechanism at a time point of a large clone size would increase the chance for a B-cell to pick up a mutation which confers higher affinity.

Stepwise accumulation of somatic mutations

The result of the sequence analysis for one of the germinal centres is shown in Fig.1. The data are presented in a form of a genealogical tree based on a stepwise accumulation of somatic mutations. Each sequence is indicated by a shaded circle. If we regard single A->G and T->C exchanges as PCR artefacts then three sequences are probably unmutated. All other sequences carry a mutation in the first complementarity region 1 (CDR1) at position 34 which changes His to Asn. In addition most sequences have a silent mutation at position 94 of CDR3. Altogether up to 10 somatic mutations have been introduced during the time this clone has been expanded in the germinal centre. In contrast in other germinal centres (data not shown) only three to four mutations per sequence were seen. This result together with the broad range in the somatic mutation frequency within a

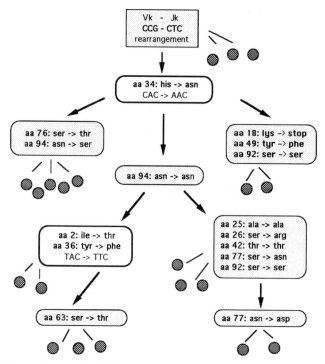

Figure 1. Intraclonal diversification in a single phOx specific germinal centre

single germinal centre indicates that the hypermutation mechanism is activated in different B-cells for different periods of time.

Affinity selection in germinal centres

It has been demonstrated that an exchange at position 34 of the VκOx1 L-chain from His to Asn increases the affinity of the phOx specific antibodies by a factor of 10 (Berek and Milstein, 1986). In most of the high affinity antibodies this mutation is accompanied by a second mutation exchanging Tyr to Phe in framework 2. The analysis of phOx specific germinal centres showed that in all germinal centres where the B-cell repertoire had been diversified by the hypermutation mechanism those mutations were present in the sequenced L-chains. This is in contrast to germinal centres of nitro-phenyl specific B-cells (Jacob et al., 1991 and Jacob and Kelsoe, 1992) were the mutation confering high affinity could not be detected.

In the germinal centre shown in Fig 1 all mutated sequences have the exchange at position 34. In addition in 5 sequences the substitution in framework 2 from Tyr to Phe (indicated by a clear box) was found. In another germinal centre all sequences carried these two exchanges (data not shown) pointing to an extremely high efficiency of the affinity selection in germinal centres.

The silent mutation in position 94 of the CDR3 has often been observed in phOx specific antibodies and this position is thought to be a hot spot for somatic mutations. The crystal structure of a phOx specific antibody shows that amino acid exchanges in the CDR3 of the VkOx1 L-chain may interfere with binding to the hapten phOx (Alzari et al., 1990). Not surprisingly the exchanges seen at this position are predominantly silent. The five sequences which have an exchange to Ser in that residue may be derived from B-cells of lower affinity.

The genealogic tree shows that the exchange from His to Asn must have been introduced approximately at the timepoint when the hypermutation mechanism became activated, otherwise not all sequences would show this substitution. For other germinal centres analysed the same observation was made (data not shown). These results suggest that B-cells of higher affinity have a proliferative advantage over other cells leading to a repertoire dominated by cells expressing this particular mutation.

REFERENCES

Alzari, P.M., Spinelli, S., Mariuzza, R.A., Boulot, G., Poljak, R.J., Jarvis, J.M., and Milstein, C., 1990, Three-dimensional structure determination of an anti-phenyloxazolone antibody: the role of somatic mutation and heavy/light chain pairing in the maturation of the immune response, EMBO J. 9: 3807.

Berek, C, and Milstein, C., 1986, Mutation drift and repertoire shift in the maturation of the immune response, Immunol. Rev. 96: 23.

Berek, C., Berger, A., and Apel, M., 1991, Maturation of the immune response in germinal centers, Cell 67: 1121.

Jacob, J., Kelsoe, G., Rajewsky, K., and Weiss, U., 1991, Intraclonal generation of antibody mutants in germinal centres, Nature 354: 389.

Jacob, J., and Kelsoe, G., 1992, In situ studies of the primary immune reponse to (4-hydroxy-3-nitrophenyl)acetyl. II A common clonal origin for periarteriolar lymphoid sheath-associated foci and germinal centers, J. Exp. Med. 176: 679.

Weigert, M., 1986, The influence of somatic mutation on the immune response, Prog. in Immunol. VI: 138.

ACKNOWLEDGMENTS

M. Ziegner is supported by the Deutsche Forschungsgemeinschaft.

CYTOKINE RESPONSIVENESS OF GERMINAL CENTER B CELLS

Vincent K. Tsiagbe, Sucheta Chickramane, Ashok R. Amin,
Joanne M. Edington, and G. Jeanette Thorbecke

Dept. of Pathology and Kaplan Comprehensive Cancer Center
New York University School of Medicine
New York, NY 10016

INTRODUCTION

Because tumors often represent differentiation-arrested stages of
normal cell development, the study of tumor cells frequently provides
information about their normal cellular counterparts. This is
particularly true for lymphoid cells and it is for that reason that,
many years ago, we undertook to study the the germinal center (GC)
derived lymphomas of SJL mice. The properties of these lymphomas,
misnamed "RCS", are summarized in table 1 and were previously reviewed
(Ponzio et al., 1986).

Table 1. Features of SJL lymphomas.

---

1) High incidence in SJL mice: > 90% by 13 months of age
2) Accompanied by serum paraproteins: IgG1 > IgA > IgG2a >> IgG3 > IgG2b
3) Originally called "reticulum cell sarcoma (RCS)" because of mixed
   cell type: now clearly identified as B cell lymphomas
4) B cell markers, including the GC specific CD77, isotype-switched Ig
   genes
5) Generally do not make intact Ig, usually some free k chain
6) Subject to reversed immunological surveillance: host CD4 T cell
   dependent: anti-CD4 treatment prevents lymphoma development
7) Are stimulated to grow by cytokines produced by CD4 T cells in
   response to RCS

STUDIES ON SJL LYMPHOMA CELLS

The cytokine requirements of these lymphomas were analyzed in bulk
culture and in a colony forming assays (CFU) in soft agar. In the
presence of excess IL-1, the additional RCS growth-stimulating cytokines
provided by the activated lymph node T cells were identified as IL-5 and
IFN-gamma by the neutralizing effects of mAbs added to the CFU assay

In Vivo Immunology, Edited by E. Heinen *et al.*
Plenum Press, New York, 1994

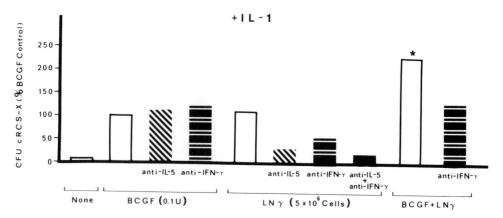

Fig. 1. Colony formation in soft agar by RCS-X cells in the presence of low molecular weight human BCGF (Cellular Products, Buffalo, NY), γ–irradiated SJL lymph node cells (LN γ) or the combination of these. These cultures contained 10 U/ml of IL-1, which was shown previously to increase responsiveness of RCS-X cells to BCGF and IL-5. The synergy between BCGF and LN cells is abrogated by the addition of anti–mIFN-γ (13 μg/ml). The effect of LN cells alone is partially neutralized by anti–mIL-5 and by anti–mIFN-γ, and virtually completely by the combination of these two mAbs, suggesting that a major factor contributed by the LN cells is IL-5 (From Lasky et al, 1988 and Lasky and Thorbecke, 1989).

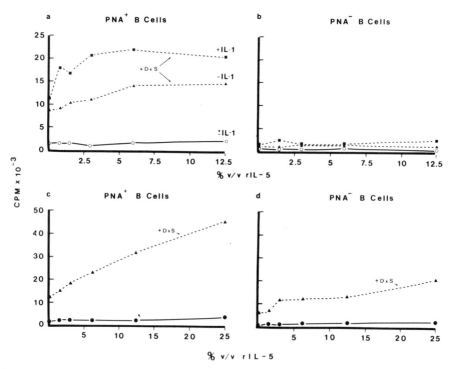

Fig. 2. Proliferation induced by dextran sulfate (10 μg/ml) and IL-5 in PNA+ and PNA− B cells. The cells were isolated from brachial SJL immune LN, draining the injection site of 3 μg trinitrophenylated B. abortus given in the front footpads 7–8 days earlier. The results in the top panels show that IL-1 (10 U/ml) enhances the response of PNA+ B cells to IL-5 (Data from Rabinowitz et al, 1990).

208

between gamma-irradiated SJL lymph node cells and human BCGF was abrogated by the anti-IFN-gamma, suggesting that the human BCGF provided an IL-5 like effect. No other cytokines had any detectable effect on RCS growth in vitro (Lasky et al., 1988). Further studies on these lymphomas have shown that the SJL T cells they stimulate all bear Vß16+, and that the stimulatory surface moiety on the RCS cells is an MMTV-LTR-ORF similar to the M-locus antigens (Tsiagbe et al., 1993a and b). One interpretation of our results is that this mmtv-LTR is not expressed on resting or activated SJL B cells except in GC, causing GC cells to become abnormally stimulatory for Vß16+ SJL T cells. We are at present testing this possibility. No evidence has been obtained for an abnormal gene translocation in the lymphoma cells causing this mmtv gene to become active (Tsiagbe et al., 1993b).

STUDIES ON GERMINAL CENTER CELLS

Turning our attention to the cytokine requirements of normal GC cells in SJL mice, we found that the B cells from immune LN taken at the peak of GC development and adherent to peanut agglutinin (PNA) coated dishes, or "PNA+" cells, respond much better to IL-5 in costimulation with dextran sulfate than do PNA− B cells (Fig. 2). In addition, this response was augmented in the presence of IL-1 (Fig. 2; top) and not by IL-4 (Rabinowitz et al., 1990). In costimulation with dextran sulfate or chondroitin sulfate C, IL-4 also caused greater proliferation in PNA+ than in PNA− B cells (Table 2). The response to anti-IgM with IL-4 was approximately equal in PNA+ and PNA− cells and was not enhanced by IL-5 (Rabinowitz et al., 1990).

Table 2. Responses of PNA+ and PNA− B cells to chondroitin sulfate C.

Stimuli Added To Culture	^{3}H-Thymidine Incorporation by	
	PNA+ B Cells	PNA− B Cells
None	176 ± 110	199 ± 47
IL-4	844 ± 95	531 ± 244
IL-5	165 ± 41	206 ± 54
Chondroitin Sulfate C	332 ± 65	310 ± 62
Chondr. S. C + IL-4	3557 ± 307	1331 ± 263
Chondr. S. C + IL-5	494 ± 95	562 ± 194

Chondroitin sulfate used at: 2 mg/ml; IL-4 at: 25 U/ml. n=4-10.

COMPARISON BETWEEN GERMINAL CENTER AND PERITONEAL B CELLS

Studies by others have shown that costimulation of normal splenic or peritoneal B cells with dextran sulfate provides a good assay for IL-5 (Wetzel, 1989). In view of the fact that SJL mice have few CD5+ B cells, we examined the response to IL-5 of peritoneal cells from BALB/c mice. Indeed, in bulk cultures a good response was found to dextran sulfate with IL-5 in BALB/c but not in SJL peritoneal cells (Rabinowitz et al., 1990). Similar results were obtained in CFU assays (Fig. 3). However, a remarkable difference was observed between PNA+ and peritoneal B cells in the response to IFN-gamma. IFN-gamma strongly

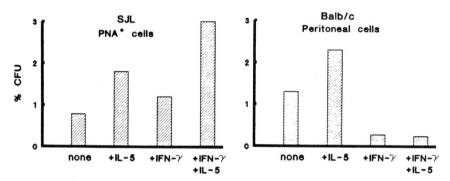

Fig. 3. Effect of cytokines on colony formation in soft agar by SJL PNA[+] B cells and BALB/c peritoneal B cells. Note the stimulating effects of IL-5 on both types of B cells, and the opposite effects of IFN-γ (Data from Tsiagbe et al., 1992).

inhibited the colony formation by peritoneal B cells, while a synergy was observed between IL-5 and IFN-gamma for PNA[+] B cells from SJL lymph nodes (Fig. 3), similar to that seen earlier with RCS cells. Our initial expectation that the study of the SJL lymphomas would provide insight into the properties of GC cells seems, therefore, to have been correct.

DISCUSSION

It has been known since the early 1980's that a special population of CD4[+] T cells is present in GC, both in lymph nodes in the mouse and in the human tonsil (Rouse et al., 1982; Poppema et al., 1981). In man, these cells are partially activated, expressing CD38 and CD69, but not CD25 (IL-2R), CD71 (transferin-R) or HLA-DR (Toellner et al., 1993; Bowen et al., 1991). CD40-ligand expression on these cells has been described by Lederman et al (1993). They belong to the helper memory T cell subset, in that they express CD45RO (Bowen et al., 1991) and they express CD57, a marker that is usually expressed on NK cells, but only on a small subset of T cells (Porwit-Ksiazek et al., 1983).

It is of some interest to determine which cytokines are produced locally in GC, because the simultaneous need for IL-5 and IFN-gamma by the GC B cells would suggest that the T cells in these sites might not have differentiated into Th1 or Th2 subsets. On isolation of CD57[+] T cells from human tonsils, Nahm and coworkers found that these cells did not secrete cytokines in response to pokeweed mitogen (PWM) stimulation (Bowen et al., 1991). In contrast, they consistently contained mRNA for IL-4 prior to stimulation, which decreased after stimulation with PWM (Butch et al., 1993). In addition, they occasionally contained mRNA for IL-10, TNF-alpha and IFN-gamma, suggesting that they indeed produced cytokines characteristic for both the Th1 and Th2 subsets. Toellner et al (1993) have confirmed these findings on isolated CD4[+]CD57[+] human T cells and found, in addition, that they contained mRNA for IL-2. In as much as the murine equivalent of CD57 has not been identified, isolation of GC T cells in the mouse is not feasible. However, in situ staining for cytokines has not resulted in the detection of IL-4, IFN-gamma or IL-2 within follicles 7 days after footpad injection of antigen (Bogen et al., 1993). In preliminary studies in our laboratory, employing in situ hybridization with cytokine riboprobes, the majority of the cytokine producing cells are, indeed, present in the paracortex. However, some IL-4 and IL-5 producing cells are also seen within GC on day 7 after antigen stimulation. Further studies are needed to determine whether continued local cytokine production by the T cells in GC is essential to GC B cell proliferation, and whether the initial impulse of the B cells to proliferate in GC comes from a contact between precursor B cells and T cells in or outside of GC.

REFERENCES

Bogen, S.A., Fogelman, I., and Abbas, A.K. 1993. Analysis of IL-2, IL-4 and IFN-gamma-producing cells in situ during immune responses to protein antigens. J. Immunol. 150:4197.

Bowen, M.B., Butch, A.W., Parvin, C.A., Levine, A., and Nahm, M.H. 1991. Germinal Center T cells are distinct helper-inducer T cells. Human Immunol. 31, 67.

Butch, A.W., Chung, G-H., Hoffmann, J.W., and Nahm, M.H. 1993. Cytokine expression by germinal center cells. J. Immunol. 150:39.

Ponzio, N.M., Brown, P.H., and Thorbecke, G.J. 1986. Host–tumor interactions in the SJL lymphoma model. In: International Reviews of Immunology, Lynch, R.G. ed. Harwood Acad. Publ., N.Y. vol. 1: 263.

Lasky, J.L., and Thorbecke, G.J. 1989. Characterization and growth factor requirements of SJL lymphomas. II. Interleukin 5 dependence of the in vitro cell line, cRCS-X, and influence of other cytokines. Eur. J. Immunol. 19:365.

Lasky, J.L., Ponzio, N.M., and Thorbecke, G.J. 1988. Characterization and growth factor requirements of SJL lymphomas. I. Development of a B cell growth factor (BCGF) dependent in vitro cell line, cRCS-X. J. Immunol. 14:679.

Lederman, S., Yellin, M.J., Inghirami, G., Lee, J.J., Knowles, D.M., and Chess, L. 1992. Molecular interactions mediating T-B lymphocyte collaboration in human lymphoid follicles. Roles of T cell-B-cell-activating molecule (5c8 antigen) and CD40 in contact-dependent help. J. Immunol. 149:3817.

Poppema, S., Bahn, A.K., Reinherz, E.L., McCluskey, R.T., and Schlossman, S.F. 1981. Distribution of T cell subsets in human lymph nodes. J. Exp. Med. 153:30.

Porwit-Ksiazek, A., Ksiazek, T, and Riberfeld, P. 1983. Leu 7[+] (HNK-1[+]) cells. I. Selective compartmentalization of Leu 7[+] cells with different immunophenotypes in lymphatic tissues and blood. Scand. J. Immunol. 18:485.

Rabinowitz, J.L., Tsiagbe, V.K., Nicknam, M.H., and Thorbecke, G.J. 1990. Germinal center cells are a major IL-5 responsive B cell population in peripheral lymph nodes engaged in the immune response. J. Immunol. 145:2440.

Rouse, R.V., Ledbetter, J.A., and Weissman, I.L. 1982. Mouse lymph node germinal centers contain a selected subset of T cells – the helper phenotype. J. Immunol. 128:2243.

Toellner, K-M., Scheel, D., Reiling, N., Sprenger, R., Pidun, I., Flad, H.D., and Gerdes, J. 1993. In: 11th International Conference on Lymphoid Tissues and Germinal Centres in Immune Reactions, Abstract 10.6:117.

Tsiagbe, V.K., Asakawa, J., Miranda, A., Sutherland, R.M., Paterson, Y., and Thorbecke. 1993 . Syngeneic response to SJL follicular center B cell lymphoma (reticular cell sarcoma) cells in Vß16[+]CD4[+] T cells. J. Immunol. 150:5519.

Tsiagbe, V.K., Yoshimoto, T., Asakawa, J., Cho, S.Y., Meruelo, D., and Thorbecke, G.J. 1993. Linkage of superantigen-like stimulatin of syngeneic T cells in a mouse model of follicular center B cell lymphoma to transcription of endogenousmammary tumor virus. EMBO J. 12:2313.

Wetzel, G.D. 1989. Interleukin 5 regulation of peritoneal Ly-1 B lymphocyte proliferation, differentiation and autoantibody secretion. Eur. J. Immunol. 19:1701.

THE DIFFERENCES IN SURVIVAL AND PHENOTYPE BETWEEN CENTROBLASTS AND CENTROCYTES

Yong-Jun Liu, Clarisse Barthelemy, Odette de Bouteiller, and Jacques Banchereau

Schering-Plough, Laboratory for Immunological Research
27 chemin des Peupliers, 69571, Dardilly, France

INTRODUCTION

Affinity maturation of T cell-dependent antibody responses is achieved by two basic mechanisms within the germinal centers (G.C) : somatic mutation in Ig V genes (1-4) and subsequent positive selection based on the affinity for antigen binding (5). Since all these experiments were performed on mouse or human total G.C. B cells, there are several further questions needed to be addressed now: a) at what stage is somatic mutation machinery operating ? b) are somatic mutations and selection occuring at the same time or does selection occur after mutation? is there a negative selection at certain stages of G.C. reaction, to deal with auto-reactive B cell clones generated by somatic mutations ? Isolation of G.C. B cell subsets seems to be a key step to answer these questions. Classically, G.C. are divided into a dark zone and a light zone (6). The dark zone contains centroblasts which are large pyroninophilic or basophilic cells. Their nuclei are large round with multiple nucleoli. The light zone contains centrocytes which are large to medium sized cells and they have nuclei with distinct clefts (7). Using these criteria, the survival of these two types of G.C. B cells were studied during a short-term culture and they were finally isolated by centrifugal elutriation.

TOTAL GERMINAL CENTER B CELLS CONTAIN LESS THAN 10% CENTROBLASTS

Total G.C. B cells were isolated from tonsil B cells by depleting IgD+ and CD39+ B cells as described before (5). The percentage of centroblasts and centrocytes were quantified based on the morphology (Fig 1a) from 6 tonsil samples. The results show that total germinal center B cells contain 7% to 10% cells which have the morphological characteristics of centroblasts: pyroninophilic cytoplasms and round nuclei with multiple nucleoli.

CENTROBLASTS SURVIVE LONGER THAN CENTROCYTES

It was previously shown that germinal center cells die rapidly by apoptosis (Apo) when placed into tissue culture (5). This process resulted in 40% of cell loss within 6 hours, 75% of cell loss within 16 hours and over 95% of cell loss after 48 hours culture. We repeated these experiments in 6 tonsil samples. The result shows that the centrocytes (CC) were preferentially lost during the culture while many centroblasts (CB) survived for 16 hours. Thus, within the viable cell populations at 6 hours and 16 hours culture, the percentages of centroblasts were greatly increased. At 4 hours culture, the percentage of centroblasts increased from less than 10% to about 20% and at 16 hours culture nearly all the viable cells were centroblasts (Fig 1a, b, c).

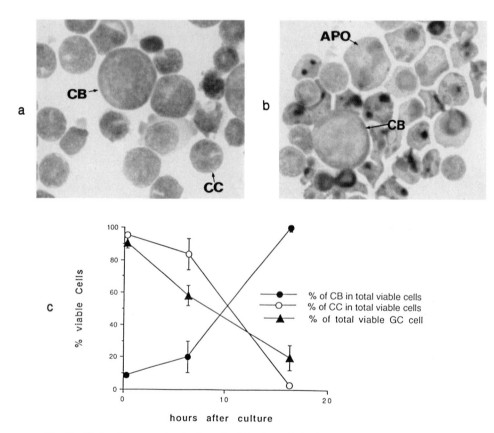

Fig 1. Selective survival of centroblasts. a): before culture; b) 16 hours after culture; c) quantitative results from 6 tonsil samples.

ISOLATION OF GERMINAL CENTER CENTROBLASTS

Germinal center B cells were separated into different fractions by elutriation using an induction drive centrifuge (model J2-21M, Beckman). This was performed at constant flow pressure with variable centrifugation rates. Different cell fractions were collected for 15 minutes at centrifugation rates of 3000 (rpm), 2900, 2800, 2700, 2600, 2500, 2400, 2300, 2200, 2100, 2000, 1900, 1800, 1700, 1600 and 1500. The morphology of the cells in each fraction is shown in Fig 3. Fractions 2000 to 1500 represent 2% of total GC cells recovered. They are very big basophilic cells with large round nuclei which have multiple nucleoli (Fig 2a). Fraction 2100 represents 9% of total GC recovered and they are big basophilic cells, some have round nuclei with multiple nucleoli and some have nuclei with clear cleft. Fractions 2200 and 2300 represent 19% of total GC cells recovered, they are medium large basophilic cells and have nuclear cleft (Fig 2b). Fractions 2500 and 2400 represent 21% of total GC cells recovered. They are non-bosophilic medium sized cells, and contain nuclei with clear cleft (Fig 2c). Fractions 2600 and 2700 represent 23% of total GC cells recovered. They are small to medium sized non-basophilic cells (Fig.2d). Many of them have nuclear cleft. Fraction 2800 represents 26% of total germinal center B cell recovered, which are small centrocytes.

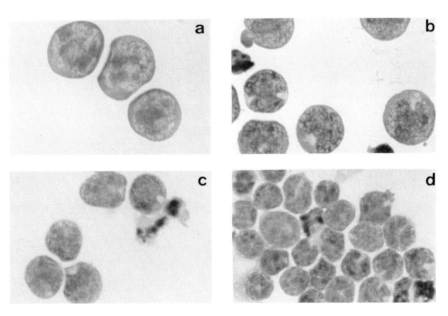

Fig 2. Giemsa staining of germinal center B cell subsets (1000x).

SURFACE PHENOTYPE OF GERMINAL CENTER B CELL SUBSETS

The expression of CD3, CD20, CD38, CD75 and sIg were analysed by FACS (Fig 3). All populations failed to express CD3 but were positive for CD20 and CD38, which indicates that these cells are germinal center B cells. They all express low levels of sIg kappa chain and lambda chain compared with CD38 low IgD+ high density B cells. Interestingly, Fraction 2000 to 1500 expresses higher level of CD75 compared with other cell fractions. These cells also express stronger nuclear proliferating antigen Ki67 compared with germinal center B cells which have nuclear clefts (not shown).

DISCUSSION

Germinal center centroblasts can be recognized in isolated form based on morphological criteria which represent less than 10% of total germinal center B cells. These cells can stay alive a little bit longer than centrocytes during in vitro culture.

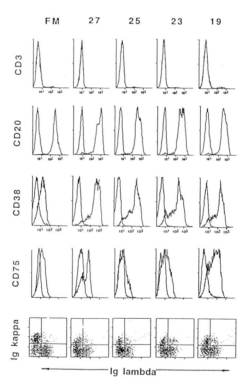

Fig 3. FACS phenotypic analysis of follicular mantle B cells (FM) and different germinal center B cell fractions (27, 25, 23 and 1900 rpm) derived from elutriation.

Subsequent isolation and phenotypic analysis confirm that these very big basophilic cells with multiple nucleoli are germinal center B cells, which are sIg low, CD3- CD20+ CD38+. The high expression of sCD75 and nuclear Ki67 antigens suggested that these cells may locate in the basal dark zone of the germinal center, one of the five germinal center compartments identified by a resent immunohistological study by Hardie et al (8). In this study, classical dark zone was divided into a basal dark zone and an apical dark zone. The basal dark zone contains centroblasts which express high levels of CD75 and Ki67 antigens. The apical dark zone contains large basophilic centrocytes, which express low levels of CD75 and Ki67 antigens compared with the centroblasts in the basal dark zone. These large basophilic centrocytes in the basal light zone have the characteristics of the germinal center cells isolated in fraction 2300 to 2100. The medium and small sized non-basophilic centrocytes (fractions 2800-2400) may be located in the basal light zone and apical light zone. Interestingly, apoptotic cells were mainly identified in the apical dark zone and basal light zone but not in the basal dark zone and apical light zone. This is consistent with our in vitro finding that the very big basophilic centroblasts can stay alive a little longer than centrocytes. This suggests that the positive selection may operate only on centrocyte stage but not on centroblast stage. MacLennan and Gray 1986 (9) proposed that somatic mutaion and positive selection are operating separately on centroblast stage and centrocyte stage respectively. The advantage of this strategy is to allow to generate large clone size and diversity by clonal expansion and somatic mutation in the basal dark zone of the germinal center, which will be selected later in the basal dark zone and light zone.

ACKNOWLEDGMENTS

We thank Muriel Vatan and Nicole Courbiere for editorial assistance, M-Clotilde Rissoan, Pascale Chomarat for technical help.

REFERENCES

1. Jacob, J., Kelsoe, G., Rajewsky, K, and Weiss, U., 1990, Intraclonal generation of antibody mutants in germinal centres. *Nature*. 354:389.

2. Weiss, U., and Rajewsky, K., 1990, The repertoire of somatic antibody mutants accumulating in the memory compartment after primary immunization is restricted through affinity maturation and mirrors that expressed in the secondary response. *J. Exp. Med.* 172:1681.

3. Berek, C., Berger, A., and Apel, M., 1991, Maturation of the immune response in germinal centers. *Cell.* 67:1121.

4 Leanderson, T., Källberg, E., and Gray, G., 1992,. Expansion, selection and mutation of antigen-specific B cells in germinal centers. *Immunol. Rev.* 126:47.

5 Liu, Y. J., Joshua, D.E., Williams, G.T., Smith, C.A., Gordon, J., and MacLennan, I.C.M., 1989, Mechanism of antigen-driven selection in germinal centres. *Nature*. 342:929.

6. Nieuwenhuis, P., and Opstelten, D., 1984, Functional anatomy of germinal centres. *Am. J. Anat.* 170:421.

7. Stein, H., Gerdes, J., and Mason, D.Y., 1982, The normal and malignant germinal centre. *Clin. Haematol.* 11:531.

8. Hardie, D.L., Johnson, G.D., Khan, M., and MacLennan,. I.C.M., 1993, Quantitative analysis of molecules which distinguish functional compartments within germinal centers. *Eur. J. Immunol.* 23:997.

9. MacLennan, I., and D. Gray, D., 1986, Antigen-driven selection of virgin and memory B cells. *Immunol. Rev.* 91:61.

IN VIVO LOCALISATION PATTERNS AND CELL-CELL INTERACTIONS OF CYTOKINE PRODUCING T-CELLS AND SPECIFIC ANTIBODY FORMING B-CELLS

Eric Claassen, Alfons van den Eertwegh, Marjan van Meurs and Wim Boersma

Dept. Immunology and Medical Microbiology, TNO-Medical Biological Lab.
POB 5815, 2280 HV, Rijswijk, The Netherlands

INTRODUCTION

Because of its central position in the bloodstream and the large amount of migrating lymphocytes, the spleen plays a central role in the primary defense against bloodstream infections. Two critical functions of the spleen can be recognized: it serves as a large phagocytic filter and it is a major antibody producing organ[1]. Although the spleen participates significantly in host defense mechanisms, it is not essential for life. Nevertheless, its removal increases the risk on overwhelming infections by bacteria with polysaccharide capsules, e.g. *Streptococcus pneumonia, Neisseria meningitidis or Haemophilus influenza*[2]. After primary i.v. immunization, the spleen is the major site of antibody production[3]. Since eight times more lymphocytes recirculate via the spleen than via all lymph nodes together[4], it is most likely that the entire antigen-specific B- T-cell repertoire is available in the spleen. The complex anatomical organization of the spleen with distinct compartments containing specialized cell types provides a unique micro-environment allowing cell-cell interactions which are essential for the initiation and continuation of various immune responses[5] (fig. 1). To fully understand the role of

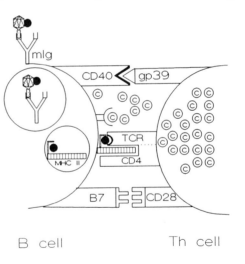

Figure 1 Cognate interaction between B and T cells. B-cells capture, process and present antigen to Th-cells (costimulated by B7-CD28), activated Th express gp39 and cytokines.

the spleen in the immune response it is obviously necessary to look at this organ in a functional *in vivo* way. This means that one should switch from conventional phenotyping of immunocompetent cells to a more functional characterisation (e.g. resting vs activated). In looking at B-cells one should for example clearly separate membrane-Ig positive, memory and plasma cells. The latter group can be further subdivided by looking at the antigen specificity of the produced antibodies. For this purpose we developed new methodology for the detection of antigen specific antibody forming B-cells (AFCs) in tissue sections. By double staining we could also simultaneously determine the isotype of these AFCs (reviewed in: 6).

In Vivo Immunology, Edited by E. Heinen *et al.*
Plenum Press, New York, 1994

ANTIGEN UPTAKE AND LOCALISATION IN THE MURINE SPLEEN

We recently demonstrated that thymus-independent type-2 antigens (TI-2 antigen) localize in splenic follicles within 1 h after administration[7]. Detection of 2,4,6-trinitrophenyl (TNP) haptenated antigen in cryostat sections of murine spleens was performed with a high-affinity TNP-specific monoclonal antibody conjugated to β-galactosidase. Follicular localization of (TNP)-Ficoll was not antibody mediated. In case of high-dose

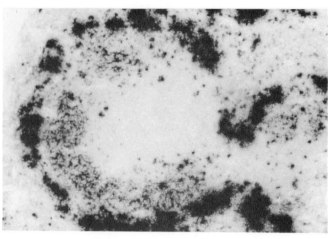

Figure 2 Localisation of TNP-ficoll in murine spleen 7 hrs after i.v. administration of the antigen. Note concentration of antigen in marginal zone macrophages and on follicular B-cells.

administration we observed a relatively large amount of TI-2 antigen in marginal zone macrophages. However, after low-dose administration we observed a preferential localization of TNP-Ficoll in the splenic follicles. Within minutes after injection the TI-2 antigen localized in the marginal zone, attached to marginal zone macrophages and B cells. Twenty minutes after injection antigen was also detected in the follicles and gradually accumulated there until 7 h after injection (fig. 2). Thereafter, the amount of follicular antigen gradually decreased but was still detectable up to 14 days after immunization. The follicular localization of TNP-Ficoll was complement dependent in contrast to the binding to and uptake by macrophages. Haptenated thymus-dependent (TD) antigen localized exclusively in the red pulp macrophages. *In vivo* macrophage elimination drastically increased the amount of TNP-Ficoll in the follicles, and enhanced the humoral immune response at low doses of antigen[8]. Moreover, complement deprivation of mice abrogated the localization of TI-2 antigen in the follicles, and led to a decreased humoral TI-2 immune response. In conclusion, we demonstrated for the first time that TI-2 antigen localize in follicles. This provided further evidence that B cells and follicular localized antigen play an important role in the induction of humoral TI-2 immune responses, and that marginal zone macrophages actually obscure the antigen from the immune system. Presentation of the antigen most probably occurs in the follicular areas either by B-cells or by follicular dendritic cells.

T AND B CELL ACTIVATION IN TD IMMUNE RESPONSES

The activation of B cells is a complex mechanism, reviewed by Noelle and Snow[9]. Briefly, TD antigens bind to B cells expressing complementary mIg receptors (fig. 1). The crosslinking of the Mig does not result in B cell activation, but may be a signal for the B cell to process the selected antigen and present it to T cells, probably in the context of B7 and CD28. Casten and Pierce observed 100-1000 fold increase in the capacity of B cells to present cytochrome-c to a T cell hybridoma when the antigen was covalently coupled to anti-Ig[10]. The potent activity of the cytochrome-c-antibody conjugates appeared to be due to the B cell targeting features of the conjugated Ig. The recognition of complexes of processed antigens and MHC on the B cell by T cells is responsible for the initial class II restricted, antigen-specific, physical interaction between T and B cells. These T and B cells form conjugates which are stabilized by the binding of ICAM-1 to LFA-1 and CD4[+] to monomorphic domains of the class II proteins. This interaction induces T cell activation, resulting in the expression of novel surface proteins on the membranes. These newly expressed membrane proteins on activated Th cells together with resident Th membrane proteins form the major growth stimulus for B cells. Recently, Noelle et al. demonstrated that blocking of the prominent Th surface molecules, LFA-1, CD4, ICAM-1, CD3 or the TCR did not inhibit the capacity of activated Th cells to induce B cell cycle entry[11]. In contrast, CD40-Ig fusion proteins or antibodies specific to the CD40 ligand, blocked B cell activation by activated Th cell, suggesting that the CD40 molecule expressed by B cells, is the receptor of the Th cell activation antigen (see van den Eertwegh et al., this volume). This activation antigen was identified as a 39 kD protein that was selectively expressed on activated Th cells[11]. The initial B cell activation by activated Th cells, requires no soluble factors and induces enhanced B cell RNA synthesis ($G_0 \rightarrow G_1$). After activation B cells develop the competence to respond to cytokines, which are produced by activated T cells. These cytokines act solely or predominantly at different steps in the B cell activation pathway. Cytokines, like IL-1, IL-2 and IL-4, support the growth of activated B cells, while others, such as IL-4, IL-5, IL-6 and IFN-γ participate as differentiation factors[12]. The above described experiments imply that T-B cell conjugate formation is an important event for the induction of TD immune responses. This interaction is not a short event but requires a contact for at least 48 h *in vitro* to obtain the maximum proliferative response of B cells[13]. In addition, cytokine production by T cells was found to require the continuous presence of the stimulating signal *in vitro*[14], suggesting that for the generation of an effective immune response T-B cell conjugate formation is required for at least 24 to 48 hours. We demonstrated these T-B conjugates *in vivo* and showed that they are predominantly found in the outer-PALS and around the terminal arterioles in the murine spleen[15 & vd Eertwegh, this volume]

IN SITU DETECTION OF CYTOKINE PRODUCING T-CELLS

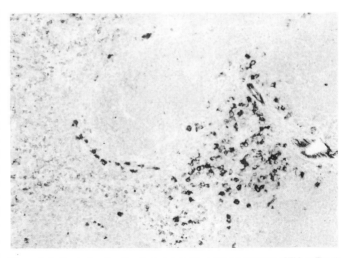

A number of *in situ* hybridization studies have determined the localization and amount of cytokine gene activity in organs. However, they have not shown the actual presence of cytokine-protein in these tissues. For the demonstration,characterization and localization of cells producing cytokine-proteins immunohistochemical techniques are very powerful[16]. Using indirect immunofluorescence techniques, Cleveland et al.[17] found an increased *in vivo* IFN-γ production in spleens 6

Figure 3 Antibody forming B-cells (grey) and juxtaposed cytokine (IFN-γ) T-cells (black), cells localise in outer-PALS and around terminal arterioles and not in follicles, marginal zone or red pulp.

days after the induction of graft versus host disease. IFN-γ was proven to be T cell dependent and derived from donor T cells. IFN-γ activity was mainly observed in the PALS and less frequently in the red pulp. In contrast, *in vitro* evaluation of IFN-γ activity showed no increased IFN-γ production by suspended spleen cells, this discrepancy was due to the *in vitro* mixing of different spleen cell populations, which essentially changed the microenvironment of the potential IFN-γ-producing cells. We investigated the activity of IFN-γ-producing cells in murine spleens 3 weeks after i.p. immunization with heat-killed Bacille Calmette Guerin (BCG)[18]. The IFN-γ-PC were detected immunohistochemically and localized in small clusters of 2-5 cells in the T-cell dependent areas like PALS and the coaxial sheaths of lymphoid tissue surrounding the terminal arteriolar branches. Only after i.v. injection of ConA in BCG primed mice, high levels of IFN-γ were detected in sera, whereas in non-BCG primed mice no increase in IFN-γ production was observed. Apparently, immunohistochemical techniques provide insight in the local *in vivo* activity of IFN-γ-PC in the immune response to BCG, which is not reflected by raised systemic IFN-γ levels. In another study we investigated IFN-γ-producing cells during immune responses against a variety of TI-2 antigens *(TNP-Ficoll, TNP-HES and Dextran B1355)*[19]. The maximum frequency of IFN-γ-producing cells was at 5-7 days after immunization, as confirmed by an IFN-γ-specific ELISA spot assay. At the peak of the response 40% of the IFN-γ-producing cells were CD4[+], 50% CD8[+] and 10% NK cells. *In vitro* experiments suggested that IFN-γ can down-regulate the humoral immune response against TNP-Ficoll[24]. Therefore, we performed a double staining for TNP-specific AFCs and IFN-γ-producing cells. We found TNP-specific AFCs in the same compartments as IFN-γ-producing cells with part of the TNP-AFCs was juxtaposed to IFN-γ-producing cells (fig. 3), suggesting intimate contact and possibly a regulating role of IFN-γ in TI-2 immune responses. However, *in vivo* treatment of mice with anti-IFN-γ antibodies after haptenated-Ficoll immunization only slightly inhibited the IgG2a anti-hapten response[20]. Svetic et al. examined the cytokine gene expression in spleens of mice after injection of GαIgD[21]. Although cytokine mRNA levels and rates of cytokine secretion are not well correlated[22], this study gave an indication which cytokine genes were expressed at various time points after GαIgD injection. We conducted an additional immunohistochemical study, in which we investigated the activity and profile of cytokine producing cells in the *in vivo* context[23]. BCBA.F1 mice were injected i.v. with RαIgD and killed after 36 h to 11 days. At day 3 and 4 high frequencies of IL-4 producing cells were observed around the terminal arterioles. In addition high frequencies of IL-2 producing cells were found in the same compartment. The number of IFN-γ-producing cells reached its

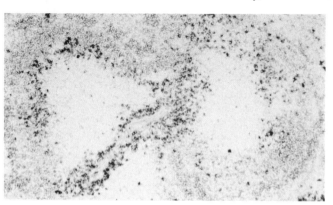

Figure 4 Rabbit-Ig-specific antibody forming B-cells localised in Outer-PALS of murine spleen after immunisation with α-IgD, IgM bearing resting B-cels found in follicles and marginal zone.

maximum at day 3, but was low as compared to the number of IL-4 producing cells. The kinetics of IL-2-producing cells in the spleen resembled the IL-2 gene activity as observed before[21], peaking at day 3 and subsequently declining. In both studies a high activity of IL-4 was observed 4 days after immunization. However, we observed a decrease of the number of IL-4 protein producing cells 5 days after immunization, whereas IL-4 mRNA levels were still high 6 days after immunization. In both studies maximum IFN-γ activity (mRNA or protein) was markedly less then the maximum observed IL-4 activity. In contrast to other antigens (TNP-Ficoll[24], TNP-KLH), we observed in the immune response to RαIgD, that cytokine production was preceding the development of specific AFCs of which the maximum frequency was observed at day 7 (fig. 4). We extended initial observations by Finkelman et al.[25], who demonstrated that IgG1 was the principal isotype of AFCs at day 7 after GαIgD injection. The precursors of IgG1 secreting B cells at day 7 were newly generated IgD[+] B cells, rather than B cells that were initially activated by anti-IgD antibody[26]. This suggested that newly generated B cells derived from the bone marrow, will bind RαIgD and present it from day 2 to 4 to Rabbit-specific T cells producing IL-4. This interaction results in isotype switching of the B cell into IgG1 or IgE and eventually to the differentiation of AFCs with the IgG1/IgE isotype. Double staining for cytokines revealed that cells with a Th0 (IL-2 and IL-4; Fig. 3m, or IL-4 and IFN-γ), Th1 (IL-2 and IFN-γ) and Th2 (IL-4) profile were all active during this immune response. Nevertheless, the dominance of the type 2 pathway appears to direct the isotype selection (IgE/IgG1) of the humoral immune response after RαIgD injection.

CONCLUSIONS AND PROPOSAL FOR ACTIVATION ROUTES IN THE SPLEEN

TI and TD antigens arrive predominately in the marginal zone of the spleen after i.v. injection. Particulate antigens will also be taken up and processed by macrophages in the marginal zone. The macrophages will transfer the processed antigen to B cells (□) in the marginal zone, or migrate into the while pulp and transfer the antigen to DC (☆) in the inner PALS. Alternatively the DC pick up the antigen and subsequently migrate into the PALS of the spleen. Upon contact with antigen, non-antigen specific T cells (○) leave the clusters formed by IDC and T cells, while antigen-specific T cells are activated to proliferate. B cells which bind soluble or processed antigens migrate from the marginal zone into the adjacent outer parts of the PALS. On arrival in the PALS, B cells encounter numerous T cells, among which are T cells of the appropriate antigen-specificity activated by IDC, migrating in an opposite direction. The counter flow of antigen-specific B and T cells optimizes the chance that these two cell types will interact with each other. Physical contact of the T cells with B cells (○□) will activate T cells to express new surface antigens, which will be the first growth

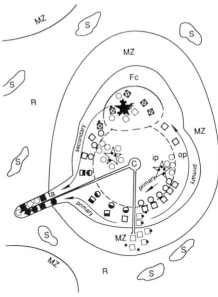

Figure 5 Activation and migration of immune cells in the spleen during immune responses. MZ = marginal zone, F = follicle, Fc = F-corona, ip = innerPALS, op = outerPALS, R = redpulp, S = sinus, ta = terminal arteriole.

stimulus for B cells. T cells will also produce cytokines (●) which will regulate the proliferation and differentiation of B cell into AFCs (■). All these cell-cell interactions most likely occur during their migration from the outer PALS along the sheaths of lymphoid tissue surrounding the terminal arterioles towards the red pulp (Fig. 5). After all these interactions B cells eventually differentiate into AFCs producing specific antibodies which will form complexes with circulating antigen. A small proportion of the antibody-antigen complexes will be trapped by FDC (★) and retained there for long periods of time, providing a microenvironment for B cell affinity maturation and involved in generation and maintenance of B cell and T cell memory[27].

REFERENCES

1. J.F. Bohnsack, and E.J. Brown. The role of the spleen in resistance to infection, *Annu. Rev. Med.* 37:49 (1986).
2. E. Claassen,, A. Ott, C.D. Dijkstra, W.J.A. Boersma, C. Deen, N. Kors, M.M. Schellekens, and N. Van Rooijen. Marginal zone of the murine spleen in autotransplants: Functional and histological observations in the response against a thymus independent type-2 antigen, *Clin. Exp. Immunol.* 77:445 (1989).
3. G. Koch, B.D. Lok, A. Oudenaren, and R. Benner. The capacity and mechanism of bone marrow antibody formation by thymus independent antigens, *J. Immunol.* 128:1497 (1982).
4. R. Pabst, and J. Westerman. The unique role of the spleen and its compartments in lymphocyte migration, *Res. Immunol.* 142:339 (1991).
5. E. Claassen. Histological organisation of the spleen: implications for immune functions in different species, *Res. Immunol.* 142:315 (1991).
6. E. Claassen, K. Gerritse, J.D. Laman, W.J.A. Boersma. New immuno-enzyme-cytochemical stainings for the *in situ* detection of epitope specificity and isotype of antibody forming B-cells in experimental and natural (auto)immune responses in animals and man, *J. Immunol. Methods* 150:207 (1992).

7. A.J.M. Van den Eertwegh, J.D. Laman, M.M. Schellekens, W.J.A. Boersma and E. Claassen. Complement mediated follicular localization of T-independent type 2 antigens: the role of marginal zone macrophages rivisited, *Eur. J. Immunol.* 22:719 (1992).
8. E. Claassen, Q. Vos, A. Ott, M.M. Schellekens, W.J.A. Boersma. Role of the splenic marginal zone in the removal of, and immune response against, neutral polysaccharides, *in*: Lympathic Tissues and In Vivo Immune Responses, B. Imhof, S. Berrih-Aknin, S. Ezine, ed., Marcel Dekker, New York, (1991).
9. R.J. Noelle, and E.Ch. Snow. Cognate interactions between helper T cells and B cells, *Immunol. Today* 11:361 (1990).
10. L. Casten, and S.K. Pierce. Receptor-mediated B cell antigen processing. Increased antigenicity of a globular protein covalently coupled to antibodies specific for B cell surface structures, *J. Immunol.* 140:404 (1988).
11. R.J. Noelle, M. Roy, D.M. Shepherd, I. Stamenkovic, J.A. Ledbetter, and A.A. Aruffo. Novel ligand on activated helper T cells bind CD40 and transduces the cognate activation of B cell, *Proc. Nat. Acad. Sci. USA.* 89:6550 (1992).
12. A.K. Abbas, M.E. Williams, H.J. Burstein, T.L. Chang, P. Bossu, A.H. Lichtman. Activation and functions of CD4$^+$ T cell subsets, *Immunol. Rev.* 123:5 (1991).
13. M.R. Kehry, L.C. Yamashita, and P.D. Hodgkin. B cell proliferation and differentiation mediated by Th cell membranes and lymphokines, *Res. Immunol* 141:421 (1990).
14. R. Swoboda, U. Bommhardt, and A. Schimpl. Regulation of lymphokine expression in T cell activation; I. Rapid loss of interleukin-specific RNA after removal of the stimulating signal, *Eur. J. Immunol.* 21:1691 (1991).
15. A.J.M. Van den Eertwegh, R.J. Noelle, M. Roy, D.M. Shepherd, A. Aruffo, J.A. Ledbetter, W.J.A. Boersma and E. Claassen. *In vivo* CD40-gp39 interactions are essential for thymus dependent humoral immunity. I. *In vivo* expression of CD40 ligand, cytokines and antibody production delineates sites of cognate T-B cell interactions, *J. Exp. Med.* 178:xxx (1993).
16. A.J.M. Van den Eertwegh and E. Claassen. T cells in the spleen: localization, cytokine production and cell-cell interactions. Forum of Immunology, *Res. Immunol* 142:334 (1991).
17. M.G. Cleveland, C.R. Annable, G.R. Klimpel. *In vivo* and *in vitro* production of IFN-β and IFN-γ during graft vs host disease, *J. Immunol* 141:3349 (1988).
18. A.J.M. Van den Eertwegh, M.J. Fasbender, W.J.A. Boersma and E. Claassen. *In vivo* detection, kinetics and characterization of interferon-gamma producing cells during a thymus dependent immune response: an immunohistochemical study, *in*: Lymphatic Tissues and In Vivo Immune Responses, B. Imhof, S. Berrih-Aknin, and S. Ezine, ed., Marcel Dekker Inc., New York (1991).
19. A.J.M. Van den Eertwegh, M.J. Fasbender, M.M. Schellekens, A. Van Oudenaren, W.J.A. Boersma and E. Claassen. *In vivo* kinetics and characterization of IFN-γ-producing cells during a thymus independent immune response, *J. of Immunol.* 147:439 (1991).
20. F.D. Finkelman, J. Holmes, I.M. Katona, J.F. Urban, M.P. Beckmann, L.S. Park, K.A. Schooley, R.L. Coffman, T.R. Mosman, and W.E. Paul. Lymphokine controle of in vivo immunoglobulin isotype selection, *Ann. Rev. Immunol.* 8:303 (1990).
21. A. Svetic, F.D. Finkelman, Y.C. Jian, C.W. Dieffenbach, D.E. Scott, K.F. McCarthy, A.D. Steinberg, and W.C. Gause. Cytokine gene expression after *in vivo* primary immunization with goat antibody to mouse IgD antibody, *J. Immunol* 147:2391 (1991).
22. A. Kelso, A.B. Troutt, E. Maraskovsky, N.M. Gough, M.H. Pech, and J.A. Thomson. Heterogeneity in lymphokine profiles of CD4$^+$ and CD8$^+$ T cells and clones activated *in vivo* and *in vitro*, *Immunol. Rev.* 123:85 (1991).
23. A.J.M. Van den Eertwegh, S. Ganesh, W.J.A. Boersma, and E. Claassen. In vivo activity of cells with different cytokine profile after immunization with an antibody to IgD, *in*: Cytokines: Basic Principles and Clinical Applications, S. Romagnani, T.R. Mosmann, and A.K. Abbas, ed., Raven press, New York (1992).
24. J.J. Mond, and M. Brunswick. A role for IFN-γ and NK cells in immune responses to T cell-regulated Antigens Types 1 and 2, *Immunol. Rev.* 99:105 (1987).
25. F.D. Finkelman, C.M. Snapper, J.D. Mountz, and I.M. Katona. Polyclonal activation of the murine immune system by a goat antibody to mouse IgD. IX. Induction of a polyclonal IgE response, *J. Immunol.* 138:2826 (1987).
26. F.D. Finkelman, D.K. Goroff, M. Fultz, S.C. Morris, J.M. Holmes, and J.J. Mond. Polyclonal activation of the murine immune system by an antibody to IgD; X. Evidence that the Precursors of IgG1-secreting cells are newly generated membrane IgD$^+$ B cells rather than the B cells that are initially activated by anti-IgD antibody, *J. Immunol* 145:3562 (1990).
27. A.J.M. Van den Eertwegh, W.J.A. Boersma, and E. Claassen. "Immunological functions and *in vivo* cell-cell interactions of T-cells in the spleen", *Critical Reviews in Immunology* 11:337 (1992).

DHEAS ENHANCES GERMINAL CENTER RESPONSES IN OLD MICE

Rebecca E. Caffrey[1], Zoher F. Kapasi[2], Stephen T. Haley[1], John G. Tew[2] and Andras K. Szakal[1]

[1]Department of Anatomy, Division of Immunobiology, Medical College of Virginia/VCU, Richmond, Virginia

[2]Department of Microbiology and Immunology, Medical College of Virginia/VCU, Richmond, Virginia

INTRODUCTION

Antigen (Ag) transport leads to the formation of the Ag retaining FDC-reticulum.[1] Studies have demonstrated that in old (23 month) mouse lymph nodes, Ag transport is defective and only a small fraction of the expected Ag transport sites develops.[2] The Ag transport sites that develop, form atrophic discontinuous pathways of globular structures. The Ag transport deficit corresponds to a similar deficit in the number of FDC-retaining reticula by day 1-3 after antigenic challenge. Follicular dendritic cells that develop are ultrastructurally atrophic, retain little Ag, and produce no iccosomes. In recent studies, we examined the capacity for germinal center development in old mice with a deficit of FDC Ag-retaining reticula. Germinal center development was monitored by image analysis utilizing the peanut agglutinin (PNA) binding feature of germinal center B cells histochemically with PNA-horseradish peroxidase (HRP) conjugates.[3] The results showed a marked age-related depression of germinal center development. Interestingly, the ratio of FDC-reticula to germinal center numbers remained 1:1, similarly to that shown for young immune mice.[3] These ratios support the concept that germinal center development in immune mice requires Ag-retaining FDC, an observation in complete agreement with the more recent *in vitro* data.[4] Thus the lack of capacity of old mice to produce germinal centers reflects age-related defects associated with antigen transport and FDC development.

Germinal centers are sites of memory B cell proliferation and affinity maturation in response to the stimulating antigen retained on the dendrites of FDC in the FDC-reticulum.[5-7] Consequently, FDC and germinal center development are important in the maintenance of long term humoral immunity.[8] Recently, we showed that in mice with an age-related depression of humoral immunity, FDC reticula and germinal center development could be reconstituted with equal efficiency using bone marrow and thymus transplants or bone marrow transplants alone.[9]

Age-associated changes in antibody responses were, more recently, shown to be reversed by dehydroepiandrosterone (DHEA) treatments.[10] DHEA and its sulfate ester (DHEAS) are the most abundant circulating adrenal steroids. DHEA is metabolized from DHEAS through the action of the enzyme DHEA sulfatase which is present in various tissues, including the macrophages of a number of lymph nodes.[11] DHEA through its intracellular receptor binding by T cells appears to influence the immune system.[12]

Our objective for the present study was to test the hypothesis that DHEA and/or DHEAS administration is capable of influencing FDC-reticulum development and, consequently, the development of lymph node germinal centers. This hypothesis appeared reasonable because DHEA acts through T cells by regulating T cell lymphokine production (i.e., IL-2[13] and IL-6[14]) and proliferation both of which are needed for T and B cell collaboration a requisite[15] of FDC-reticulum development.

Quantitation of PNA positive germinal centers showed that, subsequent to subcutaneous injection of DHEAS in the nape of the neck, the antigen-specific lymph node germinal center responses were significantly enhanced and essentially doubled in comparison to young controls within a period of six days after antigenic challenge of immune mice.

MATERIALS AND METHODS

Animals. C57BL/6 female mice of ages 6-8 wks and 21 mo were housed in a virus-free environment and given water and food *ad libitum*.

DHEA/DHEAS adminitration and immunization. Mice were passively immunized i.p. with 0.75 ml of horseradish peroxidase (HRP) specific rabbit antiserum. The following day (at appr. 21hrs after passive immunization) the mice were injected with 0.1 ml vehicle of DMSO or 0.1 ml DMSO containing 100 μg of DHEA or DHEAS subcutaneously in the nape of the neck. Three hours following this DHEA/DHEAS injection (at 24hrs), mice were challenged in all four footpads with 5μg of HRP (Type VI, Sigma).

Histochemistry. For the histochemical localization of the antigen, HRP, and PNA-HRP conjugates used for germinal center labeling at day 6 after hind and fore footpad injection of HRP (5 μgm/0.05 ml in saline), the animals were fixed by intracardiac perfusion as described previously.[3] Axillary, brachial and popliteal lymph nodes were serially sectioned at 50 μm thickness on a vibratome. For antigen localization and the PNA-HRP labelling of germinal centers the sections were developed in a DAB/H_2O_2 substrate.[15]

Image Analysis. To determine the *number* of germinal centers per lymph node, each PNA positive germinal center was identified and followed from beginning to end on serial sections. To determine the *volume (size)* of a germinal center, each section was evaluated using a Bioquant System IV (R&M Biometrics, INC., Nashville, TN.) as described.[15] The third parameter calculated was *compartment size*, defined as the sum of the volumes of all germinal centers per lymph node. Compartment size reflects of both the number and volume of the germinal centers. Since variations in germinal center numbers are often compensated by appropriate changes in germinal center size, compartment size is a good indicator for group comparisons. Significant differences were calculated according to Student's *t* test ($p \leq 0.05$ was considered significant).

RESULTS

Lymph nodes from four groups of passively immunized mice were evaluated. The first group was represented by young adults that received no hormone therapy and was only injected with the antigen, HRP; the second group of mice was vehicle (0.1 ml DMSO) injected, 21 mo old controls; the third group of mice was DHEA injected 21 mo old mice and the fourth group of mice was DHEAS injected 21 mo old mice. From each group of

4-6 mice, the draining axillary, brachial and popliteal lymph nodes were evaluated. Among these lymph nodes, the axillary and brachial lymph nodes were in the proximity of the DHEA(S) injection (nape of the neck) and were expected to be influenced by the hormone treatment. The popliteal lymph node, located at a distance from the DHEA(S) injection site [not draining DHEA(S)], was expected to serve as a negative control.

To exclude measurements of any germinal centers induced by environmental antigens (not associated with a HRP+ FDC-reticulum), it was important that all germinal centers quantitated be associated with a HRP-retaining FDC-reticulum (*de novo* germinal centers).

The results were calculated and plotted according to: 1. mean number of germinal centers (Fig. 1A), 2. mean germinal center size (Fig. 1B), and 3. mean germinal center compartment size (Fig. 1C). As a comparison, to evaluate the efficiency of the hormone treatment, a bar graph was also constructed to show germinal center numbers and compartment size for young adults and DHEAS treated old mice (Fig. 1D).

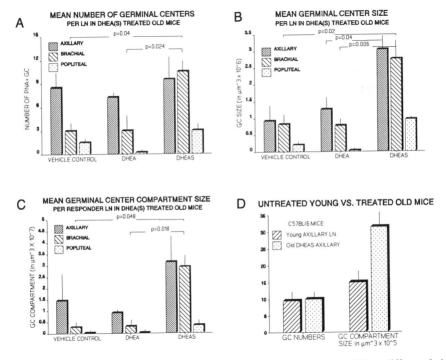

Figure 1. Effects of DHEA and DHEAS on the germinal center response of three different draining lymph nodes in 21 month old, passively immunized C57BL\6 female mice 6 days after antigenic challenge [6 days + 3 hours post DHEA(S)]. Error bars represent the standard error of the mean.

The data showed no significant enhancement of germinal center parameters in DHEA-treated old mice in any of the three types of lymph nodes examined (Fig. 1A-C). In the DHEAS group, a significant increase in germinal center numbers was detectable in comparison to vehicle controls in the brachial lymph node (Fig. 1A). Although no increase in germinal center numbers occurred in the axillary lymph nodes (except in the brachial nodes), mean germinal center size doubled after DHEAS treatment. Brachial lymph nodes after DHEAS-treatment showed significant increases in both numbers and in size. Increases in the numbers and size of popliteal nodes was not significant (Fig. 1B). The observed increases in germinal center numbers and size which figure into the calculation of the germinal center compartment size resulted in a significant 2-10 fold increases in values of axillary and brachial nodes over the vehicle controls (Fig. 1C). A trend for increase was also notable for the popliteal lymph node. The efficiency of stimulation of old lymph nodes by DHEAS is shown in Figure D. Although at this time this comparison is only available for axillary lymph nodes of young controls and old DHEAS-treated mice, the data shows that, in terms of compartment size (numbers did not change; see Fig. 1A), the capacity of axillary lymph nodes to produce germinal centers was successfully reconstituted. In fact, the compartment size in the axillary lymph node more than doubled (Fig. 1D).

DISCUSSION

Treatment of aged mice with DHEA and DHEAS is known to reverse age-related trends that culminate in immunodepression.[10] In the present study, we tested the hypothesis that DHEA/DHEAS treatments will also restore the capacity of old mice, known to have a $\geq 90\%$ deficit of FDC and germinal center development,[3] to produce normal germinal center responses. The data obtained support our contention and showed that DHEAS is capable of restoring germinal center development.

This preliminary study investigated the effects of DHEA and its sulfated form on old mice and showed that DHEAS significantly enhanced the germinal center response in two (axillary and brachial) of the three types of lymph nodes examined. When DHEAS effects on the axillary germinal center response of 21 month old mice were compared to the axillary germinal center response of young adults, the germinal center response in old mice under DHEAS influence clearly exceeded that of the response of non-DHEAS-treated young mice. Since compartment size reflects changes in both germinal center numbers and size and since germinal center numbers did not exceed that of young adults, the 50% excess in compartment size represents a 50% increase in germinal center size and consequently, in B memory cells.[3,8] Although, no special efforts were made at this time to quantitate FDC-reticulum development, we did make sure that the germinal centers quantitated could be associated with FDC-reticula in the adjacent sections. In the secondary antibody response, FDC-reticula and its associated retained antigen are known to be functional in the induction of germinal centers and an FDC-reticulum to Germinal center ratio of 1:1 is typically maintained.[3] The observations here clearly indicated that, at least in the brachial lymph nodes, DHEAS was able to reconstitute the capacity for the alternative antigen transport pathway. Regarding the axillary lymph node, although no increase in germinal center numbers occurred, germinal center size was significantly stimulated, an important effect that reflects a greater than twofold increase in potential B memory cells.

The lack of effect of the active form of the hormone, DHEA, was conspicuous. In contrast, DHEAS, the metabolically inactive form, was highly effective in the axillary and brachial lymph nodes; however, it did not effect the popliteal lymph nodes significantly. It is likely that DHEA, due to its short half life (between 30-60 min),[16] was inactivated by the time (3 hrs latter) the lymph nodes were stimulated by the injection of antigen. Conversely, DHEAS has a half life of 8-11 hours[16] and was not degraded before it could be converted to its active form, DHEA, by the activity of the enzyme DHEA sulfatase, present in increased quantities in secondary, non-mucosal lymphoid tissues such as lymph nodes.[16] Lymph node macrophages contain substantial endogenous DHEA sulfatase activity and may transport the active form of the hormone to local T cells through which DHEA has been shown to effect the immune system.[16] This information supports the contention that for stimulation of draining lymph nodes via subcutaneous routes the use of DHEAS is more desirable. The lack of DHEAS effect on the popliteal lymph nodes is not surprising and it confirms the expected drainage route from the nape of the neck.

Evidence indicates that FDC-reticulum development is dependent on the proper interaction between B and T cell populations and may be mediated by B and/or T cell lymphokines.[15] Evidence is also available which shows that DHEA achieves its effect on the immune system through a DHEA-binding receptor complex in T cells and the subsequent restoration of the capacity of old T cells to produce appropriate quantities of IL-2[13] and IL-6.[14] Therefore, the mechanisms of DHEAS-mediated repair of age-related defects in FDC[2] and germinal center[3] development include the conversion of DHEAS to DHEA and may involve the reestablishment of appropriate IL-2/IL-6 levels and T-B cell ratios and interactions required for the development of FDCs and associated germinal centers.

Acknowledgement

This work was supported by National Institutes of Health grants AG 05374 and AI 17142.

References

1. A.K. Szakal, K.L. Holmes, and J.G. Tew, Transport of immunecomplexes from the subcapsular sinus to lymph node follicles on the surface of nonphagocytic cells, including cells with dendritic morphology, *J. Immunol.* 131:1714 (1983).
2. A.K. Szakal, J.K. Taylor, J.P. Smith, M.H. Kosco, G.F. Burton, and J.G. Tew, Morphometry and Kinetics of antigen transport and developing antigen retaining reticulum of follicular dendritic cells in lymph nodes of aging immune mice, *Aging: Immunol. and Inf. Dis.* 1:7 (1988).
3. A.K. Szakal, J.K. Taylor, J.P. Smith, M.H. Kosco, G.F. Burton, and J.G. Tew, Kinetics of germinal center development in lymph nodes of young and aging immune mice. *Anat. Rec.* 227:475 (1990).
4. M.H. Kosco, E. Pflugfelder, and D. Gray, Follicular dendritic cell-dependent adhesion and proliferation of B cells in vitro, *J. Immunol.* 148:2331 (1992).
5. J.G. Tew, M.H. Kosco and A.K. Szakal, The alternative antigen pathway. *Immunology Today* 10:229 (1989).
6. A.K. Szakal, M.H. Kosco and J.G. Tew, Microanatomy of lymphoid tissue during humoral immune responses: Structure function relationships. *Ann. Rev. Immunol.* 7:91, (1989).
7. I.C.M. MacLennan and D. Gray, Antigen-driven selection of virgin and memory B cells. *Immunol. Rev.* 91:61-85, (1986).
8. J.G. Tew, M.H. Kosco, G.F. Burton and A.K.Szakal, Follicular dendritic cells as accessory cells, *Immunol. Rev.* 117:185 (1990).
9. Z.F. Kapasi, J.G. Tew and A.K.Szakal, Germinal center development and the secondary antibody response following bone marrow and thymus transplants in old mice, *Aging: Immunol. and Inf. Dis.* 4:(2):*In press* (1993).
10. R.A. Daynes and B.A. Araneo, Prevention and reversal of some age-associated changes in immunologic responses by supplemental dehydroepiandrosterone sulfate therapy, *Aging: Immunol. and Inf. Dis.* 3:(3):135, (1992).
11. R.A. Daynes, B.A. Araneo, T.A. Dowell, K. Huang, D. Dudley, Regulation of murine lymphokine production *in vivo*. III. The lymphoid tissue microenvironment exerts regulatory influences over T-helper cell function, *J. Exp. Med.* 171:979 (1990).
12. A.W. Meikle, R.W. Dorchuck, B.A. Araneo, J.D. Stringham T.G. Evans, S.L. Spruance and R.A. Daynes, The presence of a dehydroepiandrosterone-specific receptor binding complex in murine T cells, *J. Steroid Biochem.* 42:293 (1992).
13. R.A. Daynes, D.J. Dudley and B.A. Araneo, Regulation of murine lymphokine production *in vivo*. II. Dehydroepiandrosterone is a natural enhancer of interleukin 2 synthesis by helper T cells, *Eur. J. Immunol.* 20:793 (1990).
14. R.A. Daynes, B.A. Araneo, W.B. Ershler, C. Maloney, Gang-Zhou Li and Si-Yun Ryu, Altered regulation of IL-6 production with normal Aging, *J. Immunol.* 150:5219 (1993).
15. Z.F. Kapasi, G.F. Burton, L.D. Shultz, J.G. Tew and A.K. Szakal, Induction of follicular dendritic cell development in severe combined immunodeficiency mice: Influence of B and T cells. *J. Immunol.* 150:2648 (1993).
16. A.W. Meikle, R.A. Daynes and B.A. Araneo, Adrenal androgen secretion and biologic effects, *Endocr. and Matabol. Clinics of North America* 20: 381 (1991).

CELLULAR ORIGIN OF FOLLICULAR DENDRITIC CELLS

Zoher F. Kapasi,[1,2] Marie H. Kosco-Vilbois,[2] Leonard D. Shultz,[4]
John G. Tew,[1] and Andras K. Szakal[3]

Departments of [1]Microbiology/Immunology and [3]Anatomy/Immunobiology
Medical College of Virginia, Virginia Commonwealth University
Richmond, Virginia 23298, U.S.A.
[2]Basel Institute for Immunology, Basel, Switzerland
[4]The Jackson Laboratory, Bar Harbor, Maine, U.S.A.

INTRODUCTION

Follicular dendritic cells (FDC) are found in follicles of all secondary lymphoid organs. These FDC bind and retain immune complexes on the surface of their dendrites and serve as a long term repository for unprocessed antigen which is believed to maintain both B cell memory and secondary antibody responses.[1] The origin of this unique cell type has not been unequivocally established. Several authors have studied the ontogenic development of FDC in lymphoid organs of rat,[2,3,4] mouse[5] and rabbit.[6] Based on a number of morphological similarities these investigators suggest that FDC are a differentiated form of fibroblastic reticulum cells. On the basis of enzyme histochemical studies on human FDC, Rademakers et. al.[7] suggest FDC to be a differentiated form of mesenchymal cells. Based on studies with mouse radiation chimeras, Humphrey et al.[8] concluded that follicular dendritic cell (FDC) precursors are not derived from the bone marrow. In this study, chimeras maintained for over a year continued to express H-2 antigens of host phenotype on the FDC. We have confirmed Humphrey's observation (Kosco and Burton et. al., unpublished observations). However, in our studies an essential control failed. FDC are radioresistant and were not eliminated by doses of irradiation that exceeded 1200 R. Clearly the lymphocytes and macrophages were eliminated by high doses of irradiation but functional FDC were still present in the lymph nodes (Burton et al., unpublished). Thus it may be argued that on account of the radioresistant nature of FDC, host FDC were not eliminated from the recipients and their presence may have inhibited donor FDC from developing normally.

Some data supports the concept that FDC are derived from the bone marrow. For example, the antigenic phenotype of FDC is very compatible with cells of bone marrow origin. Cell surface markers that FDC bear in common with bone marrow derived cells include: ICAM-1, Class II, common leukocyte antigen, C3b receptors and Fc receptors (both FcγRII & FcεRII).[1] Furthermore, antigen transport cells, which morphologically appear to develop into FDC, are reactive with the monoclonal antibody produced against FDC (FDC-M1) and bind immune complexes like FDC.[1] The antigen transport cells appear to be of monocytic origin.[9] In addition, Parwaresch et al.[10] demonstrated that the mAb KiM4 with its highly restricted reactivity to FDC also reacts with an endogenous peroxidase-positive mononuclear blood subset. These authors suggest that KiM4+ mononuclear cells are possibly circulating precursors of FDC. The fact, that the mAb KiM4 was originally raised against a highly purified fraction of the homogenous histiocytic cell line, U-937 closely related to monocytes, is a further argument for the monocyte/macrophage origin of FDC.

Severe combined immunodeficient (SCID) mice lack functional B and T cells[11] and we have recently shown that they also lack FDC.[12] We reasoned that the SCID mouse would provide a useful model to study the origin of FDC since the problem of eliminating radioresistant FDC could be bypassed. Studies from other laboratories have demonstrated that SCID mice accept xenogeneic transplants.[13,14] The objective of the present study was determine if FDC were of bone marrow origin by using this SCID mouse model. In the present study SCID mice were reconstituted with F_1 (Balb/c x C57BL/6) bone marrow, rat bone marrow or rat fetal liver cells. We then looked for rat FDC in the recipients or FDC bearing the donor (C57BL/6) class I molecules. We report here that FDC of the donor phenotype can be found using the SCID mouse model.

MATERIALS AND METHODS

Animals

Newborn or 6-8 weeks old homozygous mutant C.B.17-scid/scid (SCID) and F_1 (Balb/c x C57BL/6) mice were obtained from The Jackson Laboratory, Bar Harbor ME. Lewis rats (6-8 weeks old) and pregnant Lewis rats (day 16 gestation) were purchased from Harlan Laboratories, Indianapolis, IN. The animals were housed in a specific pathogen free environment and given food and water ad libitum.

Cell Transfers For Reconstitution

Prior to cell transfer, SCID mice were irradiated with 300 rads to facilitate reconstitution. Bone marrow (BM) cells were obtained from femurs and tibias of F_1 mice and Lewis rats. Rat fetal liver cells were obtained by homogenizing the fetal livers between frosted ends of slides. For reconstitutions, 6-8 weeks old SCID mice received i.v. $2x10^7$ murine BM or $5x10^7$ rat fetal liver cells suspended in 200 μl of Hank's balanced salt solution supplemented with HEPES (25mM) and gentamicin (50 μg/ml). Newborn SCID mice received 10^7 rat BM or rat fetal liver cells i.p.

Immunohistochemistry

The mouse-anti-rat FDC specific mAb ED5[15] (a generous gift from Dr. C.D. Dijkstra), was used to detect rat FDC. Mouse FDC were detected by unconjugated or biotynylated rat-anti-mouse FDC reactive mAb, FDC-M1.[16] Biotynylated anti H-2K^b and anti H-2K^d mAbs were obtained from Pharmingen. The following second step reagents were used, fluorescein conjugated rat anti-mouse F(ab')2 IgG (H+L) and mouse anti-rat F(ab')2 IgG (H+L) (Jackson Immunoresearch), Streptavidin-FITC and streptavidin-texas red (Southern Biotechnology). Lymph nodes and spleen from reconstituted SCID mice were immediately embedded in Tissue Tek II O.C.T. compound and frozen on dry ice. Sections were then cut at 6-8μm thickness with a cryostat and mounted onto poly-L-lysine coated slides. After fixing in cold acetone for 30 seconds and air drying for one hour, immunohistochemistry was performed by incubating these sections with different primary antibodies in phosphate buffered saline (PBS) with 1% BSA for 2 hrs. at room temperature. The sections from F_1 bone marrow reconstituted SCID mice were incubated simultaneously with anti class I antibodies and FDC-M1. The sections were washed three times in PBS over a period of 15 mins and incubated in optimal dilutions of secondary reagents for 1 hr. at ambient temperature. The sections were then washed and mounted in Mowiol and Dabco (Fluka) and photographed. Negative controls of sections incubated with only second step reagents or with inappropriate isotype specific antibodies were negative.

RESULTS

Six to eight weeks after reconstituting SCID mice with rat bone marrow or fetal liver cells and four to six months after F_1 bone marrow cell transfer, spleen and lymph nodes were harvested, sectioned and analyzed for FDC of both the donor and host phenotype. The findings are summarized in Table 1.

Table 1. Phenotype of FDC in chimeric animals

Cell Transfers	Monoclonal Antibodies	Phenotype of FDC reticula in different sites		
Rat BM → SCID	FDC-M1	-	+	+
	ED5	+	-	+
Rat FL → SCID	FDC-M1	-	+	n.s.
	ED5	+	-	n.s.
F_1 → SCID	FDC-M1 H-2H^d	+	+	n.a.
	FDC-M1 H-2K^b	-	+	n.a.

Rat BM = Rat bone marrow; Rat FL = Rat fetal liver; n.a. = Not applicable; n.s. = Not seen

Clearly reconstituting mice with rat bone marrow or fetal liver was sufficient to elicit the maturation of murine FDC in both the lymph nodes and the spleen. However, FDC reticula in some sites did not react with the murine FDC marker FDC-M1 but did react with the rat FDC specific marker ED5. Furthermore, as indicated in the third column under "Phenotype of FDC reticula in different sites" in Table 1, some reticula contained both rat and mouse FDC. Of seven rat bone marrow reconstituted SCID mice, 3 clearly showed the presence of ED5+ FDC reticula in lymph nodes and spleens. Similarly, 1 of 5 SCID mice reconstituted with rat fetal liver cell reconstituted SCID mice also had rat FDC in their lymphoid organs. The FDC-M1 positive FDC were not reactive with ED5 indicating that the mAb ED5, as reported previously,[15] does not crossreact with mouse FDC. Similarly, the ED5 positive cells did not crossreact with the mAb FDC-M1. In some rat reconstituted mice that lacked rat FDC, it did not appear that the rat cells had successfully engrafted. In others there were sites where a few ED5 positive cells appeared to be present in follicles but the typical large FDC reticula were not apparent and the animals were scored as negative.

In some sites in the F_1 bone marrow reconstituted SCID mice, it appeared that FDC reticula only showed the presence of host class I molecules, however, in numerous sites FDC reticula also bore donor class I molecules. The presence of host FDC is not surprising since these cells are radiation resistant. The best we could hope for would be a significant number of FDC also bearing the donor phenotype and this was achieved.

DISCUSSION

The major finding reported here is that bone marrow or fetal liver contains FDC precursors. The presence of donor class I molecules on FDC in F_1 bone marrow reconstituted SCID mice and ED5 positive FDC in rat BM or rat fetal liver reconstituted SCID mice strongly supports the bone marrow as an origin for FDC. Furthermore, the data suggests the possibility that FDC may be of hematopoietic origin and experiments are underway to see if FDC might be members of the myeloid lineage.

The radioresistant nature of FDC makes it difficult to eliminate these cells in mice and it is possible that in previous radiation chimera studies[8] the persistence of host FDC inhibited or markedly diluted the donor FDC in the tissue. SCID mice lack FDC[12] and therefore the problem of eliminating host FDC at the outset can be bypassed. Recently, we showed that transferring B and T cells can induce FDC development in SCID mice suggesting the presence of FDC precursors in these mice. [12] The fact that rat bone marrow cells would support the development of murine FDC, noted in the present study, further supports the concept that FDC precursors are present in SCID mice. Since in ontogeny FDC do not appear until about 3 weeks after birth, we reasoned that transferring rat BM or fetal liver cells to newborn SCID mice would give an advantage to donor over host FDC precursors in the differentiation pathway leading to mature FDC. In the present study we noted that a given follicle tended to have either donor or host FDC predominating although there were follicles with both cell types. The presence of host FDC is not surprising considering that SCID mice have FDC precursors and these can develop into FDC under the influence of syngeneic or xenogeneic B and T cells. Nevertheless, the presence of FDC bearing donor phenotype was apparent and this is the major finding reported here.

ACKNOWLEDGMENTS

This work was supported by the National Institutes of Health Research Grants AG 05374, AI 17142, and AI 30389. The Basel Institute for Immunology was founded and is supported by F. Hoffmann-La Roche Ltd., Basel, Switzerland.

234

REFERENCES

1. J.G. Tew, M.H. Kosco, G.F. Burton, and A.K. Szakal, Follicular dendritic cells as accessory cells, *Immunol.Rev.* 117:185 (1990).
2. C.D. Dijkstra, N.J. Van Tilburg, and E.A. Dopp, Ontogenetic aspects of immune complex trapping in rat spleen and popliteal lymph nodes, *Cell Tissue Res.* 223:545 (1982).
3. A. Villena, A. Zapata, J.M. Rivera-Pomar, M.G. Barrutia, and J. Fonfua, Structure of non lymphoid-cells during the postnatal development of the rat lymph nodes, fibroblastic reticulum cells and interdigitating cells, *Cell Tissue Res.* 229:219 (1983).
4. C.D. Dijkstra, E.W.A. Kamperdijk, and E.A. Dopp, The ontogenetic development of the follicular dendritic cell. An ultrastructural study by means of intravenously injected horseradish peroxidase (HRP)-anti-HRP complexes as marker, *Cell Tissue Res.* 236:203 (1984).
5. P. Groscurth. Non-lymphatic cells in the lymph node cortex of the mouse. II. Postnatal development of the interdigitating cells and the dendritic reticular cells. *Path. Res. Pract.* 169:235 (1980).
6. U. Heusermann, K.H. Zurborn, L. Schroeder, and M.J. Stutte, The origin of the dendritic reticulum cell. An experimental enzyme-histochemical and electron microscopic study on the rabbit spleen, *Cell Tissue Res.* 209:279 (1980).
7. L.H.P.M. Rademakers. Follicular dendritic cells in germinal centre development, *Res. Immunol.* 142:257 (1991)
8. J.H. Humphrey, D. Grennan, and V. Sundaram, The origin of follicular dendritic cells in the mouse and the mechanism of trapping of immune complexes on them, *Eur.J.Immunol.* 14:859 (1984).
9. A.K. Szakal, K.L. Holmes, and J.G. Tew, Transport of immune complexes from the subcapsular sinus to lymph node follicles on the surface of nonphagocytic cells, including cells with dendritic morphology, *J.Immunol.* 131:1714 (1983).
10. M.R. Parwaresch, H.J. Radzun, A.C. Feller, K.P. Peters, and M.L. Hansmann, Peroxidase-positive mononuclear leukocytes as possible precursors of human dendritic reticulum cells, *J.Immunol.* 131:2719 (1983).
11. G.C. Bosma, R.P. Custer, and M.J. Bosma, A severe combined immunodeficiency mutation in the mouse, *Nature.* 301:527 (1983).
12. Z.F. Kapasi, G.F. Burton, L.D. Shultz, J.G. Tew, and A.K. Szakal, Induction of functional follicular dendritic cell development in severe combined immunodeficiency mice: influence of B and T cells, *J.Immunol.* 150:2648 (1993).
13. J.M. McCune, R. Namikawa, H. Kaneshima, L.D. Shultz, M. Lieberman, and I.L. Weissman, The SCID-hu Mouse: Murine model for the analysis of human hematolymphoid differentiation and function, *Science.* 241:1632 (1988).
14. C.D. Surh, and J. Sprent, Long term xenogeneic chimeras-Full differentiation of rat T and B cells in SCID mice, *J.Immunol.* 147:2148 (1991).
15. S.H.M. Jeurissen, and C.D. Dijkstra, Characteristics and functional aspects of nonlymphoid cells in rat germinal centers, recognized by two monoclonal antibodies ED5 and ED6, *Eur.J.Immunol.* 16:562 (1986).
16. M.H. Kosco, E. Pflugfelder, and D. Gray, Follicular dendritic cell-dependent adhesion and proliferation of B cells in vitro, *J.Immunol.* 148:2331 (1992).

GERMINAL CENTERS DEVELOP AT PREDILICTED SITES IN THE CHICKEN SPLEEN

Suzan H.M. Jeurissen and E. Marga Janse

Central Veterinary Institute, Department of Virology
P.O. Box 365, 8200 AJ Lelystad, The Netherlands

INTRODUCTION

Recently the various compartments of the chicken spleen were investigated for their role during the induction and effector phase of the humoral immune response against T-cell dependent antigens (1). In general, all events in the chicken spleen occurred at similar timepoints and at similar sites as they do in the mammalian spleen. For example, antigen-specific antibody-containing cells were first detected in peri-arteriolar T cell sheaths (PALS) and later in the red pulp (2). The induction of the response was found to occur in the complex of ellipsoid, peri-ellipsoid B lymphocyte sheath (PELS) and surrounding macrophages, which is therefore the functional analogue of the mammalian marginal zone with its sinus, B lymphocytes and non-lymphoid cells (3).

The precise site and moment, however, that germinal centers (GC) are induced in the chicken spleen during a humoral immune response, are unknown. Primary B cell follicles, where GC develop in the mammalian spleen, do not exist. In contrast, mature germinal centers, which are encapsulated, are located next to arteries and arterioles, thus in T cell areas. Recently, we described monoclonal antibody CVI-ChNL-74.3 that recognizes follicular dendritic cells (FDC) in mature GC (3). Although chicken FDC do not have such long and slender processes, these cells functionally represent FDC as they trap autologous and heterologous immune complexes (3, 4). In addition, monoclonal antibody CVI-ChNL-74.3 recognized clusters of dendritic cells next to arteries and arterioles (3). As this is exactly the site where germinal centers develop, we hypothesized that these clusters of 74.3-positive cells represent immature FDC. To study whether during a humoral immune response GC are indeed induced at the site of these clusters, chickens were immunized and various days later germinal centers were recognized as clusters of B cells in active cell cycle. In the present study, germinal centers always developed around the clusters of CVI-ChNL-74.3-positive dendritic cells, which therefore indeed represent precursor FDC.

MATERIALS AND METHODS

Animals

White Leghorn strain A chickens were bred and kept under specific-pathogen-free conditions. At the age of 4 weeks, groups of 3 chickens were injected i.v. with 200 µg trinitrophenyl conjugated keyhole limpet hemocyanine (TNP-KLH). After 1, 2, 3, 4, 5, 6, and 7 days, the chickens were injected i.v. with 5 mg 5-bromo-2'-deoxiuridine (BrdU; Sigma Chemical Co., St. Louis, MO, USA). Three hrs later, spleens were removed, frozen in liquid nitrogen, and used for 8 µm cryostat sections.

Simultaneous Detection of Splenic Cell Populations, Anti-TNP Antibody-Containing Cells, and BrdU-Positive Cells

Cryostat sections were fixed in pure acetone for 10 min. First, slides were incubated overnight at 4 °C with alkaline-phosphatase conjugated TNP (4). Second, they were incubated for 45 min with mouse monoclonal antibodies specific for splenic cell populations and then with peroxidase conjugated rabbit-anti mouse Ig (Dakopatts, Glostrup, Denmark). Subsequently, the alkaline phosphatase activity was visualized with Fast Blue BB base (blue color), whereas the peroxidase activity was visualized with diaminobenzidine (brown color). Third, slides were treated with 0.035 N NaOH for 10 min and 5% HAc for 1 min to expose and partially degrade the DNA. This also served to terminate the immunoenzymatic reactions which had taken place on the slides previously. The slides were then incubated with mouse anti-BrdU (MoBu-1; 5; a kind gift of Dr. L. de Ley) followd by peroxidase conjugated rabbit anti-mouse Ig (Dakopatts). The peroxidase activity was visualized with amino-ethylcarbazole (red color).

Monoclonal antibodies

Monoclonal antibodies with the following specificities were used: HIS-C1, B lymphocytes (6); HIS-C12, IgM (6); CVI-ChNL-68.2, ellipsoid-associated dendritic cells (7); CVI-ChNL-74.3, follicular dendritic cells (3); MoBu-1, BrdU (5).

RESULTS AND DISCUSSION

At all timepoints, clusters of dendritic stromal cells in T-cell areas next to arterioles were stained by monoclonal antibody CVI-ChNL-74.3 (Fig. 1a). In these young chickens, only few follicular dendritic cells were found in mature (encapsulated) germinal centers. At days 1 and 2, many single BrdU-positive cells were found in the white and the red pulp, but no clusters of BrdU-positive cells. From day 3 on, clusters of BrdU-positive cells were located next to arteries and arterioles. These clusters of BrdU-positive cells were double stained with HIS-C1, specific for B cells. Therefore, these clusters of BrdU- and HIS-C1-positive B-cells represent developing germinal centers. The localization of the developing germinal centers was not related to the sheaths of CVI-ChNL-68.2-positive ellipsoid-associated dendritic cells (EADC). This result might be surprising as in lower vertebrates, like toads and turtles which lack germinal centers, these EADC have been suggested to represent FDC as they trap immune complexes (8, 9). In the chicken, however, these EADC are only involved in the handling of all kinds of antigens, including immune complexes, when they enter the white pulp from the blood (10). From there most antigens are distributed over specific compartments and immune complexes are selectively trapped in germinal centers.

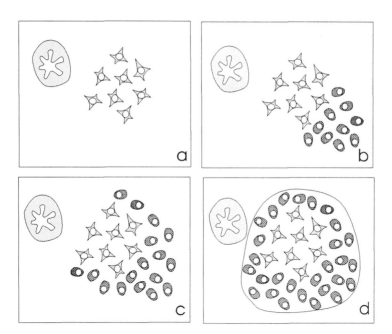

Fig. 1. Schematic diagram of the development of germinal centers during a primary immune response. a) Next to an arteriole, clusters of CVI-ChNL-74.3-positive dendritic cells are located. b) The first BrdU-positive B cells localize on one site of the clusters of dendritic cells. c). Later, BrdU-positive B cells obtain the form of a horseshoe around the dendritic cells. d). In fully developed germinal centers, BrdU-positive B cells surround CVI-ChNL-74.3-positive follicular dendritic cells.

In addition, the development of germinal centers was unrelated to the plasmacellular reaction as well. After immunization with KLH-TNP, the first anti-TNP antibody-containing cells were detected at day 2. Their number increased considerably at days 3 and 4, then decreased again at days 5 and 6, whereas they were not detected anymore at day 7. The anti-TNP antibody-containing cells were located in foci, comparable to those described in the mammalian spleen after primary immunization (2, 11). First anti-TNP antibody-containing cells were located in T-cell areas, but most of them were found in the red pulp. Never, anti-TNP antibody-containing cells were detected in or near developing germinal centers. Therefore, the site of germinal center development is unrelated to that of the simulataneously induced antigen-specific plasma cells. Using computer-aided restruction of a sectioned spleen, germinal centers and foci of plasma cells were elegantly shown to lack physical communication in the mouse spleen (11). From day 4 on, TNP-specific extracellular antibodies were sporadically detected in newly formed germinal centers. These antibodies represented immune complexes trapped by FDC. As these immune complexes were only found two days after the first newly developed germinal centers, they do not seem to play an important role in the induction of germinal centers. This result coincides with those of Kroese et al. obtained in mammals. In lethally irradiated and reconstituted rats, germinal centers develop 2 days before the capacity to trap immune complexes is restored (12). It is to be expected that, like in mammals, trapped immune complexes are important in the memory formation in the chicken as well.

The induction site of germinal centers seems to be directed by pre-existing stromal cells as clusters of BrdU-positive cells were always associated with clusters of

CVI-ChNL-74.3-positive cells. The first detectable small round clusters of BrdU-positive cells were located adjacent to the clusters of CVI-ChNL-74.3-positive cells (Fig. 1b). In a latter stage (day 3-5), larger clusters of BrdU-positive cells obtained the form of a horse-shoe. In the middle of the horse-shoe, the CVI-ChNL-74.3-positive cells were located (Fig. 1c). The clusters of BrdU-positive cells that increased in size even further, started to resemble mature germinal centers. In these germinal centers (from day 4 on), BrdU-containing germinal center B cells completely surrounded the CVI-ChNL-74.3-positive follicular dendritic cells (Fig. 1d). Interestingly, cells in the middle of the germinal center had not incorporated BrdU during the three previous hours. These cells were thus not mitotically active and might resemble centrocytes, whereas the BrdU-positive cells might represent centroblasts. Liu and coworkers have demonstrated that centrocytes are derived from centroblasts, which were in cell cycle during the previous 12 hours (13).Although morphologically, a light zone of centrocytes and a dark zone of centroblasts, as described in mammalian germinal centers, can not be discriminated in the chicken, the functional differences between the two cell types seems to be present as well.

The results of this study show that germinal centers selectively develop around clusters of CVI-ChNL-74.3-positive dendritic cells in T-cell areas. These clusters therefore represent precursor FDC. Studies with monoclonal antibodies and electron-microscopy have shown striking similarities between FDC and pericyte-like mesenchymal cells along arterioles in mice and humans as well (14, 15). Although many other components, such as complement factor C3 and adhesion molecules, can not be ruled out to be important as well, CVI-ChNL-74.3-positive cells seem to be decisive during the induction of germinal centers. In further studies we will investigate whether the ability to form germinal centers is reflected by the ontogenic development of CVI-ChNL-74.3-positive cells.

CONCLUSIONS

In an unstimulated spleen, many clusters of CVI-ChNL-74.3-positive stromal cells are found near arteries and arterioles. During a humoral immune response, newly developing germinal centers, which consist of BrdU-incorporating B cells, are located next to clusters of CVI-ChNL-74.3-positive cells. During the development, germinal center B cells grow around the clusters of CVI-ChNL-74.3-positive cells untill they completely surround them. In mature germinal centers, CVI-ChNL-74.3-positive cells can trap immune complexes on their surface; these cells are now follicular dendritic cells. Therefore, the clusters of CVI-ChNL-74.3-positive stromal cells represent the precursor cells of follicular dendritic cells. As these clusters of CVI-ChNL-74.3-positive cells are already present before immunization, germinal centers thus develop at pre-dilicted sites in the chicken spleen.

REFERENCES

1. Jeurissen, S.H.M. The role of various compartments in the chicken spleen during an antigen-specific humoral response. Immunology, in press
2. Van Rooijen, N., Claassen, E. & Eikelenboom, P. Is there a single differentiation pathway for all antibody-forming cells in the spleen? Immunol. Today 7: 193-196, 1986
3. Jeurissen, S.H.M., Claassen, E. & E.M. Janse. Histological and functional diffe-rentiation of non-lymphoid cells in the chicken spleen. Immunology 77: 75-80, 1992

4. Claassen, E., Gerritse, K., Laman, J.D. & Boersma, W.J.A. New immunoenzyme-cytochemical stainings for the in situ detection of epitope specificity and isotype of antibody forming B cells in experimental and natural (auto)immune responses in animals and man. J. Immunol. Meth. 147: 207-216, 1992

5. Harms, G., van Goor, H., Koudstaal, J., de Ley, L. & Hardonk, M.J. Immunohisto-chemical demonstration of DNA-incorporated 5-bromodeoxyuridine in frozen and plastic embedded sections. Histochemistry 85: 139-143, 1986

6. Jeurissen, S.H.M., Janse, E.M., Ekino, S., Nieuwenhuis, P., Koch, G. & de Boer, G.F. Monoclonal antibodies as probes for defining cellular subsets in the bone marrow, thymus, bursa of Fabricius, and spleen of the chicken. Vet. Immunol. Immunopathol. 19: 225-238, 1988

7. Jeurissen, S.H.M., Janse, E.M., Kok, G.L. & de Boer, G.F. Distribution and function of non-lymphoid cells positive for monoclonal antibody CVI-ChNL-68.2 in healthy chickens and those infected with Marek's Disease Virus. Vet. Immunol. Immunopathol. 22: 123-133, 1989

8. Baldwin, W.M. & Cohen, N. A gaint cell with dendritic cell properties in spleens of anuran amphibian Xenopus laevis. Devel. Comp. Immunol. 5: 461-473, 1981

9. Kroese, F.G.M. & van Rooijen, N. Antigen trapping in the spleen of the turtle, Chrysemys scripta elegans. Immunology 49: 61-68, 1983

10. Jeurissen, S.H.M., Janse, E.M. & de Boer, G.F. Antigen handling by nonlymphoid cells in the chicken spleen. In: Lymphatic tissues and in vivo immune responses (Eds B.A. Imhof, S. Berrih-Aknin & S. Ezine). Marcel Dekker Inc., p. 771-775, 1991

11. Jacob, J., Kassir, R. & Kelsoe, G. In situ studies of the primary immune response to (4-hydroxy-3-nitrophenyl)acetyl. I. The architecture and dynamics of responding cell populations. J. Exp. Med. 173: 1165-1175

12. Kroese, F.G.M., Wubbena, A.S. & Nieuwenhuis, P. Germinal center formation and follicular antigen trapping in the spleen of lethally X-irradiated and reconstituted rats. Immunology 57: 99-104, 1986

13. Liu, Y-J, Zhang, J., Lane, P.J.L., Chan, E.Y-T. & MacLennan, I.C.M. Sites of specific B cell activation in primary and secondary responses to T cell-dependent and T cell-independent antigens. Eur. J. Immunol. 21: 2951-2962, 1991

14. Rademakers, L.H.P.M. Follicular dendritic cells in germinal centre development. Res. Immunol. 142: 257-260, 1991

15. Terashima, K., Dobashi, M., Maeda, K. & Imai, Y. Cellular components involved in the germinal centre reaction. Res. Immunol. 142: 263-268, 1991

EXPRESSION AND FUNCTION OF DRC-1 ANTIGEN

Alain L. Bosseloir, Nadine Antoine, Ernst Heinen, Thierry DeFrance,*
Henk Schuurman,** and Léon Simar

Laboratory of Human Histology
University of Liège
4020 Liège
Belgium
*Institut Pasteur
Lyon
France
**Academish Centrum
Utrecht
The Netherlands

INTRODUCTION

Immune responses are generated by a series of cellular interactions which occur in distinct microenvironments. The germinal centre (GC) plays a central role in B cell proliferation and differentiation as well as in generating the secondary immune response. The architecture of the GC is designed to support cell-to-cell interactions[1,2].

In 1983, Naiem et al. produced a monoclonal antibody (type IgM, K) with which they successfully immunolabelled the germinal centres on cryosections. This antibody recognizes a follicular dendritic cell membrane antigen called DRC-1. A slight signal was mentioned on the mantle and marginal zone[3]. In immunofluorescence experiments, spleen and tonsillar B and T lymphocytes appeared DRC-1 negative[3,4]. Terashima et al.[5] have distinguished, by immunoelectron microscopy, three DRC-1 positive cells: type A (in the germinal centre), type B (in the corona), type C (outside the follicle). DRC-1 positive mononuclear cells were encountered in the peripheral blood of some autoimmune disease patients. In a recent study, one-third of EBV-B cells lines revealed DRC-1 expression and approximately 90% of CD20 positive tonsillar cells and 50% of the blood CD20 positive cells reacted with DRC-1[6].

We have focused on the phenotype of cells expressing the DRC-1 antigen and analysed its function and modulation by cytokines and activators.

MATERIALS AND METHODS

Reagents

Rabbit anti-human immunoglobulins coupled to polyacrylamide beads were purchased from Biorad Laboratories (Richmond, CA) and used at a final dilution of 1/600. Staphylococcus aureus Cowan I (SAC) was purchased from Calbiochem-Behring Corporation (La Jolla, CA) and used at a final concentration of 0.005% (v/v). Purified IL-2 was purchased from Amgen Biologicals (Thousand Oaks, CA) and was used at 10 U/ml throughout the study. Purified recombinant IL-10 was a generous gift from Dr. J. Banchereau (Shering-Plough, France) and was used at a final concentration of 100 ng/ml. IL-4 was used as a 0.5% dilution of a culture supernatant of Cos 7 cells transfected with the human IL-4 cDNA clone kindly provided by Dr. A. Minty (Sanofi, France). PMA were purchased from Sigma (St Louis, MO) and used at a final concentration of 10ng/ml.

Antibodies

Table 1 shows the mab used in this study. FITC and PE-conjugated streptavidin were from Becton Dickinson (Moutain View, CA).

Cultures

All cultures were grown in RPMI 1640 medium supplemented with 10% selected heat-inactivated FCS, 2 mM L-glutamine, 100 U/ml penecillin, 100 ug/ml streptomycin, and 2% Hepes (all from GIBCO BRL Laboratories, Grand Island, N.Y.). For proliferation and differentiation, B cells were dispensed at 5×10^4 or 1×10^5 cells per well into 96-well microtiter trays at a final culture volume of 0.1 ml for proliferation and 0.2 ml for differentiation assays. DNA synthesis was determined by pulsing the cells with [^{3}H] thymidine for the last 16 h of the culture period. IgG and IgM levels were determined in 7-to-10-day culture supernatants by standard ELISA techniques as described elsewhere[7]. For modulation of DRC-1 antigen expression, B cells were dispensed at 6×10^5 cells per well into 24-well microtiter trays at a final culture volume of 1.4 ml. Cytokines and polyclonal B cell activators were added at the onset. DRC-1 expression was determined in 2-day cultures.

Immunofluorescence staining

The cells were incubated with the anti-DRC-1 mab and with an appropriate conjugate. For two-color analysis, cells labelled with anti-DRC-1 mab were stained with PE-conjugated anti-CD3 or CD19 or CD14 mab. Irrelevant IgM and PE-conjugated IgG were used for control tests. The cells were analysed with a FACScan (Becton Dickinson, Mountain Vieuw, CA).

Immunoenzymatic staining

DRC-1 positive cells were identified on cytocentrifuge preparations of B cell populations by enzyme cytochemistry. After 10 min. fixation in acetone at -20°C, the slides were incubated with anti-DRC-1 mab, Goat anti-mouse IgM biotinylated antibodies and steptABComplex HRP (DAKO). Peroxidase activity was visualized by incubation with the AEC substrate solution in acetate buffer, pH=4.9. Cells were counterstained with haematoxylin and embedded in Eukitt (Kindler).

Cells

Tonsillar and blood mononuclear cells were separated by the standard Ficoll/Hypaque gradient method and were then subjected to rosetting with SRBC. Non-rosetting cells were labelled with anti-T cell (anti-CD2 and anti-CD3) mabs and subsequently incubated with magnetic beads coated with anti-mouse IgG antibodies (Dynal, Oslo). Residual T cells were removed by applying a magnetic field for 2x5min. For T cell isolation, the SRBC were lysed.

Table 1. List of antibody reagents used

Antibody reagent	Cluster designation	Major cell reactivity
UCHT1/PE[a]	CD3	T cells
HD37/PE[a]	CD19	B cells
Tük4/PE[a]	CD14	Monocytes/Macrophages
DRC-1[a]	-	FDC
G28-5[b]	CD40	B cells
mouse IgM[c,d]	-	-
GAM/IgM/FITC	-	-
RAM/IgM/biot	-	-
mouse IgG/PE	-	-

Reagents were derived from [a]Dakopatts, Glostrup, Denmark; [b]kindly provided by Dr. E.A. Clark (University of Washington, Seattle, WA); [c]Gamma, Liège, Belgium; [d]Sigma, St Louis, MO; [e]Becton Dickinson, Mountain View, CA.

RESULTS

Specificity of DRC-1 antigen expression

These experiments were performed on different isolated cells and cell lines. We showed that eighty-five to ninety percent of blood and tonsillar B cells express DRC-1 antigen (Fig. 1). We observed no difference in fluorescence intensity or in numbers of cells between subsets of B lymphocytes (IgD$^+$ and IgD$^-$ B cells)(data not shown). Table 2 shows DRC-1 expression on T lymphocytes, monocytes/macrophages, and cell lines. All CD3 T cells were

DRC-1 negative, but we observed a variable percentage of positive Daudi cells. BL-2 cells never expressed the antigen. Raji cells gave a high and constant percentage of DRC-1 expression. We have also investigated DRC-1 expression on chronic leukemic lymphocytes (B-CLL) and acute leukemic lymphoblasts (B-ALL). B-ALL were not labelled by anti-DRC-1 antibody (five cases observed), eighty to ninety percent of B-CLL expressed DRC-1 antigen.

After immunoperoxidase staining, the density of DRC-1 expression was heterogenous; a polar localization and labelling between adjacent cells were then apparent (not shown).

Influence of anti-DRC-1 mab on B cell proliferation and differentiation

Highly purified tonsillar B cells were activated by PMA and incubated with anti-DRC-1 antibody (Fig. 2). We showed that the antibody (0 to 1.92 ug/ml) induced a significant decrease in the proliferative activity but the effect was not dose-dependent. Unrelated mouse IgM failed to produce this effect. The decrease was not observed on IL-4 or IL-10/CD40 mab activated B cells (data not shown).

To assess differentiation, we measured the IgG and IgM levels by ELISA in B supernatants of cells activated by SAC/IL-2 in the presence of anti-DRC-1 antibody (0 to 1.92 ug/ml). Addition of mab did not modify the capacity of B cells to produce IgG or IgM . The same results were obtained with activated T cell and B lymphocyte co-cultures (data not shown).

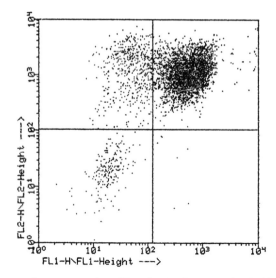

Figure 1. Dual-parameter fluorescence plots of B-cells. B cells were stained with PE-conjugated anti-CD19 (vertical axis) and with anti-DRC-1 antibody, anti-mouse IgM biotinylated antibody revealed by FITC-streptavidin (horizontal axis).

Modulation of DRC-1 antigen

We investigated the possibility of modifying DRC1 expression with different cytokines (IL-4 or IL-10) and activators (PMA, anti-Ig or anti-CD40 mab), used alone or in combination. No significant variations of DRC1 expression were observed.

Table 2. Immunofluorescence analysis of DRC-1 antigen expression. Different cell lines were stained with anti-DRC-1 mab revealed by FITC-GAM or PE-GAM antiserum.

CELLS	% of DRC1[+]
Blood T lymphocytes[1]	0
Tonsillar T lymphocytes[1]	0
Activated T lymphocytes[1]	0
Blood B lymphocytes[1]	90
Tonsillar B lymphocytes[1]	85-90
Monocytes/Macrophages[1]	0
DAUDI	0-50
JIJOYE	40-60
BL-2	<1
RAJI	80-90
HL-60	0

1. Dual-parameter fluorescence analysis (CD3 for T cells, CD19 for B cells and CD14 for monocytes/macrophages).

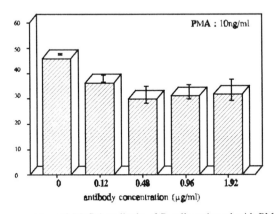

Figure 2. Proliferative response to anti-DRC-1 antibody of B cells activated with PMA .
1×10^5 purified B cells were cultured with anti-DRC-1 antibody (0 to 1.92 ug/ml). Mouse IgM was used as a control. The figure is representative of four experiments. [^{3}H] TdR incorporation levels were assessed on day 2 following a 16-hour pulse. The mean incorporation rates for triplicate wells are shown with the corresponding S.D.

DISCUSSION

In this study, we show that blood and tonsillar B lymphocytes are DRC-1 positive. Tumor B cell lines gave variable DRC-1 expression. Our study on leukemic cells shows that DRC-1 expression distinguishes chronic leukemic lymphocytes (B-CLL) from acute leukemic lymphoblasts (B-ALL), since all B-CLL are labelled with anti-DRC-1 antibody whereas the B-ALL don't express DRC-1 antigen. DRC-1 expression thus seems to depend on B cell activation or differentiation. However, we failed to modulate DRC1 expression on B cells by use of cytokines and polyclonal activation. Our results suggest that DRC-1 plays a role in intercellular contacts. This was also suggested by our previous observations on the effects of anti-DRC1 mab on cell adhesion to follicular dendritic cells[8]. DRC-1 appears to play a role during proliferation of B cells but not in their terminal differentiation into Ig-secreting cells. It is possible, however, that the antibody we use does not effectively block its entire active part.

ACKNOWLEDGMENTS

The authors wish to thank M. Jackers and A.M. Greimers for their expert technical assistance and Dr. Boniver, Dr. M. Evrard and Dr. D. Malaise for the supply of tonsils. They are grateful to Dr. Ed. Clark, University of Washington, for providing the anti-CD40 (G28-5) antibody, . This work was supported by the Belgian FNRS and the "Fonds anticancérologique" of Liège.

REFERENCES

1. E. Heinen, C. Lilet-Leclercq, D.Y. Mason, H. Stein, J. Boniver, D. Radoux, C. Kinet-Denoel and L.J. Simar, Isolation of follicular dendritic cells from human tonsils and adenoids. II. Immunocytochemical characterization, Europ. J. Immunol. 14:267 (1984).
2. K. Inaba, M.D. Witmer and R.M. Steinman, Clustering of dendritic cells, helper T lymphocytes, and histocompatible B cells during primary antibody responses in vitro, J. Exp. Med. 160:858 (1984).
3. M. Naiem, J. Gerdes, Z. Abdulazis, H. Stein and D.Y. Mason, Production of a monoclonal antibody reactive with human dendritic reticulum cells and its use in the immunohistological analysis of lymphoid tissue, J. Clin. Pathol. 36:167 (1983).
4. G.D. Gordon, L. Deborals, N. Hardie, R. Ling and I.C.M. Maclennan, Human follicular dendritic cells (FDC): a study with monoclonal antibodies (MoAb), Clin. Exp. Immunol. 64:205(1986).
5. K. Terashima, K. Ukai, R. Tajima, F. Yuda and Y. Imai, Morphological diversity of DRC1 positive cells: human follicular dendritic cells and their relatives, Adv. Enj. Med. Biol. 237:157(1989).
6. H. K. Parmentier, J.A. Van der linden, J. Krijnen, D.F. Van Wichen, L.H. Radermakers, A.C. Bloem and H.J. Schuurmann, Human follicular dendritic cells : isolation and characteristics in situ and in suspension, Scand. J. Immunol. 33:441(1991).
7. T. Defrance, B. Vanbevliet, J. Pene and J. Banchereau, Human recombinant IL-4 induces activated B lymphocytes to produce IgG and IgM, J. Immunol. 141:2000 (1988).
8. E. Louis, B. Philippet, B. Cordons, E. heinen, N. Cormann, C. Kinet-Denoel, M. Braun and L.J. Simar, Intercellular contacts between germinal centre cells. Mechanisms of adhesion between lymphoid cells and follicular dendritic celss, Acta Oto-Rhino-Laryng. Bel. 43:297 (1989).

B CELL DIFFERENTIATION AND MUCOSAL IMMUNITY

THE APPENDIX FUNCTIONS AS A MAMMALIAN BURSAL EQUIVALENT IN THE DEVELOPING RABBIT

P. D. Weinstein,[1,2] R. G. Mage,[2] and A. O. Anderson[1]

[1]ARD, USAMRIID, Ft. Detrick, Frederick, MD 21702 and
[2]LI/NIAID, NIH, Bldg. 10, Rm 11N311, Bethesda, MD 20892

ABSTRACT

In this paper we present genomic DNA sequence and histological evidence that the appendix is a site of diversification of the rabbit's primary antibody repertoire. By 6 weeks after birth, the B cell follicular regions of the rabbit appendix and the distribution of the resident lymphoid cells bear a strong morphological resemblance to similar regions within two primary lymphoid tissues, the chicken bursa and the sheep ileal Peyer's patch. However, similarities between the rabbit appendix, chicken bursa and sheep ileal Peyer's patch end as these animals reach adulthood. The rabbit appendix undergoes morphological and cellular distribution changes as it matures taking on the appearance of a secondary lymphoid tissue, while the sheep ileal Peyer's patch and the chicken bursa both involute. We determined DNA sequences of PCR amplified rearranged variable region genes from germinal center B cells of 6 week old rabbits isolated from several different appendix dark zones and light zones. There was a trend toward a higher degree of diversification from the germ-line VH gene DNA sequence in dark zones than light zones. It is likely that both gene conversion and somatic hypermutation are responsible for the nucleotide changes we observed. Our findings suggest that the rabbit appendix functions as a mammalian bursal equivalent early in development. As the rabbit matures, the appendix appears to evolve into a secondary lymphoid tissue resembling secondary GALT in appearance and possibly in function.

INTRODUCTION

Productive rearrangement of three distinct genetic elements, VH, DH, and JH, at the genomic DNA level is necessary before a heavy chain variable region can be transcribed and translated. The rabbit contains approximately 100 distinct VH genes, all of which belong to the VHIII gene family. Of these VH genes, the one located at the 3' end of the locus, VH1, is used by rabbit B cells 80-95% of the time (1, 2). This preferential utilization of one VH gene makes it possible to analyze and sequence the rearranged heavy chain variable region DNA in most rabbit B cells irrespective of the cells' antigen specificity. In addition, Becker and Knight have shown that diversification of this rabbit VH sequence can occur through gene conversion (1).

B cells mature over time through several stages of development within various lymphoid tissues. Antigen specific responses take place within secondary lymphoid tissues such as the spleen, lymph nodes, and jejunal Peyer's patch (JPP). The follicular regions in which these reactions occur are known as germinal centers (GC) (3). While in GC, B cells can go through affinity maturation, which at the genomic DNA level leads to changes in V gene nucleotide sequences by a process known as somatic hypermutation. Another kind of GC which is not necessarily antigen specific can occur in primary lymphoid tissues like the chicken bursa and the sheep ileal PP (SIPP), both of which are gut associated lymphoid tissues (GALT). These GC are concerned with the diversification of the antibody repertoire of B cells which have already gone through DNA rearrangements utilizing a limited number of V genes. The mechanism used to alter the DNA sequence of light chain variable region genes of SIPP B cells is somatic hypermutation (4); the rearranged VH and VL genes in the chicken bursa are diversified by both gene conversion and somatic hypermutation (5). GC of secondary lymphoid tissues contain CD4 T cells, while those of primary lymphoid tissues are not (6).

During the 1960's several groups proposed that the rabbit appendix, a GALT, might be a mammalian bursal equivalent. Contributing to this belief were experiments in which appendectomized rabbits were found to have lower antibody titers in response to antigen challenge, fewer circulating lymphocytes in the peripheral blood and reduced lymphoid development in peripheral lymphoid tissue. The observed decrease in the B cell pool could not be solely explained by the loss of B cells located in the appendix at the time of its removal (7-10). In this study we present new evidence that the rabbit appendix appears to be a primary lymphoid tissue which acts as a site where the initial diversification of the rearranged VH1 gene takes place. We have found that early after birth the rabbit appendix has many morphological and cellular distribution similarities with the chicken bursa and the SIPP. In addition, we have found that rabbit appendix GC B cells are probably changing their genomic DNA variable region sequences by both somatic hypermutation and gene conversion. However, unlike the chicken bursa and SIPP, the rabbit appendix does not involute by 8-14 months. Instead the rabbit appendix undergoes several changes, one of which may be a change in function.

MATERIALS AND METHODS

Animals

Mixed breed rabbits of the VH1a2 (F-I) haplotype were bred and raised in our own allotype derived pedigreed colonies. Rabbits were sacrificed at 1 day; 2, 4, 6, and 9 weeks; 4, 5, and 9 months; and 1, and 4 years and relevant tissues removed.

Immunohistochemistry

Tissues were frozen in OCT compound and 7 μm sections cut on a cryostat. Tissues were allowed to air dry, and stored in a desiccator cabinet until used. Sections were stained using a previously described avidin biotin method (11). When the primary reagents were non-biotinylated mouse anti-rabbit IgM, and mouse anti-rabbit IgA monoclonal antibodies, a second step antibody was used, biotinylated goat anti-mouse IgG (Southern Biotechnologies, Birmingham, AL). In addition we used biotinylated mouse anti-rabbit CD4 and biotinylated mouse anti-rabbit CD8 monoclonal antibodies (Spring Valley Laboratories, Sykesville, MD).

PCR Amplification and Sequencing of Rabbit Appendix B Cell Variable Region Genes

Germinal center cells from semi-thin sections of 6 week old rabbit appendix stained with succinylated wheat germ agglutinin, were isolated using an Eppendorf micromanipulator and DNA extracts were prepared from isolated cells (12). This was followed by two sets of PCR amplifications with Taq DNAP (Perkin Elmer Cetus, Branchberg, NJ) using primers for the leader exon and a J consensus region, followed by hemi-nesting with primers specific for a highly conserved sequence in framework region 2 and the J consensus region. PCR amplified DNA was purified, cloned into pUC 18, and used to transform library efficiency DH5α (BRL, Gaithersburg, MD). Positive bacterial clones were isolated and their DNA sequenced by the dideoxy chain termination method, labeling with ^{35}S-dATP and using the Taq Track (Promega Biotech., Madison, WI) or the Circumvent DNA sequencing kit (NEB, Beverly, MA).

RESULTS

Histological Analysis of Rabbit Appendix Development

At one day after birth the rabbit appendix is populated by IgM positive B cells, but contains no organized follicular lymphoid structures, in contrast to the chicken bursa and the SIPP. GC can be detected by 2 weeks after birth and these GC contain both IgM and IgA positive B cells. CD4 positive, but not CD8 positive T cells are located in the inter-follicular regions of the rabbit appendix at two weeks after birth. However, no CD4 positive T cells were detected in GC or the dome regions of the rabbit appendix, a feature associated with GC of primary but not secondary lymphoid tissues. The rabbit appendix reaches its maximal size by 6 weeks after birth. At this time, CD4 positive T cells are detected in the interfollicular regions of the rabbit appendix, but these cells continue to be absent from GC and the dome regions where many IgM and IgA positive B cells can be found. The GC of the 6 week old rabbit appendix is very similar in morphology to GC found in the chicken bursa and the SIPP. All three lymphoid tissues have GC that are tall and thin, with a dark zone that surrounds the light zone on every side except the luminal one (8, 13). These three lymphoid tissues also have follicle associated epithelium (FAE), the site where antigen is actively transported from the lumen of the gut into the tissue, and pointed dome regions that protrude into the gut lumen (8, 13, 14).

Starting at 9 weeks after birth, and continuing until adulthood the rabbit appendix undergoes several morphological and cellular distribution changes. First, CD4 positive T cells begin to infiltrate the dome region. Then at 4-5 months, CD4 positive T cells are found to occupy the luminal side of GC light zones. Complete population of all regions of GC occurs by 12 months after birth. At the same time that the population of the rabbit appendix B cell follicular regions by CD4 positive T cells commences, morphological changes are initiated. Around 4-5 months after birth, the FAE and dome regions begin to lose their pointed shape and round off with the consequent enlargement of the cellular traffic zones and the FAE in relation to the other regions of the appendix. By adulthood these regions of the rabbit appendix complete their transformations and resemble similar regions of the rabbit and mouse JPP, both of which are secondary lymphoid tissues. The GC also undergo morphological changes during this time as they shrink by 50-60% and broaden out. The net result of these cellular distribution and morphological changes is a lymphoid tissue in the adult that does not resemble the same organ of the young rabbit.

Variable Region DNA Sequence Analysis of Rabbit Appendix GC B Cells

Appendix B cells were isolated from 6 week old rabbits from the two primary compartments of the GC, the dark zone and the light zone, to examine whether DNA sequence diversification of the antibody repertoire was occurring. The rationale for isolating GC B cells at 6 weeks after birth came from our observations that the rabbit appendix GC reached their peak in size, and closely resemble similar sites in both the chicken bursa and the SIPP at this time.

All variable region DNA sequences that we have cloned and sequenced in this study appear to have utilized VH1. Dark zone GC B cells were found to contain rearranged variable regions with a high degree of sequence diversity when compared to the germ-line VH1 DNA sequence (Fig. 1). Most of the base pair changes were found in complementarity determining regions (CDR), but several nucleotide changes were detected in framework regions (FR). In contrast, variable regions from light zone GC B cells were closer to the germ-line VH1a2 DNA sequence. Those light zone VH sequences which contained base pair changes, tended to be less diversified than comparable dark zone B cell sequences (Fig. 1). Both dark zone and light zone GC B cells probably diversify their variable region genomic VH1 DNA sequences through gene conversion and somatic hypermutation. Changes in VH sequences have been found to result in almost exclusively amino acid replacements, with only a few silent substitutions. Finally, within an individual section, dark zones and light zones appear to contain cells which originated from only a few progenitor cells (Fig. 1).

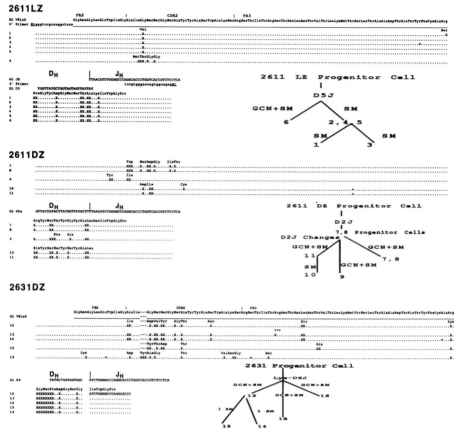

Figure 1. Representative examples of rearranged VH gene sequences of cloned PCR amplified DNA from a light zone (LZ) and dark zones (DZ) of a single GC of a 6 week old rabbit appendix. A full paper with all the sequences from several GC is in preparation. The 5' and 3' primers used in the second hemi-nesting reaction are shown in lower case letters (see Materials and Methods). Evolutionary trees of the clonally related VH gene sequences are shown for each set. Abbreviations are: GCN, gene conversion; SM, somatic mutation. 2631 DZ is from the same GC as 2611 LZ and 2611 DZ, but was taken from a section approximately 7 μm from 2611 DZ. Dots (....) signify identity with germline VH1a2 or known closest DH and JH sequences, dashes (---) signify gaps inserted to align sequences. Almost all DNA base pair changes led to amino acid replacements; Xs represent replacement changes and + silent changes; (***) indicates a change that generated a stop codon. Note the greater diversity of rearranged VH gene sequences from B cells collected from 2611 DZ and 2631 DZ compared to 2611 LZ.

DISCUSSION

Our data suggest that the rabbit appendix is a mammalian bursal equivalent during the early stages of neonatal development. At 6 weeks of age the rabbit appendix has many of the morphological, and cellular distribution characteristics associated with both the chicken bursa and the SIPP. The most important of these is the lack of CD4 T cells in the rabbit appendix GC. The general morphology of the rabbit appendix, with its pointy dome and tall thin GC with dark zones enveloping light zones is very similar to these regions of the chicken bursa and SIPP. In addition, by approximately six weeks of age, all three lymphoid tissues reach their peak in both gross anatomical and GC follicle size, and the rearranged V genes in B cells are undergoing somatic diversification (7, 13).

The rabbit appendix also has several features which appear to make it unique. At birth both the chicken bursa and the SIPP contain GC, while the rabbit appendix has no organized follicular structures. The development of GC in the rabbit appendix appears to be antigen dependent, unlike the chicken bursa and SIPP, which develop GC in the absence of antigen. However, antigen is necessary in order for the GC of the SIPP to reach their maximal sizes (15). DNA sequences from GC of fetal SIPP have few changes from the germ-line DNA sequence (4). Therefore, even in sheep the genetic diversification mechanism may be stimulated by exposure of the B cells to environmental antigens. The exact nature of the antigens responsible for driving these GC is unknown, but we have found remnants of bacteria in the rabbit appendix which leads to the suggestion that bacterial antigens, B cell mitogens, or superantigens may play a role. We plan to determine the degree of antigen specificity of B cells undergoing diversification in rabbit appendix GCs in future experiments.

The variable region diversity we find in rabbit appendix GC probably results from both somatic hypermutation and gene conversion with most of the changes localized within the CDR. It is striking that in rabbit appendix GC B cell sequences there is a marked preponderance of amino acid replacement changes. These changes may be indicative of a diversification process by gene conversion, and not affinity maturation by somatic hypermutation because we find very few silent nucleotide changes in the variable region DNA sequences that have been examined. Indeed, antibody diversification and affinity maturation must be different. Affinity maturation is a fine tuning process to yield a better antibody against a specific antigen responsible for initiating an individual GC B cell response. The multiple amino acid changes we see in the rearranged variable region DNA sequences of rabbit appendix GC B cells suggest that the antigen binding specificity of many of these clonally related cells may be changing. Thus, antibody diversification is a more likely explanation of our results. In the future we plan to examine whether a similar diversification process is occurring for light chain genes in the rabbit appendix early in life.

The rabbit appendix goes through a gradual process of change leading to a tissue in the adult animal that has little similarity to the appendix of a neonate. This change is in contrast to the chicken bursa and the SIPP, both of which involute by 8-14 months. The end result of the morphological and cellular distribution changes that the rabbit appendix goes through is the development of a lymphoid tissue that now resembles a JPP, a known secondary lymphoid tissue. The increase in both FAE surface area covering each follicle and the number of cells trafficking through the adult appendix are consonant with the idea that antigen-specific lymphocyte responses are occurring rather than the primary diversification we suggest occurs in the young rabbit appendix. If such functional changes have indeed occurred in the adult rabbit appendix, there may be a stage when primary and secondary lymphoid functions coexist.

ACKNOWLEDGEMENTS

We thank Drs. J. Jacob and G. Kelsoe (Univ. MD-Baltimore, School of Medicine) for teaching us their technique for isolation of cells from semi-thin sections for PCR and DNA sequence analysis. We also thank Glendowlyn O. Young-Cooper and Cornelius Alexander for help with maintenance and preparation of animals and Drs. M. Fitts, H. T. Chen, P. Fuschiotti and R. Pospísil (LI/NIAID, NIH, Bethesda, MD) for helpful discussions.

REFERENCES

1. Becker, R. S. and K. L. Knight, Cell, 63:987 (1990).
2. Allegrucci, et al., Eur. J. Immunol., 21:411(1991).
3. Anderson, A. O., Immunophysiology of lymphocytes, organization of lymphatic tissues, pp 14-45 *in:* "Immunophysiology. The Role of Cells and Cytokines in Immunity and inflammation," J. J. Oppenheim and E. M. Shevach, eds. Oxford University Press, New York (1990).
4. Reynaud, C. A., et. al., Cell, 64:995 (1991).
5. Reynaud, C. A., et. al., Cell, 59:171 (1989).
6. Aleksandersen, M., et. al., Immunology, 70:391 (1990).
7. Sutherland, D. E. R., et.al., Proc. Soc. Exp. Biol. Med., 115:673 (1964).
8. Cooper, M. D., et al., Int. Arch. Allergy, 33:6 (1968).
9. Cooper, M. D., et. al., The Lancet, 1388 (1966).
10. Archer, O. K., et al., Nature, 200:337 (1963).
11. Weinstein, P. D. and J. J. Cebra, J. Immunol ., 147:4126 (1991).
12. Jacob, J., et. al., Nature, 354:389 (1991).
13. Landsverk, T., Acta Path. Microbiol. Immunol. Scand., 92:77 (1984).
14. Reynolds, J. D. and B. Morris, Eur. J. Immunol., 13:627 (1983).
15. Reynolds, J. D. and B. Morris, Eur. J. Immunol., 14:1 (1984).

DEVELOPMENT OF COMPONENTS OF THE MUCOSAL IMMUNE SYSTEM IN SCID RECIPIENT MICE

John J. Cebra,[1,2] Nicolaas A. Bos,[2] Ethel R. Cebra,[1,2]
Christopher F. Cuff, [1] Gerrit Jan Deenen,[2] Frans G. M.
Kroese,[2] and Khushroo E. Shroff[1]

[1]Department of Biology, University of Pennsylvania,
 Philadelphia, PA 19104-6018
[2]Department of Histology and Cell Biology, University
 of Groningen, NL-9713 EZ Groningen, NL

INTRODUCTION

We have used adoptive transfer of congenic lymphoid cells from different tissue sources into severe combined immunodeficient (SCID) mice to: (1) compare the contributions of B1 B cells from the peritoneal cavity (PeC) and B2 B cells from Peyer's patches (PP) to the pool of splenic (Spl) IgM plasma cells and mesenteric lymph node (MLN) and gut lamina propria (LP) IgA plasma cells, and (2) assess the potential of T cell precursors from bone marrow (BM) and PP to give rise to α/β TCR+, CD8+ T cells in the intraepithelial leukocyte (IEL) compartment upon oral infection with enteric reovirus.

METHODS

Cell Transfers

Cells from lymphoid tissue taken from congenic BALB/c (Igh[a]) and/or CB.17 (Igh[b]) mice were transferred intraperitoneally into CB1.17 SCID recipients. Cells from the IEL space were recovered as described[1] and recipient mice were orally infected with reovirus as detailed[1,2].

Immunohistochemical Analysis of Cells

Cell suspensions were stained for analysis by fluorescence-activated cell sorting (FACS) or after deposition on slides as cytospots and fixation using (1) labeled MAbs against IgM^a (DS.1) or IgA^a (HY16) Igh allotype followed by polyclonal labeled anti-IgM or -IgA isotypes respectively, or (2) MAbs against α/β or γ/δ TCR (hamster) followed by labeled anti-CD8 and anti-hamster Abs. Labeled peanut agglutinin (PNA) was used to detect germinal center (GC) B cells and MAb against bromodeoxyuridine (BrdU) (85.2) followed by labeled polyclonal anti-mouse IgG1 was used to detect incorporation of BrdU in DNA after administering BrdU via drinking water to recipients for 6-7 days.

RESULTS

Development of B Cells in SCID Recipients

Analysis by FACS of both Spl and PeC cells recovered 108, 125, and 231 days after transfer from recipients of either PeC cells alone or of mixtures of PP and PeC cells showed that most B cells found at these sites have the characteristics of B1 B cells (see Bos et al., this Volume). Almost all of the recovered B cells are surface IgM-high IgD-low, CD5 (Ly1)-intermediate and bear the IgM-allotype of the PeC cell source.

The co-transferred PeC and PP B cells differed in expression of Igh-locus controlled allotype markers. Thus, their plasma cell progeny could be identified and relatively quantitated long after cell transfer. We found that the plasma cell progeny of the PeC B cells predominated in the Spl at times of 10, 15, 28, 44, 88, and 108 days after transfer of initial ratios of PP:PeC of 2:1, 3:1, and 2:3 -- typically these acounted for 75-100% of the splenic IgM plasma cells. Examination of IgA plasma cells in MLN and intestinal LP of these same recipients showed that PP and PeC B cell sources made a more balanced contribution to the pool of IgA plasma cells developing in the SCID hosts. At earlier times after cell transfer, especially in recipients of higher ratios of PP:PeC B cells, IgA plasma cells derived from the PP source tend to predominate (75-80%). However, even after longer periods (28-108 days after transfer) IgA cells derived from either source remain rather evenly balanced (50-65%). This finding is not consistent with the view that B1 cells from PeC are self-renewing while B2 cells ordinarily must be replaced by precursors from BM. What considerations could explain this unexpected finding? Some possibilities that are not mutually exclusive include: (1) that the B2-cell source generates or contains long-lived memory cells that persist for months, for instance IgM-IgD-IgA+ B cells, and these would not be detected in PeC or Spl by FACS analysis for IgM-low, IgD-high B cells; (2) that B1-like contaminants in the B2-cell source account for long-term contributions to the IgA-plasma cell pool; (3) that a small inoculum of B2 cells would be dispersed recipient-wide and could not be detected by typical analyses for IgM-low IgD-high B2 cells in any given lymphoid tissue, even though the total numbers of these cells may

Table 1. Incorporation of BrdU by IgA-plasma-blasts[1] in mesenteric lymph nodes of SCID/SCID mice following transfer of PeC cells[2] .

days after transfer	# BrdU+/cytoplasmic IgA+	% BrdU+
148	145/200	73
148	158/200	79
148	40/44	91
231	88/124	71

[1] IgA plasmablasts comprised about 17% of total nucleated cells
[2] An inoculum of 5 x 10[6] PeC transferred per recipient

remain equivalent to the B1 B cells that mostly remain in the PeC and in a Spl that never becomes more than 20% of normal size.

In the course of these studies, we never observed the development of PPs in the small intestine, even after 231 days following cell transfer, even though the MLN and LP accumulated abundant plasma cells. The gradual hypertrophy of the MLNs observed in SCID recipients suggest that these may be the sites where IgA plasmablasts are generated. Table 1 indicates that at 148 and 231 days after transfer of PeC cells, IgA plasma cells account for a significant proportion of the nucleated cells in MLN and most of these incorporate BrdU (71-91%) over a 6-7 day period. This observation in-dicated that such MLN cells may be productive fusion partners for making IgA hybridomas derived from either B1 or B2 B cells (see Bos et al., this Volume).

In an effort to constitute PP with GCs de novo in SCID mice we trans-ferred 25 x 10[6] BM cells. If reovirus was administered orally 12 weeks later, easily detectable PP developed within 12 days with GC (11% PNA-high B cells compared with 1.4% in non-infected recipients).

Development of CD8+ T Cell Subsets in the IEL Compartment of SCID Recipients

We have found that the IEL population of antigen-free or germ-free (GF) mice constitutively contains about 19-22% γ/δ TCR+, CD8+ T cells but only about 6-10% α/β TCR+ CD8+ cells[3]. Conventionally-reared mice typically display 12% and 60% of these subsets in their IEL population respectively[3]. If GF mice are orally infected with reovirus, within 10 days a marked increase in CD8+ T cells occurs in the IEL space and most of these cells are α/β TCR+ and many are virus-specific cytotoxic T cell precursors[2] (see Figure 1).

If SCID mice are given 10[7] PP cells and then orally infected with reovirus one day later, a significant population of T cells (53% of total) appears in the IEL space within 3 weeks. Almost all of these (50% of total) are α/β TCR+.[2] The development of these α/β TCR+ T cells in the IEL space is dependent on the reovirus infection[2]. Finally, we have also found that the same SCID recipients of BM cells whose PP development was described above also display a reovirus-dependent appearance of α/β TCR+, CD8+ T cells (41% of total) in their IEL compartment within 12 days after infection following 12 weeks after cell transfer.

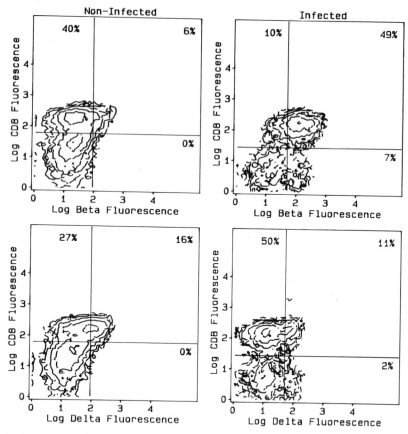

Figure 1. Changes in IEL populations following reovirus infection in germ-free mice. Germ-free BALB/c mice were inoculated with 1 x 10[7] plaque-forming units of reovirus serotype 1/Lang. Ten days after infection, IEL were isolated and analyzed by two-color immunofluorescence.

SUMMARY

Co-transfers of B1 and B2 B cells into immunoincompetent SCID mice indicate that both subsets can contribute IgA plasma cell progeny to the MLN and LP of the mucosal immune system. The MLN appear to be a major site for the generation of IgA-blasts in these mice.

Our findings that GF mice colonized with commensal gut bacteria such as Morganella morganii display transient GC reactions in their PPs and generate local, specific IgA responses[4] and that hybridomas made from B1 PeC B cell-derived IgA blasts react with a proportion (3-11%) of the organisms comprising the normal intestinal flora (Bos et al., this Volume) also are consistent with a normal role for both B1- and B2-derived IgA cells in the intestinal LP -- perhaps in limiting bacterial translocation and in diminishing continous antigenic stimulation by bacterial antigens. The relative contributions of B1- and B2-derived IgA plasma cells remains to be assessed in immunocompetent, physiologically normal mice.

Use of SCID mouse recipients of well-defined subsets of B- and T-cells, should permit identification of those cell mixtures required for:

(1) the development of functional PP which display preferred isotype switching to IgA expression during their GC reactions[5], and

(2) the development of Ag-specific primed or memory cytotoxic CD8+ T cells in the IEL compartment.

ACKNOWLEDGEMENTS

This work was supported by grants AI-17997 and AI-23970 from the National Institute of Allergy and Infectious Diseases, USA and the I.R.S., Leiden, the Netherlands .

REFERENCES

1. S.D. London, J.J. Cebra, and D.H. Rubin, Intraepithelial lymphocytes contain virus-specific, MHC-restricted cytotoxic cell precursors after gut mucosal immunization with reovirus serotype 1/Lang, *Regional Immunol.* 2:98 (1989).

2. C.F. Cuff, C.K. Cebra, D.H. Rubin, and J.J. Cebra, Developmental relationship between cytotoxic α/β T cell receptor-positive intraepithelial lymphocytes and Peyer's patch lymphocytes, *Eur. J. Immunol.* 23: 1333 (1993).

3. D.C. Hooper, E.H. Molowitz, N.A. Bos, V.A. Ploplis, and J.J. Cebra, Spleen cells from antigen-minimized mice are superior to spleen cells from germ-free and conventional mice in the stimulation of primary in vitro proliferative responses to nominal antigens, *Inter. Immunol.* in press

4. K. E. Shroff and J. J. Cebra, Development of mucosal humoral immune responses in germ-free mice, *in::* "Recent Advances in Mucosal Immunity", J. R. McGhee, J. Mestecky, H. Tlaskalova, and J. Sterzl, eds., Plenum Press, New York, (1993), in press.

5. P.D. Weinstein and J.J. Cebra, The preference for switching to IgA expression by Peyer's patch germinal center B cells is likely due to the intrinsic influence of their microenvironment. *J. Immunol.* 147: 4126 (1991).

MANY NEWLY FORMED T LYMPHOCYTES LEAVE THE SMALL INTESTINAL MUCOSA VIA LYMPHATICS

Hermann J. Rothkötter, Claudia Hriesik, and Reinhard Pabst

Centre of Anatomy, -4120-
Medical School of Hannover
D-30623 Hannover
Germany

INTRODUCTION

As in other species in the pig many lymphocytes are produced in the Peyer's patches (PP)[1,2] and in the lamina propria of the gut mucosa[3]. It is not known how many of the newly formed cells stay in these compartments and how many emigrate via lymphatics to other organs. Newly formed cells emigrating from the intestinal wall undergo further maturation and finally reach the effector compartments of the mucosal immune system (for review see [4,5]). The mechanisms of the lymphoblast migration in the mucosal immune system have been studied by injection of cell suspensions from PP, mesenteric lymph nodes or the thoracic duct. In these suspensions all cells in the S-phase of the cell cycle had been labelled in vitro with ^{3}H-thymidine[6,7]. However, the suspensions contained lymphocytes which would normally not migrate or cells from other organs than the gut when the thoracic duct lymph was used. The emigration kinetics of newly formed lymphocytes from the gut mucosa under physiological conditions are not known.

The aim of the present study was to determine how many newly formed T and Ig[+] lymphocytes really leave the small intestinal mucosa per hour. The thymidine analogue bromodesoxyuridine was used as a label for newly formed cells. Lymphocytes leaving the gut wall were obtained using a recently developed pig model[8].

MATERIAL AND METHODS

The experiments were carried out in 13 Göttingen minipigs. Five animals served as control, in 8 animals all mesenteric lymph nodes (mLN) draining the small intestine were removed when the animals were three months old. Within a few weeks anastomoses developed between the afferent and efferent lymphatics. Three months later the main intestinal lymph duct was cannulated[8]. In control animals mLN-derived

In Vivo Immunology, Edited by E. Heinen *et al.*
Plenum Press, New York, 1994

cells were collected (efferent lymph), in the mLN-resected pigs the lymph coming from the small intestinal wall (afferent lymph) was obtained. During the experiments the animals were not restrained and had free access to food and water. The lymph was collected for 93h. The collecting flask was fixed in a bag at the right flank of the animal and was changed at least twice a day. Forty-four h after successful cannulation of the intestinal lymph duct the animals were given a single i.v. injection of the thymidine analogue bromodesoxyuridine (BrdU, 20 mg/kg body weight) to label all cells in the S-phase of the cell cycle.

The lymph samples were analysed as described before[8]. In brief, the number of lymphocytes/ml was determined in each lymph sample using a hemocytometer and phase contrast microscopy. The lymphocyte subsets were characterized by monoclonal antibodies for pig lymphocytes (CD2, CD4, CD8, pig-IgA, pig-IgM[9]) and flow cytometry. In cytospots made from lymph samples collected after the BrdU injection the lymphocyte subsets and the incorporated BrdU were determined using an immunocytochemical double stain[10]. These double stained cytospots were checked to see how many of the subset positive cells had incorporated BrdU.

RESULTS

In control and mLN-resected animals the lymph flow was comparable (18.2 ± 12.3 and 17.3 ± 7.3 ml/h, respectively). The hourly lymphocyte yield was 1.7 ± 1.1 x 10^6 in control animals. In mLN-resected animals a ~15 times higher lymphocyte output was observed (25.2 ± 21.6 x 10^6/h). In both groups the lymphocytes were mostly T cells (Tab. 1).

Table 1. Lymphocyte subpopulations in efferent (control animals) and afferent lymph (mLN-resected pigs)

subset	control			mLN-resected		
CD2+	77.0	±	13.8%	65.8	±	19.0%
CD4+	10.4	±	10.3%	33.8	±	13.1%
CD8+	55.3	±	16.2%	42.0	±	22.0%
IgA+	1.8	±	1.9%	2.2	±	1.5%
IgM+	7.8	±	6.2%	8.1	±	4.1%

In the first lymph sample collected until 4h after BrdU injection in control animals 3.1 ± 0.1% and in mLN-resected pigs 4.8 ± 1.0% of the CD2+ cells had incorporated the label. The numbers of CD8+BrdU+ cells were comparable (control: 3.9 ± 0.1%, mLN-resected: 3.6 ± 1.7%). In both animal groups many IgA+BrdU+ lymphocytes were observed (control: 16.1 ± 19.6%, mLN-resected: 52.6 ± 17.7%). In control animals 6.8 ± 5.7% of the IgM+ cells and in mLN-resected animals 24.5 ± 17.4% of the IgM+ cells were BrdU+. During the following collection periods only the amount of BrdU+ T cells increased.

In the mLN-resected animals the absolute yield/h of newly formed CD2+, CD8+, IgA+ and IgM+ cells in the gut lymph was calculated based on the lymphocyte yield/h, the lymphocyte subsets (Tab. 1) and the percentage of newly formed lymphocytes in the subsets. In all samples more CD2+BrdU+ were found than IgA+BrdU+ or IgM+BrdU+ cells (Tab. 2).

Table 2. Absolute yield of lymphoblasts x 10^6 per hour in afferent gut lymph obtained in mLN-resected animals

collection period (h)	CD2+	CD8+	IgA+	IgM+
0-4	1.0 ± 0.7	0.4 ± 0.3	0.2 ± 0.3	0.3 ± 0.3
4-11	1.9 ± 1.3	1.0 ± 0.5	0.3 ± 0.2	0.6 ± 0.3
11-24	2.1 ± 1.4	1.3 ± 0.8	0.5 ± 0.4	0.6 ± 0.5
24-35	3.2 ± 1.6	1.1 ± 0.4	0.4 ± 0.4	0.6 ± 0.2
35-48	1.3 ± 0.6	0.4 ± 0.1	0.1 ± 0.1	0.3 ± 0.2

SUMMARY

The results show that 50% of the IgA+ and 25% of the IgM+ cells that leave the gut are newly formed BrdU+ cells. However, in absolute numbers the BrdU+Ig+ lymphocytes are the smaller cell pool in the afferent lymph, 2 to 3 times more newly formed T cells were observed. The function of this unexpectedly large pool of newly formed T lymphocytes in oral immunity or tolerance has to be clarified. In a recent study Dunkley and Husband[11] reported that non-B cells play an important role for the localization of plasma cell precursors in the lamina propria of the mucosa.

So far it is unknown where the pool of newly formed T and Ig+ lymphocytes comes from. Partially they are produced in the PP. However, they may have their origin in the lamina propria of the mucosa as well as in other organs of the body. Further studies are necessary to characterize the origin and the function of the large numbers of newly produced T lymphocytes in the intestinal lymph.

REFERENCES

1. R. Pabst, F.J. Fritz, Comparison of lymphocyte production in lymphoid organs and their compartments using the metaphase-arrest technique, *Cell. Tissue Res.* 245:423 (1986).
2. R. Pabst, M. Geist, H.J. Rothkötter, F.J. Fritz, Postnatal development and lymphocyte production of jejunal and ileal Peyer's patches in normal and gnotobiotic pigs, *Immunology* 64:539 (1988).
3. H.J. Rothkötter, H. Ulbrich, R. Pabst, The postnatal development of gut lamina propria lymphocytes: number, proliferation, and T and B cell subsets in conventional and germ-free pigs, *Pediat. Res.* 29:237 (1991).
4. J. Bienenstock and A.D. Befus, The gastrointestinal tract as an immune organ, *in*: "Gastrointestinal Immunity for the Clinician," R.G. Shorter and J.B. Kirsner ed., Grune & Stratton, Orlando (1985), 1-22.
5. R. Pabst, The anatomical basis for the immune function of the gut, *Anat. Embryol.* 176:135 (1987).
6. D. Guy-Grand, C. Griscelli, P. Vassalli, The gut-associated lymphoid system: nature and properties of the large dividing cells, *Eur. J. Immunol.* 4:435 (1974).
7. M.E. Roux, M. McWilliams, J.M. Phillips-Quagliata, M.E. Lamm, Differentiation pathway of Peyer's patch precursors of IgA plasma cells in the secretory immune system, *Cell. Immunol.* 61:141 (1981).
8. H.J. Rothkötter, T. Huber, N.N. Barman, R. Pabst, Lymphoid cells in afferent and efferent intestinal lymph: lymphocyte subpopulations and cell migration. *Clin. Exp. Immunol.* 92:317 (1993).
9. J.K. Lunney, Characterization of swine leukocyte differentiation antigens, *Immunol. Today* 14:147 (1993).
10. J. Westermann, S. Ronneberg, F.J. Fritz, R. Pabst, Proliferation of lymphocyte subsets in the adult rat: a comparison of different lymphoid organs, *Eur. J. Immunol.* 19:1087 (1989).
11. M.L. Dunkley, A.J. Husband, The role of non-B cells in localizing an IgA plasma cell response in the intestine, *Reg. Immunol.* 3:336 (1991).

ANALYSIS OF IgA-PRODUCING HYBRIDOMAS DERIVED FROM PERITONEAL B1 CELLS

Nicolaas A. Bos, Judy C.A.M. Bun, Henk Bijma, Ethel R. Cebra, John J. Cebra, Gerrit Jan Deenen, Maarten J.F. van der Cammen and Frans G.M. Kroese

Dept of Histology and Cell Biology, Immunology Section, University of Groningen Oostersingel 69/I, NL-9713 EZ Groningen, The Netherlands

INTRODUCTION

In the small intestine of conventionally reared mice the number of IgA producing plasma cells is greater then the total number of plasma cells that can be found in other lymphoid tissues.[1] The produced IgA is thought to play an important role in the humoral protection against pathogens that might invade the animal at mucosal surfaces.[2] Most studies showing the role of IgA in protection involve oral or intraperitoneal immunization and subsequent analysis of antigen-specific IgA.[3] The interaction between the normal gut flora and spontaneously produced IgA, however, is much less clear. In mice that are kept under germfree conditions a very drastic reduction in the total number of IgA producing cells is observed,[4] suggesting an inductive role of the normal microflora for the IgA production. The specificity repertoire of these spontaneous IgA producing cells is largely unknown.

IgA plasma cells in the intestine are generally thought to be derived from precursor B cells that are triggered in the Peyer's patches and thereafter migrate to the lamina propria to become IgA plasma cells.[5] Recently, it has been shown that significant numbers of IgA plasma cells can be derived from B1 (formerly called Ly-1 B) cells, which reside in the peritoneal cavity.[6] B1 cells differ from conventional B cells among others in their origin, phenotype and function.[7] They have been shown to be responsible for the production of many of the multireactive, autoreactive IgM antibodies, that are encoded by germline, not somatically mutated immunoglobulin genes.[8] Whether this is also true for B1 cell derived IgA remains to be answered. In order to investigate the specificity repertoire of B1 cell derived IgA, we have transferred peritoneal cells of BALB/c mice into CB17-SCID mice. Eight months after injection only cells with the B1 phenotype are retained in these mice. We have established IgA producing hybridomas from the mesenteric lymph nodes (MLN) of such mice and analyzed them for anti-bacterial reactivity.

MATERIALS AND METHODS

Production of chimeric mice

BALB/c and CB17-SCID mice are reared and maintained at our own animal facilities. 8-12 week old CB17-SCID mice are injected intraperitoneally with 5×10^6 cells, derived from the peritoneal cavity of age-matched BALB/c mice. Animals are analyzed eight months after transfer.

Flowcytometric analysis

Spleen cell suspensions are stained with MAb specific for IgM (331.12), allotype-specific IgD (AMS 9.1) as described.[6] 30,000 cells are analyzed by flowcytometry on a Coulter Epics Elite cytofluorimeter.

ELISA-plaque assays

Intestinal lymphoid cells are isolated as described.[9] ELISA-plaque assays are performed essentially as described before.[10] PVC plates are coated with MAb specific for total IgA (71.14) or for IgAa (HY16),[11] for determination of the numbers of total and of donor-derived IgA plasma cells, respectively. Plaques are detected by goat-anti-mouse IgA coupled to alkaline phospatase (Southern Biotechnology Associates).

Hybridoma production

For hybridoma production MLN are collected from three CB17-SCID mice, eight months after injection of 5 x 10[6] BALB/c peritoneal cells. MLN cells are pooled and fused directly to Sp2/0 fusion partner cells. Growing hybridomas are screened for Ig production and, if positive, subsequently for IgA production by ELISA. IgA producing clones are subcloned in soft agar.

Staining of bacteria

Staining of bacteria is done as will be described in detail elsewhere.[12] Briefly, bacterial cell suspensions are obtained from faecal samples of untreated SCID mice or from faecal samples of a human volunteer by centrifugation of 5 gram of faeces, resuspended in 4 ml PBS, at 35 g, 20 min., 5ºC. Samples from the supernatant (containing the bacteria) are taken and incubated with culture supernatant of IgA hybridomas. As a negative control culture medium is taken and as positive control normal mouse serum (1 in 20 diluted). IgA staining of the bacteria is detected by goat-anti-mouse IgA-FITC conjugate (CALTAG). Bacteria are counterstained with 4 μg/ml propidium iodide. 20,000 bacteria are analyzed on a Coulter Epics Elite cytofluorometer.

RESULTS

Flowcytometric analysis

CB17-SCID mice, eight months after injection of peritoneal cells from BALB/c mice are analyzed for the presence of donor-derived B cells in the spleen and peritoneal cavity. Cytofluorometric analysis shows that all B cells are IgM[high] and IgD[low], both in the spleen and peritoneum (Fig. 1). This phenotype is characteristic for peritoneal B1 cells in conventional mice. All B cells are of donor-origin, since they stain with allotype-specific anti-IgD and anti-IgM MAb (Fig. 1 and data not shown).

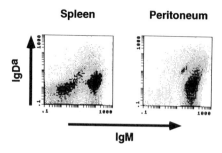

Figure 1. Cytofluorometric analysis of spleen and peritoneal cells from CB-17-SCID mice, eight months after injection of 5 x 10[6] peritoneal cells from BALB/ c mice.

Intestinal IgA-secreting cells

Intestinal lymphoid cell suspensions of CB-17-SCID mice, eight months after injection of 5 x 10^6 peritoneal cells from BALB/c mice are analyzed for numbers of total and donor-derived IgA-secreting cells by ELISA-plaque assays. The number of IgA-secreting cells of donor origin in these mice as detected by allotype-specific ELISA-plaque assays is even somewhat greater then the total number of IgA-secreting cells (Table 1).

Table 1. Number of intestinal IgA-secreting cells in CB17-SCID mice, eight months after injection of 5 x 10^6 peritoneal cells from BALB/ c mice.

Mice	Total number IgA-secr. cells (x 10^{-6})	Donor-derived IgA-secr. cells (x 10^{-6})
CB17-SCID injected with 5 x106 PerC (BALB/c)	25 ± 1[a]	49 ± 8
CB17	44	0
BALB/c	28	44

[a] Numbers represent the mean and SD of three mice. As a control the numbers of CB17 and BALB/c mice are shown.

Hybridoma production

Earlier experiments with these chimeric mice have shown that in the mesenteric lymph node of these mice many donor-derived IgA+ cells can be detected by immunofluorescence microscopy. A large proportion of these IgA+ cells are recently divided cells as shown by BrdU incorporation (see Cebra et al., this volume). On the basis of these experiments, we have fused directly MLN cells of three chimeric mice with a myeloma celline. From a total of 174 wells we have obtained 76 growing hybridomas, which are analyzed for Ig production. Eighteen of a total of 46 Ig-producing hybridomas are producing IgA (21%), as analyed by ELISA. Subcloning of the IgA hybridomas has resulted in 8 IgA-producing clones that are further analyzed.

Staining of bacteria

The specificity repertoire of the IgA hybridomas is tested by analyis of reactivity with faecal bacteria. To obtain (mainly anaerobic) bacteria that are free of endogeneous IgA, we have used faecal bacteria from untreated SCID mice. An example of the staining of SCID mouse derived faeces with hybridoma culture supernatant is shown in Fig. 2.

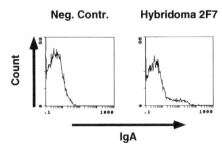

Figure 2. Histogram of staining of bacteria from faeces of SCID mice, stained with culture medium (negative control) or supernatant of hybridoma 2F7. IgA was detected with goat-anti-mouse IgA-FITC

Staining of bacterial samples with supernatant of the IgA hybridomas reveal that all IgA samples of the eight tested hybridomas stain specifically a percentage (3-11%) of bacteria derived from faeces of SCID mice (Table 2). We have also stained human faecal bacteria and seven of the eight IgA samples stain a percentage of these bacteria (Table 2). Combination of different supernatants in the staining of human faeces, reveals that the IgA samples recognize partially different subsets of bacteria (data not shown).

Table 2. Percentage of faecal bacteria from SCID mice and humans that are brightly stained with supernatant of IgA-producing hybridomas

	Hybridomas							
	1B5	2F7	2D11	1F6	3G8	3C10	3C6	2B4
% stained bacteria from SCID mice faeces	7.3[a]	6.6	3.4	3.2	7.3	6.6	5.5	11.0
% stained bacteria from human faeces	9.1	14.1	5.3	<1.0	10.8	3.2	6.7	19.9

[a]Number represent percentage bacteria that are brightly stained compared to a negative control of culture medium alone.

DISCUSSION

The B1 cell lineage in the mouse has unique phenotypic and functional properties. More importantly, in adult mice conventional B cells are replenished by bone marrow precursors, but B1 cells have selfrenewal capacity as IgM+ cells.[7] They are enriched in the peritoneal cavity, where they approximately make up half of the B cells.[7] Because of this self-renewal capacity it is to be expected that after transfer of peritoneal cells into SCID mice, B1 cells will be able to maintain in the host over long time. By the lack of donor-derived bone marrow precursors, the peritoneal conventional B cells will have less chance of long-time maintenance in the SCID recipients. This is in accordance with our finding that eight months after transfer of five million peritoneal cells into the peritoneal cavity of SCID mice, only cells with the B1 cell phenotype can be detetected both in the peritoneum and in the spleen.

These chimeric mice enabled us to confirm our previous findings in B cell depleted animals (by irradiation or anti-IgM treatment) that intestinal IgA plasma cells can originate from B1 cells.[6]

In the MLN of these chimeric mice, a large proportion of the IgA-positive cells have divided recently (see Cebra et al., this volume). This finding, in combination with the observed B1 phenotype of the B cells, makes it very likely that these IgA-positive cells are derived from B1 cells. We have immortalized such IgA-producing cells by hybridoma technology.

Intestinal IgA plays an important role in the humoral immune reponse to pathogenic microorganisms. The reactivity of IgA with the normal flora is, however, largely unknown. We have therefore analyzed our hybridomas for reactivity with the normal anaerobic bacterial flora of SCID mice. All eight IgA samples of our hybridomas stain a percentage, varying between 3 and 11%, of faecal bacteria derived from SCID mice. Faecal bacteria from human origin were stained by seven of the eight IgA samples. One hybridoma (1F6) produces IgA that stains 3% of mouse-derived faecal bacteria, but was completely negative for staining of bacteria derived from human faeces. The other IgA samples recognize populations bacteria that are present both in the human as in the mouse intestinal tract.Currently we do not know which bacteria are stained by our MAb. The very high percentage of stained bacteria, might either be explained by common determinants or by multireactivity of our MAb. This latter option would be in agreement with the observed multireactivity of B1 cell derived IgM.[13] Other properties of B1 cell derived IgM are the apparent lack of somatic mutations and N-insertions in the used Vh genes. Currently we are investigating if this property also holds for B1 cell derived IgA by cloning and sequencing the Vh genes of our hybridomas.

In conclusion, our data support the evidence that B1 cells can give rise to intestinal

IgA-producing cells. Furthermore, our data suggest that B1 cell derived IgA might play a role in the relationship of the host with the normal gut microflora.

ACKNOWLEDGEMENT

This work was financially supported by the I.R.S., Leiden, the Netherlands.

REFERENCES

1. P.J. Van der Heijden, W. Stok and A.T.J. Bianchi, Contribution of immunoglobulin-secreting cells in the murine small intestine to the 'background' immunoglobulin production, *Immunology* **62**: 551-555 (1987).
2. J.R. McGhee, J. Mestecky, M.T. Dertzbaugh, J.H. Eldridge, M. Hirasawa and H. Kiyono, The mucosal immune system: from fundamental concepts to vaccine development, *Vaccine* **10**: 75-88 (1992).
3. J. Mestecky, The common mucosal immune system and current strategies for induction of immune reponses in external secretions, *J. Clin. Immunol.* **7**: 265 (1987).
4. P.J. Van der Heijden, A.T.J. Bianchi, P.J. Heidt, W. Stok and B.A. Bokhout, Background (spontaneous) immunoglobulin production in the murine small intestine before and after weaning, *J. Reprod. Immunol.* **15**: 217 (1989).
5. S.W. Craig and J.J. Cebra, Rabbit Peyer's patches and popliteal lymph node B lymphocytes: a comparative analysis of their membrane immunoglobulin components and plasma cell precursor potential, *J. Immunol.* **114**: 492-502 (1975).
6. F.G.M. Kroese, E.C. Butcher, A.M. Stall, P.A. Lalor, S. Adams and L.A. Herzenberg, Many of the IgA producing plasma cells in the murine gut are derived from self-replenishing precursors in the peritoneal cavity, *Int. Immunol.* **1**: 75-84 (1989).
7. L.A. Herzenberg, A.M. Stall, P.A. Lalor, C. Sidman, W.A. Moore, D.R. Parks and L.A. Herzenberg, The Ly-1 B cell lineage, *Immunol. Rev.* **93**: 81-102 (1986).
8. R.R. Hardy and K. Hayakawa, Developmental origins, specificities and immunoglobulin gene biases of murine Ly-1 B cells, *Int. Rev. Immunol.* **8**: 189-207 (1992).
9. P.J. Van der Heijden and W. Stok, Improved procedure for the isolation of functionally active lymphoid cells from the murine intestine, *J. Immunol. Meth.* **13**: 161 (1987).
10. N.A. Bos, C.G. Meeuwsen, B.S. Wostmann, J.R. Pleasants and R. Benner, The influence of exogenous antigenic stimulation on the specificity repertoire of background immunoglobulin-secreting cells of different isotypes, *Cell. Immunol.* **112**: 371-380 (1988).
11. E.C. Butcher, R.V. Rouse, R.L. Coffman, C.N. Nottenburg, R.R. Hardy and I.L. Weissman, Surface phenotype of Peyer's patch germinal center cells: implications for the role of germinal centers in B cell differentiation, *J. Immunol.* **129**: 2698-2707 (1982).
12. L.A. Van der Waaij, G. Mesander, P.C. Limburg and D. Van der Waaij, Flow cytometry of non-cultured anaerobic bacteria in human faeces, *Submitted for publication*.
13. K. Hayakawa, R.R. Hardy, M. Honda, L.A. Herzenberg, A.D. Steinberg and L.A. Herzenberg, Ly-1 B cells: Functionally distinct lymphocytes that secrete IgM autoantibodies, *Proc. Natl. Acad. Sci. USA* **81**: 2494-2498 (1984).

MODULATION OF THE NEONATAL IGA RESPONSE TO ENTERIC ANTIGENS BY MATERNAL ANTIBODY

David R. Kramer and John J. Cebra

Department of Biology
University of Pennsylvania
Philadelphia, PA. USA

INTRODUCTION

Two unique features of adult gut associated lymphoid tissue (GALT) relative to other secondary systemic lymphoid tissues are the presence of chronic germinal center reactions (GCR) in the Peyer's patches (PP) and the vast numbers of plasma cells in the gut lamina propria (LP). This steady state of activation presumably results from continuous exposure to novel environmental enteric antigens, attested by the observation that germ free (GF) mice lack PP GCR and have few LP IgA plasma cells.[1] When adult GF mice are removed from their sterile environment, they are rapidly colonized by a diverse microbial flora,[2] inducing both PP GCR and the population of LP with IgA plasma cells. Likewise, a similar variety of microbes is established in the gut of newborn mice once they leave the sterile uterine environment at birth.[3] Nevertheless, despite the fact that by 7-10 days age neonatal PP structurally resemble the immunocompetent PP of adult GF mice, suckling mice lack PP GCR and contain few LP IgA plasma cells until they are weaned at 3-4 weeks age.[4] Why suckling mice are initially unresponsive to their burgeoning microbial flora is still unresolved.

Depressed systemic immune responsiveness during the neonatal period has generally been attributed to either functional immaturity in lymphoid tissues or to immunoregulatory mechanisms.[5,6] Protection from potential pathogenic agents during neonatal life is garnered by the passive transfer of maternal antibodies that may also have important immunoregulatory functions. Immunization programs leading to the development of certain anti-idiotypic antibodies in adult female mice can influence the immune repertoire and clonotypes that respond in subsequent antigenic challenge of the offspring.[7,8] In mice, like humans, particular isotypes of maternal antibodies are actively transported across the placental barrier and mother's milk is rich in IgA throughout the suckling period.[9] Deliberately prolonging suckling in mice results in delayed 'spontaneous' mucosal IgA responses compared to naturally weaned littermates.[10]

Our investigations have focused on the role that maternal antibodies play in modulating IgA responses in the neonatal PP to indigenous gut bacteria and to acute enteric reovirus infection prior to weaning. We have devised a breeding scheme to generate genetically identical, immunocompetent F1 scid/+ mice that develop in either the absence or influence of maternal antibody (see below). Through reciprocal foster rearing experiments, this scheme has permitted us to examine the relative contributions of maternal antibody acquired in utero versus after birth in milk in regulating gut IgA responses.

In Vivo Immunology, Edited by E. Heinen *et al.*
Plenum Press, New York, 1994

METHODS

We have employed a modified version of the PP tissue fragment culture developed in our laboratory that permits the assessment of the status of the ongoing in vivo humoral immune response.[11] Briefly, the small intestine is harvested, cut into 2-3 cm lengths and opened longitudinally. Segments are then washed in isotonic media containing EDTA to remove mucous and to denude the viili of epithelial cells. This procedure effectively removes all maternal antibody from the tissue while preserving the integrity of the PP and LP. PP are excised from the surrounding intestinal tissue by microdissection and $3mm^2$ small intestine (SI) fragments are prepared. The intact PP and SI fragments are then cultured in enriched hybridoma grade media under 10% CO_2 and 90% O_2 for 7 days and in vitro immunoglobulin production is measured by radioimmunoassay (RIA). Based on comparisons with data obtained from ELISPOT analyses of isolated PP and LP cells and with frequencies of IgA^+ positive cells as revealed by immunocytochemistry, and, finally with the kinetics of the serum antibody response, we believe that the data obtained from these cultures is representative of the status of the ongoing in vivo humoral immune response at the time of tissue sampling without significant in vitro differentiation (unpublished observations). In fact, since this technique does not involve the disruption of the local microenvironment these cultures may be superior to other techniques with respect to being supportive of antibody secretion by pre-committed B cells.

Animals were bred in our gnotobiotic facility, which houses breeding colonies of GF BALB/c, GF C.B20 as well as specific pathogen free (SPF) breeding colonies of C.B17 scid mice. GF BALB/c or C.B20 mice were introduced into SPF isolator units containing scid mice in order to establish similar microbial florae in the guts of the dams of both strains. Reciprocal matings of BALB/c or C.B20 mice with C.B17 scid mice were undertaken to generate genetically identical, immunocompetent, F1 scid/+ litters that were born to and reared by either immunocompetent dams (BALB/c female x C.B17 scid male) or that were born to and reared by immunoincompetent dams (C.B17 scid female x BALB/c male). To study the influence of placental versus colostral/milk maternal antibodies on the developing neonatal immune response, litters from the above mating examples were swapped within 6 hours of birth.

Reovirus experiments were conducted using third passage, CsCl purified reovirus type 1, strain lange. 10 day old mice were inoculated per os with 10^7 pfu reovirus while dams were orally immunized two weeks prior to mating with $5x10^7$ pfu reovirus. Previous experiments have demonstrated that normal adult mice completely resolve enteric reovirus infection by 10-14 days.[12]

To examine the initiation of putative antigen specific PP GCR 1 mg of BrdU dissolved in 0.1 ml saline was injected into the peritoneal cavity 6 days after oral reovirus infection. After 4 hours PP were harvested and BrdU incorporation was revealed by immunohistochemistry of 6 μm frozen sections.

RESULTS

10 day old mice are competent to initiate IgA responses in PP leading to the development of LP IgA plasma cells and PP GCR

We have examined the kinetics of reovirus specific IgA production in serum and in cultured PP and SI fragments from suckling mice following enteric reovirus infection at 10 days age. As we have previously reported for adult GF mice,[13] IgA was the only non-IgM isotype expressed by PP B cells of the immunized pups. Thus, the intrinsic preference for isotype switching to IgA in murine PP is evident as early as 10 days age. Reovirus specific IgA is first detectable in serum and in culture supernatants from PP tissue cultures as early as 3 days post infection (p.i.). This initial IgA antibody production by PP B cells reaches its maximum rate by day 6 p.i. Reovirus specific IgA is first detected in cultures of mesenteric lymph nodes 4 days p.i and in cultures of SI fragments by day 6 p.i. Since PP are known to be primary sites of the development of LP IgA plasma cell precursors[14] we believe that these kinetics reflect the time necessary for in vivo migration of B cells from the PP to the intestinal LP.

We wished to correlate the above findings with in situ proliferation of PP lymphocytes. 10 day old GF BALB/c litters were orally inoculated with reovirus and PP proliferation was assessed at 4 and 7 days p.i. by in vivo BrdU incorporation. Our immunohistochemical analyses of PP from these mice demonstrated that by 4 days p.i a substantial number of BrdU+ lymphocytes were localized to the interfollicular zone of the PP. As expected, the majority of the lymphocytes in this region are Thy-1+, yet in reovirus immunized GF pups there were also many IgM+ and IgA+ cells. Age matched non-immunized GF littermates had few BrdU+ PP lymphocytes, yet did contain some IgA positive cells. Few BrdU+ cells from either GF or reovirus immunized GF pups were found within the PP follicles at 14 days age or 4 days p.i., respectively. However, by day 7 p.i. the localization of BrdU+ cells had shifted such that the interfollicular zone now contained few BrdU+ cells, while many BrdU+ cells were found in the follicles of reovirus immunized pups (but not in GF controls). Interestingly, the lectin peanut agglutinin (PNA) which is known to bind avidly to germinal center B cells bound weakly to all PP follicular lymphocytes at 14 and 17 days age, regardless of the immune status of the pups.

Taken together these data demonstrate that the humoral immune response initiated within PP of 10 day old mice to enteric reovirus infection occurs in at least two discreet stages. Early in the response 3-6 days p.i. there is extensive proliferation of IgA+ cells in the interfollicular zone along with maximal production of virus specific IgA antibody by cultured PP. Afterwards, BrdU+ cells are localized to the PP follicles signaling the onset of the PP GCR and local antibody production within the PP begins to decline. Thus, in PP of suckling mice the humoral immune response to acute viral infection (in the absence of pre-existing specific maternal antibody) undergoes a transition from primary antibody formation to germinal center development around day 7 p.i.

Profound differences are seen in natural immunoglobulin levels in serum of non-immunized F1 scid/+ pups of scid versus normal dams

Two week old F1 scid /+ pups of normal dams contain high levels (> 50 µg /ml) of serum IgG1 and IgG2 and low levels of serum IgA (<5 µg/ml). In contrast, age-matched F1 scid /+ pups of scid dams virtually lack serum IgG1, have low levels of serum IgG2, but have high levels of serum IgA. Both groups have equally high concentrations of serum IgM and very low amounts of IgG3 and IgE. Since maternal IgG1 is passively acquired in utero and IgG2 is concentrated in mouse colostrum --murine neonatal enterocytes express an Fc gamma receptor,[9] we believe that most of the serum immunoglobulin of these isotypes in F1 scid/+ pups of normal dams is of maternal origin. Because the scid dams are incapable of providing maternal antibody to their offspring, all of the serum immunoglobulin in F1 scid /+ pups of scid dams is endogenously produced. Thus, these data indicate that in the absence of maternal antibody, neonatal mice produce substantial amounts of IgA that accumulates in the serum in the absence of deliberate antigenic stimulation. Interestingly, serum levels of IgA in F1 scid /+ pups of normal dams do not significantly increase until the onset of weaning at approximately 18-20 days. Lastly, serum IgG2 levels in F1 scid/+ pups of scid dams steadily increase between 10 and 20 days life from approximately 10 µg /ml to >40 µg/ml. This is in sharp contrast to serum IgG1 concentrations in these mice which do not appreciably increase for several weeks.

Maternal antibody is able to forestall the development of local GALT IgA responses to normal gut bacteria in their suckling offspring

PP cultures from non-immune pups of normal dams fail to produce IgA if the tissues are taken prior to 18-20 days age. Conversely, in the total absence of maternal IgA, PP and SI cultures from F1 scid/+ pups of scid dams produced IgA as early as 8-10 and 13-16 days age, respectively. At 8 days age, MLN cultures from F1 scid/+ pups of scid dams also produce copious amounts of IgA. Presently, we have not determined whether these MLN IgA responses are initiated de novo in the MLN or if these responses are from IgA pre-plasma cells from the PP that have migrated to the MLN to complete their differentiation.

We were interested in determining if the delay in IgA responses to gut bacterial antigens in suckling mice was the result of modulation by specific maternal antibodies. Towards this end, adult GF mice were monoassociated with *Proteus rettgeri*, an occasional gut commensal that naturally colonizes the neonatal gut during the first week of life.[3] After 1 month, approximately half of the mucosal IgA in *P. rettgeri* monoassociated adult mice binds to the bacterium in direct RIA. When pups are born to such monospecific associated dams, their guts are rapidly colonized by large numbers of bacteria; yet, the PP fail to produce specific IgA until after the animals are weaned off the antibody rich milk.

Maternal antibodies acquired in utero alone are unable to inhibit the initiation of specific GALT IgA responses to enteric antigens

The relative efficacy of prenatal versus postnatal maternal antibody in regulating gut IgA responses to enteric antigens was compared by swapping F1 scid/+ litters born to normal dams with F1 scid/+ litters born to scid dams. The results of these experiments were very clear: maternal antibody acquired in utero, or lack thereof, had little effect in preventing the development of the neonate's gut IgA response; while, maternal antibody provided in milk secretions was very effective. PP cultures from non-immunized F1 scid/+ pups born to normal dams but nursed by scid dams produced IgA at earlier ages than PP cultures from non-foster reared controls. And, age matched F1 scid/+ pups born to scid dams but nursed by normal dams displayed delayed IgA responses to environmental antigens relative to littermates reared by scid dams.

F1 scid/+ pups born to reovirus immune dams but nursed by either scid or normal dams develop a vigorous specific IgA response to enteric reovirus infection. However, these responses are qualitatively different than the response engendered in pups born to non-immune dams. Although maximal reovirus specific IgA responses at day 6 p.i. are equivalent, pups born to reovirus immune dams but nursed by either scid or non-immune dams produce less virus specific IgM and IgA at day 3 p.i. and contain fewer proliferating cells on day 6 p.i. than their counterparts born to non-immune dams.(Table 1)

TABLE 1. In situ proliferation and IgA expression in Peyer's patches taken from foster reared F1 scid/+ pups 6 days after enteric reovirus infection at 10 days age.

BIRTH DAM	NURSE DAM	REOVIRUS @10 DAYS	IgA+ PP CELLS	BrdU+ CELLS[1] INTER-FOLLICULAR	BrdU + FOCI[2] FOLLICULAR
SCID	SCID	NO	MANY	SOME	NO
SCID	SCID	YES	MANY	SOME	YES
BALB/C	BALB/C	NO	FEW	FEW	NO
BALB/C	BALB/C	YES	MANY	SOME	YES
REO IM	REO IM	YES	FEW	FEW	NO
SCID	REO IM	YES	MANY	SOME	YES
BALB/C	REO IM	YES	FEW	FEW	NO
REO IM	SCID	YES	MANY	SOME	+/-
REO IM	BALB/C	YES	MANY	SOME	+/-

1. Few = <10 cells/section. Some = 10-50 cells/section
2. Foci were scored as positive when >10 cells/foci of BrdU+ cells per section ; +/- = 5-10 cells/foci

Pups from reovirus immune dams or foster reared from birth by reovirus immune dams fail to mount a specific IgA response following enteric reovirus challenge at 10 days age

We previously had demonstrated that newborn mice nursed by reovirus immune dams are protected from lethal encephalitis when challenged orally with a neurotropic strain of reovirus.[15] If the mothers had been immunized by the oral route, as oppposed to parenterally, there was also a marked reduction in recoverable viral titers from the intestines of their challenged newborns. We wished to determine whether reovirus specific antibodies present in milk could inhibit the development of reovirus specific IgA responses in 10 day old mice born to and/or nursed by pre-immune dams.

Despite the incredible antigenic load (10^9 virion particles), pups nursed by pre-immune dams fail to initiate reovirus specific antibody responses in PP when challenged at an age when pups nursed by non-immune dams respond vigorously. Interestingly, F1 <u>scid</u>/+ pups born to <u>scid</u> dams but nursed on reovirus immune dams develop a "non-specific" IgA response in PP including the initiation of GCR following enteric reovirus infection at 10 days without developing a specific IgA response to reovirus (Table 1).

CONCLUSIONS

Peyer's patches present in 10 day old mice are competent to initiate specific IgA responses including germinal center reactions to enteric antigens. Postnatal transfer of maternal antibody present in milk is capable of forestalling or preventing IgA responses to enteric antigens developing in their suckling offspring, while prenatal transfer alone is not sufficient.

REFERENCES

1. Crabbe, P.A. <u>et al</u>. The normal microbial flora as a major stimulus for proliferation of plasma cells synthesizing IgA in the gut. Int. Arch. Allergy. **34**:362 (1968)
2. Cebra, J.J. <u>et al.</u> Role of environmental antigens in the ontogeny of the secretory immune response. J. Ret. Endo. Soc. s**28**:61 (1980)
3. Schaedler, R.W., Dubos, R. and R. Costelllo. The development of bacterial flora in the gastrointestinal tract of mice. J. Exp. Med. **122**:77 (1965)
4. Parrot, D. and T.T. MacDonald. The ontogeny of the mucosal immune system in rodents. in <u>Ontogeny of the Immune System of the Gut,</u> T.T. MacDonald, ed. CRC press,Inc. Boca Raton FL USA. (1990)
5. Sterzl, J. and A.M. Silverstein. Developmental aspects of immunity. Adv. Immunol. **6**:337 (1967)
6. Murgita, R.A. and H. Wigzel. Regulation of immune functions in the fetus and newborn. Prog. Immunol. **29**:54 (1981)
7. Okamoto Y. <u>et al</u>. Effect of breast feeding on the development of anti-idiotype antibody response to F glycoprotein of respiratory syncitial virus in infant mice after post-partum maternal immunization. J. Immunol. **142**:2507. (1989)
8. Ainsworth A.J. and J.E. Brown. Detection of in ovo derived anti-idiotypic antibodies I. a model for maternal-neonatal idiotype network studies. J. Immunol. **147**:910 (1991)
9. Mackenzie, N.M. Transport of maternally derived immunoglobulin across the intestinal epithelium. in <u>Ontogeny of the Immune System of the Gut,</u> T.T. MacDonald, ed. CRC press, Boca Raton FL USA (1990)
10. Van der Heijden,P.J. <u>et al</u>. Influence of the time of weaning on the spontaneous (background) immunoglobulin production in the murine small intestine. in <u>Advances in Mucosal Immunology,</u> T.T. MacDonald and S.J. Challacombe,eds. Kluwer Academic Publishers, Lancaster UK pp 479-480. (1990)
11. Logan A.C. <u>et al</u>. The use of Peyer's patch and lymph node fragment cultures to compare local immune response to *Morganella morgani*. Infect. Immun.**59**:1024 (1991)
12. London, S.D., Ruben,D.R. and J.J. Cebra. Gut mucosal immunization with reovirus serotype1/lange stimulates virus specific cytotoxic T cell precursors as well as IgA memory cells in Peyer's patches. J. Exp. Med. **165**:830 (1987)
13. Weinstein,P.D. and J.J. Cebra. The preference for switching to IgA expression by Peyer's patch germinal center B cells is likely due to the intrinsic influence of their microenvironment. J.Immunol. **147**:4126 (1991)
14. Craig,S.W. and J.J. Cebra. Peyer's patches: an enriched source of precursors for IgA producing immunocytes in the rabbit. J. Exp. Med. **134**:188 (1971)
15. Cuff, C.F. <u>et al.</u> Passive immunity to reovirus serotype 3-induced meningoencephalitis is mediated by both secretory and transplacental factors in neonatal mice. J. Virol. **64**:1256 (1990)

ANTIBODY-FORMING CELLS (AFCs) IN THE LUNG LYMPHOID TISSUE AFTER PRIMARY AND SECONDARY IMMUNIZATION THROUGH DIFFERENT ROUTES:A SEMIQUANTITATIVE ANALYSIS IN ADULT RATS USING T-DEPENDENT (TNP-KLH) AND T-INDEPENDENT ANTIGENS (TNP-LPS)

Luis Alonso, Aart van Appeldorf, Marcelino Bañuelos, Maria G. Barrutia and Agustín G. Zapata

Dept. of Cell Biology, Faculty of Biology, Complutense Univ., 28040 Madrid, Spain

INTRODUCTION

Despite pioneer reports emphasizing the mutual resemblances of the bronchus-associated lymphoid tissue (BALT) and the gut-associated lymphoid tissue (GALT), so claiming the relationship of BALT to the so-called mucosa-associated lymphoid tissue (MALT), the evidence is merely circumstantial. To date, there are important differences in the histological organization of both tissues[1,2]. The lymphoepithelium condition of the epithelium covering the lung lymphoid aggregates can only be observed in locally immunized animals and even in that situation the existence of M-like cells in the epithelium is controversial[2,3.] Moreover, germinal centers have only been reported in the BALT after extensive immunization[2].

On the other hand, attemps made by several authors to induce immune responses in the lung have lead to contradictory results. In general intratracheal (IT) immunization induces histological changes in the BALT[1,2,], but there are important differences in the local production of antibody-forming cells (AFCs). T-independent, but not T-dependent (HRP, BSA) antigens, elicited a primary immune response after IT immunization, although the antigen-specific AFCs occurred mainly in the paratracheal lymph nodes rather than in the BALT. A few AFCs found in the BALT might represent immigrant lymphoblasts specifically stimulated in other locations, principally in the lung-draining lymph nodes[1, 4]. There are only a few studies on the secondary immune reactivity in the BALT. After intraintestinal (II) priming and intratracheal (IT) boosting with HRP, no AFCs appeared in the BALT whereas, by contrast, the subcutaneous (SC) priming elicited specific AFCs in the lung after IT boosting[1]. However, using other T-dependent antigens, i.e. cholera toxin[5], TNP-KLH[1], the secondary response was stronger, principally in the site of the booster injection, when rats were II primed and IT boosted than in the reverse condition.

Therefore, the semiquantitative analysis used in the present work to evaluate the number of AFCs induced in distinct pulmonary lymphoid compartments after primary and secondary immunization throughout different routes, is an indirect way to study the relationships of lung lymphoid tissue with the mucosal and /or systemic immune system.

MATERIALS AND METHODS

2 to 2½ month old Wistar rats were immunized either with a T-dependent (TNP-KLH) or a T-independent antigen type I (TNP-LPS) antigen. Both IT and SC immunized rats received 100 µg. of each antigen whereas those II injected received 200 µg. SC immunization was done in the hindfoot pads whereas IT and II stimulated rats received the antigens directly into the lumen of the trachea and the duodenum, respectively. Animals receiving a single dose of each antigen were sacrificed 4 and 7 days later. Other groups of rats were primed with each antigen either IT, SC or II and always IT boosted 3 or 8 weeks later. These animals were sacrificed 7 days after boosting. Control rats received saline solution in each case.

From anaesthesized rats, the spleen, the lung, the Peyer's patches (PP), the paratracheal (PT), the popliteal (Po) and the axillary (Ax) lymph nodes were removed aseptically, embedded in Tissue Teck, snap-frozen in liquid nitrogen and stored at -70° C. Anti-TNP forming cells were detected using the method described by Claassen and van Rooijen (J. Immunol. Methods 75, 181, 1984). Briefly, 8 µm at random 100-200 µm serial cryosections were air-dried for 2 hours at room temperature, fixed with acetone for 10 min. and incubated overnight at 4° C with the conjugate TNP-alkaline phosphatase (TNP-AP). Control sections for endogenous AP activity were incubated with only PBS/0.1% BSA pH 7.4. AP- activity was revealed using Fast blue- BB salt and 0.25% levamisole for 25 min. at 37° C, the sections were counter-stained with haematoxylin and embedded in glycerine-gelatin. A blue reaction product indicates that the cells contain anti-TNP antibodies. To evaluate the number of anti-TNP-AFCs, 10 sections, chosen at random, of each organ/ rat were counted at low magnification on ten squares selected at random using a Zeiss grid-containing ocular. The number of positive cells was related to mm^2 organ section and marked in Tables 1 and 2 as: -, no cells; +/-, 1-10 cells; +, 11-30 cells; + +, 31-50 cells; + + +, more than 50 cells.

RESULTS

1. Numbers of anti-TNP AFCs after a single dose either of TNP-LPS or TNP-KLH (Tab. 1)

For both antigens the responses were mainly local except in II-inmunized rats, and TNP-LPS elicited, in general, better primary responses than TNP-KLH. 4 days after IT injection of a single dose of TNP-LPS numerous anti-TNP AFCs occurred in the BALT and in lesser extent in both the spleen and the axillary lymph nodes. After 7 days the number of AFCs had decreased in all the organs but the highest values still corresponded to the BALT. After SC immunization the spleen and the Po lymph nodes, which drain the site of antigen administration, showed some immune reactivity. No response was found after II administration of TNP-LPS.

At short time IT immunization with TNP-KLH induced a few numbers of AFCs in both the PT lymph nodes and the spleen, but not in the BALT. 7 days after antigen administration, however, the highest numbers of TNP-specific AFCs occurred in the BALT. Only the Po lymph nodes contained AFCs to TNP after SC administration of TNP-KLH and the IT injection of the antigen only induced a weak response in the spleen 4 days later.

Table 1. Numbers of AFCs occurring in different rat organs after primary immunization by three different routes either with a T-dependent (TNP-KLH) or a T-independent (TNP-LPS) antigen.

	I.T. 4 days		I.T. 7 days		S.C. 4 days		S.C. 7 days		I.I. 4 days		I.I. 7 days	
	LPS	KLH	LPS	KLH	LPS	KLH	LPS	KLH	LPS	KLH	LPS	KLH
BALT	+++	-	+	+	-	-	-	-	-	-	-	-
Parenchyma	-	-	-	-	-	-	-	-	-	-	-	-
Spleen	+	+/-	+/-	+/-	+/-	-	+/-	-	-	+/-	-	-
PTLN	+/-	+/-	+/-	+/-	-	-	-	-	-	-	-	-
POLN	+/-	-	+/-	-	+/-	+/-	+/-	+/-	-	-	-	-
AXLN	+	-	+/-	-	-	-	-	-	-	-	-	-
P P	+/-	-	+/-	-	-	-	-	-	-	-	-	-

2. Numbers of anti-TNP AFCs in IT primed IT boosted rats either with TNP-LPS or TNP-KLH (Tab. 2)

Contrary to primary immune response, the secondary responses were generally stronger in TNP-KLH immunized rats than in those receiving TNP-LPS. A high number of anti-TNP AFCs occurred not only in the BALT, but also in the spleen, the PT and the AX lymph nodes of rats IT boosted with TNP-KLH 3 weeks later to be primed through the same route. In rats boosted 8 weeks after priming the numbers of AFCs decreased although remained high in the BALT. In the same conditions, the response to TNP-LPS was poor in any studied organ, except in the BALT, the spleen and the Po lymph nodes of rats IT boosted 8 weeks after priming.

3. Numbers of anti-TNP AFCs in SC primed IT boosted rats either with TNP-LPS or TNP-KLH (Tab. 2)

Both antigens elicited similar responses in SC primed IT booster rats. Higher numbers of anti-TNP AFCs occurred in rats boosted 3 weeks after priming than in those receiving the second dose 8 weeks later. In both cases, however, the Po lymph nodes, which drain the site of antigenic priming, contained the highest numbers of AFCs, although good responses were found also in the spleen, the BALT, the PT and the Ax lymph nodes and the lung parenchyma.

4. Numbers of anti-TNP AFCs in II primed IT boosted rats either with TNP-LPS or TNP-KLH (Tab. 2)

As described above for IT primed rats, the secondary response elicited in II primed IT boosted rats was notably higher in animals immunized with T-dependent antigens than in those receiving TNP-LPS. In addition, the highest number of specific AFCs occurred in the BALT, and then in the PT lymph nodes, the spleen, and the lung parenchyma, whereas the elicited response to TNP-LPS involved mainly to both the PT lymph nodes and the spleen, but not to the BALT. No significant response was found in the PP of rats immunized with either of the two antigens.

Table 2. Numbers of AFCs occurring in different rat organs after priming by three different routes and intratracheal boosting either with a T-dependent (TNP-KLH) or a T-independent (TNP-LPS) antigen.

	I.T.-I.T.				S.C.-I.T.				I.I.-I.T.			
	3 weeks		8 weeks		3 weeks		8 weeks		3 weeks		8 weeks	
	LPS	KLH	LPS	KLH	LPS	KLH	LPS	KLH	LPS	KLH	LPS	KLH
BALT	+/-	++	+	+	+	+	+/-	-	+/-	+++	-	+/-
Parenchyma	-	+/-	+/-	+/-	+	+/-	-	-	-	+	-	-
Spleen	+/-	+	+	+/-	+	+/-	+	+	+/-	+	+/-	+/-
PTLN	+/-	+	+/-	+/-	+	+/-	+	+/-	+/-	++	+	+/-
POLN	-	+/-	++	+/-	++	+	+/-	+/-	+/-	+/-	+/-	+/-
AXLN	+/-	+	+/-	+/-	+/-	+	+/-	+/-	+/-	+	+/-	+/-
P P	+/-	+/-	+/-	+/-	+/-	+/-	+/-	+/-	+/-	+/-	+/-	+/-

DISCUSSION

The present results, in agreement with previous reports using similar experimental procedures[1], confirm the influence of both the type of antigen and the route of administration on the pattern of appearance of antigen-specific AFCs in different mucosa-associated and peripheral lymphoid organs. In addition, our findings support that the immune response in the pulmonary lymphoid tissue, is presumably a local phenomenon more related with the activation of the systemic immune system than of the MALT.

The stronger primary immune response to T-independent than to T-dependent antigens observed after IT immunization, had previously been related to the existence of suppressor mechanisms to T-dependent antigens in lung mediated either by suppressor T cells[1, 6] to macrophages[7]. Nevertheless, the good response observed in the BALT 7 days after IT immunization with TNP-KLH and the earlier presence (at 4 days) of a few anti-TNP AFCs in the PT lymph nodes suggest that some anti-TNP specific blasts could migrate between 4 and 7 days from the lung-draining lymph nodes to the BALT. Various authors have noted that after IT stimulation the antigen-specific reactive cells occur firstly in the lung-draining lymph node and then circulate preferentially to lung reaching the BALT via HEVs[1,2].

On the other hand, although the best immune responses after IT stimulation occur locally, other peripheral lymphoid organs, mainly the spleen and the Ax lymph nodes (but not the PP) show a consistent specific response. This lack of response in the GALT of IT stimulated rats have previously been reported by numerous authors testing different antigens[4, 5]. Also, the local response found in the lymph nodes which drain the site of antigen injection of SC stimulated rats has been observed by other authors[8], although they reported a response to TNP-KLH in the spleen, not observed on the present study. Another remarkable finding, in agreement with previous results[9], is the low response observed in the PP after antigen administration through any route, and specially after II stimulation. Other authors have claimed that orally administered soluble protein antigens may induce tolerance rather than a mucosal immune response[10] and Jeurissen et al.[9] found, as our own results indicate, that after II TNP-KLH injection, primary and secondary responses occurred in the spleen. These authors assume that, at least partially, antigens are taken up in the PP villi and transported to the spleen via blood vessels.

The observed secondary immune responses confirm in general our interpretations of the immune significance of lung lymphoid tissue. IT primed rats, boosted 3 weeks after priming exhibited stronger responses to TNP-KLH than to TNP-LPS. The reverse condition was observed in rats boosted 8 weeks after priming. In both cases, the responses are local, mainly involving the BALT, although there are also good responses in the spleen and the peripheral lymph nodes. The local response was also predominant in SC primed IT boosted rats, however, for the two studied antigens good responses were recorded in the spleen, the BALT and the PT lymph nodes, especially in those animals boosted 3 weeks after priming. Similar results were obtained by other authors[1] confirming the migration of antigen-specific blast cells from the peripheral lymph nodes to lung lymphoid tissue. Finally, the best response in II primed IT boosted rats ocurred in the lung, including the BALT as well as the PT lymph nodes, but not in the PP, confirming previous data which emphasized that some T-dependent antigens, such as cholera toxin[5] or TNP-KLH[1], elicited a stronger immune response in the site of booster injection in II primed IT boosted rats than in the opposite situation.

From these results we can conclude that whereas the II immunization induces the appearance of antigen-specific immunoreactive cells which migrate preferently to the mucosal lymphoid tissues, including the BALT, the IT administration of both T-dependent and T-independent antigens evokes a local response and the dissemination of anti-TNP specific blasts to the peripheral lymphoid organs rather than to the MALT.

REFERENCES

1. G.J. van der Brugge-Gamelkoorn, Structure and function of bronchus associated lymphoid tissue (BALT) in the rat. Ph. D. Thesis, Free University, Amsterdam (1986).
2. T. Sminia, G.J. van der Brugge-Gamelkoorn and S.H.M. Jeurissen, Structure and function of bronchus associated lymphoid tissue (BALT), *Crit. Rev. Immunol.* 9:119 (1989).
3. W. Pankow and P. von Wichert, M cell in the immune system of the lung, *Respiration* 54:209 (1988).
4. D.E. Bice and G.M. Shopp, Antibody responses after lung immunization, *Exp. Lung Res.* 14:133 (1988).
5. N.F. Pierce and W.C. Cray, Cellular dissemination of priming for a mucosal immune response to cholera toxin in rats, *J. Immunol.* 127:2461 (1981).
6. P.G. Holt and J.D. Sedgwick, Suppresssion of Ig E responses following inhalation of antigen, *Immunol. Today* 8:14 (1987).
7. E.C. Lawrence, B.J. Theodore and R.R. Martin, Modulation of pokeweed-mitogen induced immunoglobulin secretion by human bronchoalveolar cells, *Am. Rev. Respir. Dis.* 126:248 (1982).
8. F.G.A. Delemarre, E. Claasen and N. van Rooijen, Primary in situ immune response in popliteal lymph nodes and spleen of mice after subcutaneous immunization with thymus-dependent or thymus-independent (type 1 and 2) antigens, *Anat. Rec.* 223:152 (1989).
9. S.H.M. Jeurissen, E. Claasen, N. van Rooijen and G. Kraal, Intraintestinal priming leads to antigen specific Ig A memory cells in peripheral lymphoid organs, *Immunology* 56:417 (1985).
10. J. Biewenga, E.P. van Rees and T. Sminia, Induction and regulation of Ig A responses in the microenviroment of the gut, *Clin. Immunol. Immunopathol.* 67:1 (1993).

NON-LYMPHOID CELLS IN ACUTE AND CHRONIC EXPERIMENTAL INFLAMMATORY BOWEL DISEASE

Mary J.H.J. Palmen[1], Marja B. van der Ende[1],
A. Salvador Peña[2] and Emmelien P. van Rees[1]

[1]Department of Cell Biology, Div. Histology
[2]Department of Gastroenterology
Faculty of Medicine, Free University
Van der Boechorststraat 7
1081 BT Amsterdam
The Netherlands

INTRODUCTION

The etiology of inflammatory bowel disease (IBD), like Crohn's disease and ulcerative colitis remains unclear. A recurrent theme is a failure to down-regulate a local hyperreactive immune response. Autoimmunity possibly plays a role as circulating antibodies reactive against a protein in colonic epithelial cells are found in patients with ulcerative colitis (Takahasi et al., 1990). Local non-lymphoid cells like macrophages, dendritic cells and epithelial cells could be important in IBD in the pathogenesis and in the uptake and processing of antigen in affected tissue, leading to secondary bacterial infection.

Several studies indicate the involvement of macrophages and dendritic cells in IBD. Differences are found in numbers and heterogeneity of macrophages and dendritic cells between tissue obtained from patients and controls (Wilders et al., 1984; Allison et al., 1988; Seldenrijk et al., 1989). Furthermore, lamina propria macrophages obtained from mice have a suppressive effect on immune responses, whereas dendritic cells isolated from Peyer's Patches are very stimulating (Pavli et al., 1990).

Morris et al. (1989) have developed an animal model for chronic IBD, induced by a single rectal administration of 2,4,6-trinitrobenzene sulfonic acid (TNBS) in ethanol. The rats develop both clinical and histopathological symptoms of IBD, lasting for at least 8 weeks.

In the present study intestinal macrophages and dendritic cells in the acute and in the chronic phase were being studied in this animal model for IBD, using immunohisto-chemistry.

In Vivo Immunology, Edited by E. Heinen *et al.*
Plenum Press, New York, 1994

Influx of monocytes into the inflamed tissue could be an important aspect in IBD. A membrane protein involved in monocyte adherence to endothelium is complement receptor type 3 (CR3, or CD11b/CD18). The expression of CR3 is confined to macrophages, granulocytes, dendritic cells and natural killer cells (Schmitt et al., 1981; Wright et al., 1983). In rat, CR3 is being recognized by several MoAb's, i.e. ED7, ED8 and OX42 (Damoiseaux et al., 1989; Huitinga et al., 1993). It was demonstrated that treatment with MoAb ED7 and ED8 in rats resulted in a decrease of the symptoms in experimental encephalomyelitis (Huitinga et al., 1993). In the present study the role of CR3 in experimental IBD has been studied.

MATERIALS & METHODS

Induction Of Colitis

Colitis was induced in male Wistar rats by intracolonic administration of TNBS dissolved in ethanol, as described by Morris et al. (1989), with slight modifications. Under Hypnorm anaesthesia, each rat received 30 mg TNBS in 0,25 ml ethanol 40% using a catheter inserted approximately 8 cm in the colon. After administration of TNBS in ethanol, the rats were checked daily with respect to their general condition, body weight and consistency of stools. On several time points (from day 1 until day 84) after induction of colitis, rats were sacrificed. Cryostat sections of thymus, spleen, mesenteric lymph nodes, Peyer's Patches and inflamed and non-inflamed parts of the colon were made. Immunohistochemistry was performed with MoAb's ED1, ED2, ED3 recognizing macrophage subpopulations (Dijkstra et al., 1985) and Ox6, Ox19 and Ox33 (all from Serotec), to study acute and chronic stages of IBD.

ED7 Treatment In IBD

MoAb ED7 was administered on day 0 and day 3 to 7 rats. Each rat received 1.2 mg in 1 ml PBS into the tail vein. On day 0 the rats also received 30 mg TNBS in ethanol 30% locally in the colon. As a control, 7 rats were used which received PBS instead of ED7 on day 0 and 3. All rats were sacrificed on day 7, after which damage-scores of the colon were established according to Morris (1989). Immunohistochemistry was performed on cryostat sections of inflamed and non-inflamed parts of the colon. MoAb's ED1, ED2, ED3, ED7 (raised in our own laboratory), Ox6, Ox19 and Ox33 were used.

RESULTS

TNBS Model

Most animals treated with TNBS-ethanol developed both clinical and histopathological symptoms, such as diarrhea and transmural inflammation, with or without ulceration. Mean damagescores from day 1 to day 84 are shown in table 1. Colon wall thickening occurred in about 70% of the total IBD group. Sometimes we also observed giant cells and associated granulomas in the mucosa.

Histologically an influx was seen in the number of granulocytes and in ED1+ and ED2+ macrophages in the acute phase of inflammation. Furthermore, we observed a redistribution in ED2+ macrophages from the basal part of the crypts to the upper parts. After induction of TNBS-ethanol mediated colitis ED3+ cells, which normally are exclusively present in spleen and lymph nodes, were also found in low numbers in the colon. MHC class II expression, observed in the upper part of the lamina propria and on DC around the crypts, also increased (table 1). Interestingly, no MHC class II expression occurred on colonic epithelial cells during active disease. From day 7 an influx was seen in the number of T-cells and from day 14 also in the number of B-cells. From day 28, the number of granulocytes and the number of macrophages started to decline again. This was related to a reduction in damage-score. On day 84 the number of all studied cell types was the same as in control animals again, except for the number of macrophages which still was slightly increased (table 1).

Table 1. Effect of TNBS-induction on (non)-lymphoid cells and on damagescore

time in days	mφ		PMN	MHC cl.II	T-cells	B-cells	mean damagescore
0	induction	of	colitis				
1	+ + +		+ +	=	=	=	4
7	+ + + +		+ + +	+	+	=	4,9
14	+ + + +		+ + +	+ +	+ +	+	4
28	+ + +		+ +	+	+ +	+	2,8
42	+ +		+	+	+	+	3
56	+ +		+	=	+	=	2
70	+		=	=	=	=	2
84	+		=	=	=	=	1

=	number of positive cells same as in controls
+	0 - 5 positive cells per microscopic field more than in controls
+ +	6 - 10 positive cells per microscopic field more than in controls
+ + +	11 - 15 positive cells per microscopic field more than in controls
+ + + +	> 15 positive cells per microscopic field more than in controls

ED7 Treatment In IBD

After treatment with ED7 in colitis 4 out of 6 rats showed a damagescore ≤ 2, while the other 2 rats had a score > 2. The mean score in this group was 2,6. In the control group 5 out of 7 rats had a score 5 and only 2 rats had a damagescore ≤ 2. In the control group, the mean score was 4,6 (table 2).
In the ED7 treated group smaller areas of ulceration as well as a decrease in the number of ulcerations was observed. However, with respect to infiltrating macrophages and granulocytes the inflamed areas in ED7 treated rats resembled the inflamed tissue in colitis controls.

Table 2. Damagescore after ED7 treatment in IBD

ED7 treatment	1	1	2	2	5	5	
PBS controls	2	2	5	5	5	5	5

DISCUSSION

In the acute phase of TNBS-induced colitis, an enormous infiltration of macrophages and PMN's was found, which were responsible for tissue damage. On the other hand, in the chronic phase, T-cells probably play a role, and there are some suggestions that experimental IBD is T-cell mediated (Sartor et al., 1993). Furthermore TNBS looks like the contact allergen DNCB.

In rats MHC class II expression was only found on dendritic cells in the small intestine, never on epithelial cells, whereas expression of HLA-DR by colonic epithelial cells in healthy humans has been described and was enhanced in IBD-patients (Mayer et al., 1991 and Malizia et al., 1991). The role of gut epithelial cells in antigen presentation could be species dependent. Furthermore, it is possible that colonic epithelial cells are different from epithelial cells in the small intestine.

After induction of IBD, the number of Ia+ dendritic cells in the lamina propria had increased. This probably contributes to a state of local chronic inflammation. The balance between stimulatory and suppressive signals from dendritic cells and suppressive macrophages in IBD requires further attention. By manipulating subpopulations non-lymphoid cells in the animal model which is described in the present study, the role of non-lymphoid cells in IBD can be studied in vivo.

After treatment of colitis with the MoAb ED7 a reduction in the number of infiltrating granulocytes and macrophages was found. This suggests that ED7 interferes with the epitope on CR3 which is involved in the recruitment of phagocytes to inflammatory sites. Besides (partial) blockade of infiltrating macrophages and granulocytes into inflamed tissue by ED7 during IBD, this MoAb might also have interfered with other phagocyte functions which are thought to play a role in different effector functions of phagocytes in the inflamed tissue. For example, the release of H_2O_2 by primed neutrophils can be blocked by MoAb's directed against CD11b (Von Asmuth et al., 1991; Shappel et al., 1990). The release of reactive oxygen species (ROS) by infiltrating phagocytes is likely to contribute to damage of the mucosa and submucosa (Henson and Johnson, 1987). Thus, inhibition of the production of ROS by macrophages and granulocytes by ED7 could very well have contributed to the observed suppression of IBD.

REFERENCES

Allison, M.C., Cornwall, S., Poulter, L.W., Dhillon, A.P., Pounder, R.E., 1988, Macrophage heterogeneity in normal colonic mucosa and in inflammatory bowel disease, *Gut* 29: 1531-1538.

Damoiseaux, J.G.M.C. Döpp, E.A., Neefjes, J.J., Beelen, R.H.J. and Dijkstra, C.D., 1989, Heterogeneity of macrophages in the rat evidenced by variability in determinants: two new anti-rat macrophage antibodies against a heterodimer of 160 and 95 kD (CD11/CD18), *J. Leuk. Biol.* 46: 556.

Dijkstra, C.D., Döpp, E.A., Joling, P., Kraal, G., 1985, The heterogeneity of mononuclear phagocytes in lymphoid organs: distinct macrophage subpopulations in the rat recognized by monoclonal antibodies ED1, ED2 and ED3, *Immunology* 54: 589.

Henson, P.M. and Johnson, R.B., 1987, Tissue injury in inflammation. *J. Clin. Invest.* 79: 669-674.

Huitinga, I., Damoiseaux, J.G.M.C., Döpp, E.A. and Dijkstra, C.D., 1993, Treatment with anti-CR3 antibodies ED7 and ED8 suppresses experimental allergic encephalomyelitis in Lewis rat, *Eur. J. Immunol.* 23: 709-715.

Hynes, R.O., 1987, Integrins: A family of cell surface receptors, *Cell* 48: 549.

Malizia, G., Calabrese, A., Cottone, M., Raimondo, M., Trejdosiewicz, L.K., Smart, C.J., Oliva, L. and Pagliaro, L., 1991, Expression of leukocyte adhesion molecules by mucosal mononuclear phagocytes in inflammatory bowel disease, *Gastroenterology* 100: 150.

Mayer, L.D., Eisenhardt, D., Salomon, P., Bauer, W., Plous, R. and Piccinini, L., 1991, Expression of class II molecules on intestinal epithelial cells in humans: difference between normal and IBD, *Gastroenterology* 100: 3.

Morris, G.P., Beck, P.L., Herridge, M.S., Depew, W.T., Szewczuk, M.R., Wallace, J.L., 1989, Hapten-i induced model of chronic inflammation and ulceration in the rat colon, *Gastroenterology* 96: 795-803.

Pavli, ., Woodhams, C.E., Doe, W.F., Hume, D.A., 1990, Isolation and characterization of antigen-presenting dendritic cells from the mouse intestinal lamina propria, *Immunology* 70: 40-47.

Sartor, R.B., Bender, D.E., Allen, J.B., Zimmermann, E.M., Holt, L.C., Pardo, M.S., Lund, P.K., Wahl, S.M., 1993, Chronic experimental enterocolitis and extraintestinal inflammation are T lymphocyte dependent, *Gastroenterology* 104, no.4: A 775.

Schmitt, M., Mussel, H.H. and Dierich, M.P., 1981, Qualitative and quantitative assessment of C3-receptor reactivities on lymphoid and phagocytic cells, *J. Immunol.* 126: 2042.

Seldenrijk, C.A., Drexhage, H.A., Meuwissen, S.G.M., Pals, S.T., Meijer, C.J.L.M., 1989, Dendritic cells and scavenger macrophages in chronic inflammatory bowel disease, *Gut* 30: 484.

Shappel, S.B., Toman, C., Anderson, D.C., Taylor, A.A., Entman, M.L. and Smith, C.W., 1990, Mac-1 (CD11b/CD18) mediates adherence-dependent hydrogen peroxide production by human and canine neutrophils, *J. Immunol.* 144: 2702.

Takahasi, F., Shah, H.S., Wise, L.S., Das, K.M., 1990, Circulating antibodies against human colonic extract enriched with a 40 kD protein in patients with ulcerative colitis, *Gut* 31: 1016-20.

Von Asmuth, E.J.U., Van der Linden, C.J., Leeuwenberg, J.F.M. and Buurman, W.A., 1991, Involve ment of the CD11b/CD18 integrin, but not of the endothelial cell adhesion molecules ELAM-1 and ICAM-1 in tumor necrosis factor-induced neutrophil toxicity, *J. Immunol.* 147: 3869.

Wilders, M.M., Drexhage, H.A., Kokje, M., Verspaget, H.W., Meuwissen, S.G.M., 1984, Veiled cells in chronic idiopathic inflammatory bowel disease, *Clin. Exp. Imm.* 55: 461-468.

Wright, S.D., Rao, P.E., Van Vorrhis, W.C., Craigmyle L.S., Iida, K., Talle, M.A., Westberg, E.F., Goldstein, G. and Silverstein, S.C., 1983, Identification of the C3bi receptor of human monocytes and macrophages by using monoclonal antibodies, *Proc. Natl. Acad. Sci. USA.* 80: 5699.

FIVE HUMAN MATURE B CELL SUBSETS

Yong-Jun Liu, Odette de Bouteiller, Christophe Arpin,
Isabelle Durand and Jacques Banchereau

Schering-Plough, Lab. Immunological Research
27 chemin des Peupliers, BP 11
69571 Dardilly, France

INTRODUCTION

Secondary lymphoid organs display B lymphocytes at distinct stages of differentiation as a consequence of ongoing antigenic stimulation. In order to understand the molecular mechanisms which regulate B cell differentiation from virgin B cells to either memory B cells or plasma cells, it is important to isolate B cells at different stages during immune responses in vivo. The working model (Fig. 1) is based on many *in vivo* experiments on the microenvironments of B cell activations (1-3). It predicts 5 mature B cell stages. Bm1(mature B cell subsets 1) represents virgin B cells; Bm2 ligand selected B cells (4), Bm3 germinal center centroblasts, Bm4 centrocytes and Bm5 memory B cells. Here we report on the identification and isolation of these B cell subsets from human tonsils.

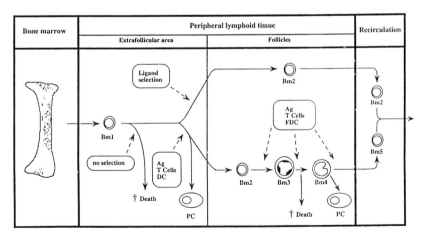

Fig 1: A working model for mature B cell differentiation in vivo during the immune response

RESULTS

Heterogeneity of B cell populations defined by multicolor fluorescence using anti-IgD, anti-CD23 and anti-CD39

Immunohistological studies have demonstrated that anti-IgD, anti-CD23 and anti-CD39 mAbs stain follicular mantle B cells and some extrafollicular B cells but not germinal center B cells (5). This immunohistological study cannot however tell us whether B cells outside germinal center represent an homogeneous IgD+CD23+CD39+ population of B cells or contain several populations of double positive or single positive B cells. Thus triple staining with anti-IgD-FITC, anti-CD23-PE and anti-CD-39-tricolor was performed on total tonsil B cells (Fig. 2). The stainings with anti-CD23 and anti-CD39 are shown in the dot plot and the expression of IgD by the cells in each region within the dot plot (Bm1 &5, Bm2, Bm 3 & 4) is shown in the histograms. The region numbers are corresponding to the B cell subset numbers which are predicted in the working model. Three non-germinal center B cell subsets were identified:
1) IgD+CD23-CD39+ (mature B cell subset 1 Bm1);
2) IgD+CD23+CD39+ (Bm2)
3) IgD-CD23-CD39+ (Bm5).
In addition, germinal center B cells were identified as IgD-CD23-CD39- (Bm3&4).

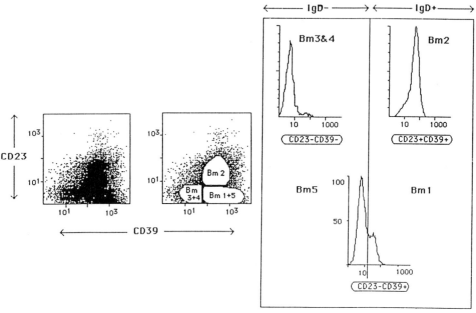

Fig. 2

Double staining with anti-IgD and anti-CD38 reveals three subpopulations of tonsillar B cells

Previous studies have shown that germinal center B cells are IgD-CD38+ and follicular mantle B cells are IgD+CD38-. In addition, germinal center B cells were shown to be CD39-. Thus the IgD-CD23-CD39+ B cell population (Bm5) identified by triple immunofluorescence staining presented in Fig 1, seems to be a distinct population of B cells which are neither CD38+ germinal center B cells nor IgD+ follicular mantle B cells. This predicts that these cells should be IgD-CD38-. In order to confirm the existence of this population of B cells, tonsil B cells were double stained with anti-CD38 and anti-IgD. Three main populations of B cells were clearly identified (Fig3a) :
1) CD38+IgD- (Bm3&4) germinal center B cells,
2) CD38-IgD+ (Bm1&2) follicular mantle B cells,
3) CD38-IgD- (Bm5) non-germinal center and non-IgD follicular mantle B cells.

Finally, the CD38+IgD+ B cells represented less than 7% of total tonsil B cells which may represent germinal center precursor cells.

Isolation and detailed phenotypic analysis of three populations of B cells defined by anti-IgD and anti-CD38 staining

In order to have a detailed phenotype and future functional studies, we have purified the three B cell populations by negative depletions using immunomagnetic beads (Fig 4). The FACS profiles of some surface markers which have different expression patterns on these three B cell populations are illustrated in Fig 3b and summarized in table 1.

1)*CD38+IgD- germinal center B cells* (Bm3 &4) were purified by depletion of IgD+ and CD39+ B cells;
2)*CD38-IgD+ follicular mantle B cells* (Bm1&2) were purified by depletion of CD38+, IgG+ and IgA+ B cells;
3)*CD38-IgD- B cells* (Bm5) were isolated by depletion of CD38+ and IgD+ B cells.

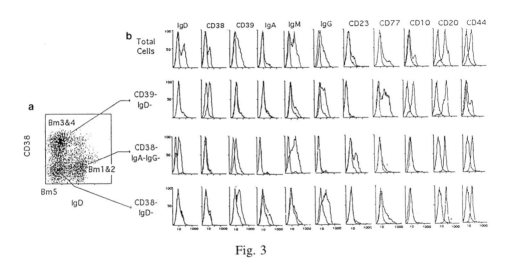

Fig. 3

Isolation of CD38+CD77+ and CD38+CD77- germinal center B cells

The above detailed phenotypic analysis shows that IgD-CD38+ germinal center B cells contain both CD77+ and CD77- B cells. This is consistent with the immunohistological finding on tissue sections showing that CD77 stain germinal center centroblasts in the dark zone but not germinal center centrocytes in the light zone. The CD38+ germinal centre B cells (Bm3&4) can be sorted into CD77+(Bm3) and CD77-(Bm4) cells (Fig 4).

Isolation of IgD+CD23+ and IgD+CD23- B cell subsets

The detailed phenotypic analysis also showed that the IgD+CD38- (Bm1&2) population contains CD23+ and CD23- cells (Fig 3) which can be sorted into CD23+(Bm2) and CD23-(Bm1) subpopulations (Fig 4).

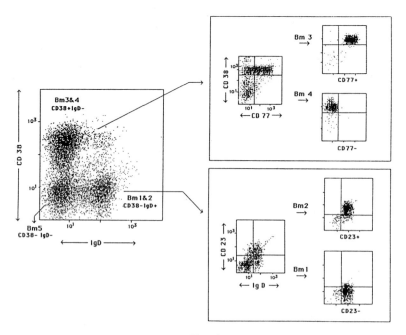

Fig. 4

Table 1. Summary of the characteristics of 5 mature B cell subsets

	Bm 1	Bm2	Bm3	Bm 4	Bm 5
Percentage in total B cells	31	13	17	15	26
Differential phenotype					
IgD	+	+	-	-	-
IgM	+	+	-	-	-
CD23	-	+	-	-	-
CD39	+	+	-	-	++
CD44	+	+	-	-	+
BCL-2	+	+	-	-	+
CD38	-	-	+	+	-
CD10	-	-	+	+	-
CD77	-	-	++	+	-
CD20	+	+	++	++	+
IgG	-	-	+	+	++
Ki67	-	-	++	+	-
Location	FM	FM	G.C DZ	G.C LZ	FM
Morphology	◎	◯	◉	◉	◎
Apoptosis during in vitro culture	-	-	+	+	-

292

DISCUSSION

The central issue raised by the present study concerns the relationships among these B cell subsets, which follow the sequence of evolution of B cells from virgin cells to memory cells (model detailed in Fig 1).

Bm1 and Bm-2

IgD+CD38- B cells (Bm1&2) have been separated into IgD+CD23- (Bm1) and IgD+CD23+ (Bm2) two subpopulations. The relationship of these two IgD+ B cell subsets and their degree of " virginity" can be questioned. It has been reported that the newly produced virgin B cells from the bone marrow are IgD+ B cells which express low or negligible levels of CD23 antigen (7). CD23 rapidly appears on peripheral sIgD+IgM+ B cells possibly following activation in peripheral lymphoid tissue (7). In vitro studies have demonstrated that a number of stimuli including anti-Ig, PMA, Ca++ ionophore, IL-4, and anti-CD40 antibody can induce and enhance the expression of CD23 antigen on IgD+IgM+ B cells (reviewed in 8). These data suggest that the Bm1(IgD+CD23-) B cells may represent the very early bone marrow derived virgin B cell which have migrated into the peripheral lymphoid tissues and have not yet received any activation signals. The Bm2 (IgD+CD23+) cells may derive from Bm1 cells after ligand selection and should thus not be considered as virgin B cells. This hypothesis is consistent with a recent study of Gu et al (4) who showed that most peripheral IgD^{high} B cells in mice are ligand selected, based on the analysis of V_H gene utilization.

Bm3 and Bm4

IgD-CD38+ germinal center B cells (Bm3&4) have been separated into CD77+(Bm3) and CD77- (Bm4) two subpopulations. Immunohistological study (9) suggests that CD77+Bm3 cells are the centroblasts in the dark zone of the germinal center while CD77- Bm4 cells are the centrocytes in the light zone of germinal center. The separation of these two germinal center B cell subsets will provide a model to study the kinetics and molecular mechanisms of germinal center reaction in relation to somatic mutation, class switching and differentiation.

Bm5

Significant numbers of B cells were found to be double negative for IgD and CD38. Detailed phenotypic analysis suggested that these cells may represent post germinal center memory B cells. First, these cells express high levels of IgG which indicates that they have already switched. Second, these cells are resting B cells since they do not express the proliferating antigen Ki67. Third, these cells express high levels of CD39 and Bcl-2 protein which cannot be detected within the germinal center.

CONCLUSION

Five mature B cell subsets from human tonsils have been identified and separated. We believe that they represent the different maturation stages from virgin B cells (Bm1) to memory B cells (Bm5). The present study demonstrates that B cells at each stages of differentiation express a distinct set of surface molecules and cell cycle status. These various sets of surface molecules may preferentially interact with distinct sets of ligands on T cells, dendritic cells and follicular dendritic cells, which are located in the different compartments of peripheral lymphoid organs.

ACKNOWLEDGMENT

We acknowledge Muriel Vatan and Nicole Courbiere for expert editorial assistance.

REFERENCES

1. **Liu, Y.-J., J. Zhang, P. J. L. Lane, E. Y.-T. Chan, and I. C. M. MacLennan**. Sites of specific B cell activation in primary and secondary responses to T cell-dependent and T cell-independent antigens. *Eur. J. Immunol. 21:2951.* (1991).

2. **Jacob, J., R. Kassir, and G. Kelsoe**. . In situ studies of the primary immune response to (4-hydroxy-3-nitrophenyl) acetyl. I. The architecture and dynamics of responding cell populations. *J. Exp. Med. 173:1165.* (1991).

3. **Gu, H., D. Tarlington, W. Müller, K. Rajewsky, and I. Förster**. Most peripheral B cells in mice are ligand selected. *J. Exp. Med. 173:1357.* (1991).

4. **Ling, N. R., I. C. MacLennan, and D. Y. Mason**. B-cell and plasma cell antigens : new and previously defined clusters. In *Leucocyte Typing III*. A. J. McMichael, ed., Oxford University Press, p. 302. (1987).

5. **Liu, Y. J., D. E. Joshua, G. T. Williams, C. A. Smith, J. Gordon, and I. C. M. MacLennan**. Mechanism of antigen-driven selection in germinal centres. *Nature. 342:929.* (1989).

6. **Kikutani, H., M. Suemura, H. Owaki, H. Nakamura, R. Sato, K. Yamasaki, E. L. Barsumian, R. R. Hardy, and T. Kishimoto**. Fce receptor, a specific differentiation marker transiently expressed on mature B cells before isotype switching. *J. Exp. Med. 164:1455.* (1986).

7. **Gordon, J., J. A. Cairns, Y.-J. Liu, L. Flores-Romo, I. C. M. MacLennan, K. U. Jansen, and J.-Y. Bonnefoy**. . Role of membrane and soluble CD23 in lymphocyte physiology. In *CD23. A novel multifunctional regulator of the immune system that binds IgE. 29*. J. Gordon, ed., Karger, Basel. p. 156. (1991).

8. **Hardie, D.L., Johnson, G.D., Khan, M, and MacLennan,. I.C.M.** Quantitative analysis of molecules which distinguish functional compartments within germinal centers. *Eur. J. Immunol.* 23: 997. (1993).

ABSENCE OF EGF RECEPTORS AND OF EGF UPTAKE IN PEYER'S PATCH DOME EPITHELIUM

Tomohiro Kato and Robert L. Owen

Cell Biology and Aging Section (151-E), Department of Veterans Affairs Medical Center, and Department of Medicine, University of California, San Francisco, 4150 Clement St., San Francisco, CA 94121, U.S.A.

INTRODUCTION

M cells (microfold cells, or membranous cells), which are located in the dome epithelium of Peyer's patches, function as antigen sampling sites for various intestinal microorganisms and antigens.[1] They differentiate from crypt stem cells,[2] but the mechanisms of regulation of M cell differentiation and migration are unknown. M cells have characteristic morphological features: short and irregular microvilli or microfolds, sparse lysosomes, endosome formation along their apical membranes, and mononuclear leukocytes enfolded in their pockets. M cells also function as antigen transporting cells, taking up various microorganisms and macromolecules from the intestinal lumen and transporting them to enfolded lymphocytes and macrophages.[3,4] Because of the wide range of enteric pathogens and commensal microorganisms taken up by M cells, it is presumed that microbial adherence to M cells depends on several factors, but these factors have not yet been defined.

Epidermal growth factor (EGF) is known to be one of the growth factors that facilitate cell differentiation and cell proliferation in many tissues in various mammalian species. In digestive organs, EGF is distributed in multiple regions including submandibular glands, stomach, duodenum, and pancreas.[5] EGF, secreted directly into the small intestine by Brunner's glands and indirectly from bile and salivary glands, is thought to maintain intestinal epithelium.[5] In the small intestine, EGF is abundant in proximal sites,[6] and EGF receptor has been biochemically demonstrated in enterocytes,[7,8,9,10] but its subcellular location is still unclear.[11,12] In cultured enterocytes, EGF receptor has been found to participate in adherence and uptake of *Salmonella* and possibly vaccinia virus.[13] Subsequently it had been suggested that EGF receptors on enterocytes might serve as attachment sites for microorganisms colonizing the mucosal surface *in vivo*.

To test the hypothesis that EGF receptor is present on the luminal surface of M cells, where it could play a role in adherence and uptake of microorganisms, or on crypt stem cells, where it could mediate M-cell differentiation, we examined the distribution of EGF receptors in mice and rats immunohistochemically. We also looked for functional evidence

In Vivo Immunology, Edited by E. Heinen *et al.*
Plenum Press, New York, 1994

of EGF receptors by examining uptake of biotin- or Texas Red-labeled EGF by dome epithelium of Peyer's patches in ligated mouse and rabbit intestinal segments.

MATERIALS AND METHODS

Materials

After peritoneal anesthesia with sodium pentobarbital, BALB/c mouse (20 - 25 g) and Sprague-Dawley rat (250 - 275 g) Peyer's patches were collected and immediately embedded in OCT compound without fixation, frozen using Freon and liquid nitrogen, and stored at –80°C prior to study.

For the detection of EGF receptor in rats, we used mouse anti-EGF receptor monoclonal antibody (MAb) (1:100 dilution; 29.1 clone, Sigma, St. Louis, Missouri). For the study of EGF uptake in mice and rabbits (New Zealand White, 2.5 – 3.0 kg), we used EGF from mouse submaxillary gland conjugated with biotin (EGF-biotin; Boehringer-Mannheim, Germany), or with Texas Red (Molecular Probes, Eugene, Oregon).

Localization of EGF receptor

For detection of the EGF receptor, immunohistochemical techniques were used with anti-EGF receptor monoclonal antibody in rats and with EGF-biotin in mice.

(i) **Rat EGF Receptor.** Rat Peyer's patch blocks were cut in 7-µm sections with a cryostat, mounted on uncoated slides, and dried completely at room temperature (RT). Sections were fixed with acetone for 10 minutes at RT prior to immunolabeling. For immunohistochemical investigation, the avidin-biotin-peroxidase system (ABC-kit, Vector, Burlingame, California) was utilized as follows: pretreat with diluted normal horse serum, and sequentially incubate in primary MAb for 1 hour at RT, biotinylated secondary antibody (Ab) from horse for 1 hour at RT, avidin-biotin-horseradish peroxidase complex (ABC) solution for 1 hour at RT, and 0.05% 3,3'-diaminobenzidine tetrahydrochloride plus 0.01% H_2O_2 (DAB/H_2O_2) in 50 mM Tris buffer (pH 7.4) for 10 minutes. For rinsing sections, phosphate-buffered saline (PBS, pH 7.4) was used. After nuclear staining with methyl green, sections were examined by light microscopy. As a control, PBS (which was used to dilute the primary MAb) was used instead of the primary MAb.

(ii) **Mouse EGF Receptor.** For the detection of mouse EGF receptor, EGF-biotin was used. Before fixation, mouse cryosections were incubated with EGF-biotin for 1 hour at 37°C. After fixation with 4% paraformaldehyde (15 minutes, 4°C) and methanol (10 minutes, –20°C), sections were incubated with ABC solution for 30 minutes at RT, and incubated with DAB/H_2O_2 in Tris buffer for 15 minutes. After nuclear staining with methyl green, sections were examined by light microscopy.

EGF Uptake

For studying the uptake of EGF by epithelium of mouse and rabbit Peyer's patches, biotin-labeled mouse EGF and Texas Red-labeled mouse EGF were used. Under peritoneal or intravenous anesthesia with sodium pentobarbital, labeled EGF was injected into ligated intestinal loops containing Peyer's patches. As a control, distilled water was injected into one loop in each animal. After incubation for 1 hour in mice and rabbits on a rotary table, loops were removed, rinsed, and embedded in OCT compound without fixation.

Seven-μm sequential sections were made with a cryostat, and fixed with acetone for 10 minutes at RT prior to immunolabeling. For the detection of biotin-labeled EGF, sections were incubated in 0.3% H_2O_2 in methanol for 30 minutes to block endogenous peroxidase, ABC solution for 1 hour at RT, and DAB/H_2O_2 in 50 mM Tris buffer for 15 minutes. After nuclear staining with methyl green, sequential sections were examined by light microscopy. For localization of Texas Red-labeled EGF, acetone-fixed cryosections were mounted and examined by fluorescence microscopy using both Texas Red and rhodamine filters.

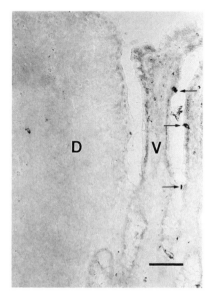

Figure 1. Rat Peyer's patch incubated *in vitro* with mouse anti-EGF receptor MAb. Lack of staining in the epithelium of the lymphoid follicle dome (D) suggests absence of EGF receptors. Some positive product (arrows) is seen in the epithelial cells of villi (V). (*bar* = 200 μm; × 60)

RESULTS

Localization of EGF Receptor

An indirect immunolocalization approach, reacting mouse anti-EGF receptor MAb with sections of rat Peyer's patch, failed to label dome epithelial cells including M cells and cells lining adjacent crypts. Only a few enterocytes in the epithelium over villi developed clear peroxidase reaction product, indicating localization of anti-EGF receptor MAb (Figure 1).

A more direct approach, looking for binding of biotin-labeled EGF to its receptor in sections of mouse Peyer's patch, also did not show any adherence to cells in the Peyer's patch follicle dome epithelium, although there was positive labeling of occasional villus enterocytes (Figure 2).

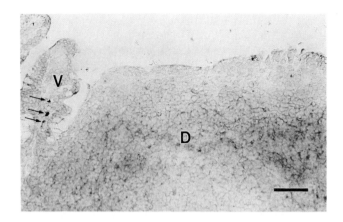

Figure 2. Mouse Peyer's patch section incubated *in vitro* with mouse EGF-biotin. No positive product is seen in the epithelium of the dome (D). Some positive product (arrows) is seen in the lamina propria of the villus (V). (*bar* = 200 μm; × 60)

EGF Uptake

In mouse, Peyer's patch dome epithelial cells did not take up luminally administered EGF-biotin (Figure 3) or EGF-Texas Red (not shown). Similarly, there was no evidence of *in vivo* EGF uptake by rabbit Peyer's patch dome epithelium (Figure 4). Only a very few enterocytes in rabbit villi were seen to have small positive spots, consistent with endocytosed EGF-biotin (not shown).

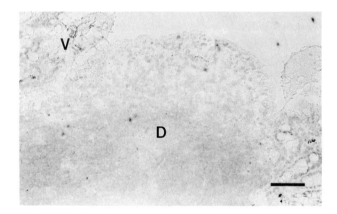

Figure 3. Mouse Peyer's patch from ligated intestinal loop incubated with EGF-biotin *in vivo*. No uptake of EGF-biotin is seen in any dome (D) epithelial cell. (*bar* = 200 μm; × 60)

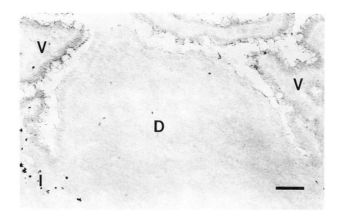

Figure 4. Rabbit Peyer's patch from ligated intestinal loop incubated with EGF-biotin *in vivo*. No positive product is seen in the epithelial cells of the dome (D) or the adjacent villi (V). Endogenous peroxidase product, which was also present in control loops, is seen in the interfollicular areas (I) flanking the dome. (*bar* = 200 μm; × 45)

DISCUSSION

M cells function as antigen transporting cells, and are initiation sites for intestinal mucosal immune responses. Along the transport pathway toward lymphocytes and macrophages that are enfolded by M cells, there are numerous endosomes in the apical cytoplasm of M cells, in which degradation and/or chemical alteration of antigens could take place.[14] Furthermore, there is evidence that M cells express class II MHC determinants.[15] These characteristics suggest that M cells might function as antigen presenting cells, as well as antigen transporting cells. Though the regulation of uptake by M cells is quite obscure, there is some information about the M-cell apical surface: compared with enterocytes, the M-cell apical surface differs in lectin distribution,[16] has an increased capacity to adsorb secretory immunoglobulin A,[17] lacks secretory component,[18] and expresses less alkaline phosphatase.[19] To date, M-cell receptors for antigen adherence have not been clearly identified.

In suckling rat ileum, EGF has been shown histochemically[20] and biochemically[21] to be transported across enterocytes and it is thought to facilitate the proliferation and migration of enterocytes.[22,23] EGF stimulates metabolism of enterocytes *in vivo* when administered into the intestinal lumen in adult rats[22] and *in vitro* when added to culture medium of cells of enterocyte origin.[24] It has been hypothesized that EGF itself may function as a microbial receptor on enterocytes, because an EGF precursor functions as the receptor for the B subunit of diphtheria toxin,[25] and because EGF facilitates adhesion to cultured cells and uptake of *Salmonella typhimurium*.[13] Consequently, we anticipated that EGF might be involved in M-cell development and in antigen uptake into M cells.

Contrary to this expectation, our histochemical study showed that in adults rodents EGF receptor was not evident in enterocytes in the villi or in any dome epithelial cells (including M cells and their stem cells in surrounding crypts). Luminally administered EGF was not taken up by any epithelial cells over Peyer's patch domes. In the normal adult intestinal environment *in vivo*, any roles of EGF and its receptor appear to be much more limited than we anticipated from the published *in vitro* data. Only under special conditions, such as in destroyed or damaged intestinal mucosal tissues, is EGF abundant and easily detected immunohistochemically.[26] Our findings indicate that in untraumatized adult intestine, local uptake of EGF is not a major factor in M-cell development, proliferation, or differentiation, that the expression of EGF receptor in intestinal epithelial cells is down-regulated in adults, and that EGF receptor is not an available site for microbial adherence to Peyer's patches *in vivo*.

ACKNOWLEDGMENTS

This work was supported by the U.S. Department of Veterans Affairs and the Northern California Institute for Research and Education.

REFERENCES

1. R.L. Owen and A.L. Jones, Epithelial cell specialization within human Peyer's patches: an ultrastructural study of intestinal lymphoid follicles, *Gastroenterology* 66: 189 (1974).
2. D.K. Bhalla and R.L. Owen, Cell renewal and migration in lymphoid follicles of Peyer's patches and cecum - an autoradiographic study in mice, *Gastroenterology* 82: 232 (1982).
3. J.S. Trier, Structure and function of intestinal M cells, *Gastroenterol. Clin. North. Am.* 20: 531 (1991).
4. T. Kato and R.L. Owen, Structure and function of intestinal mucosal epithelium, *in*: "Handbook of Mucosal Immunology," P. Ogra, J. Mestecky, M.E. Lamm, W. Strober, J. Bienenstock, and J.R. McGhee, eds., Academic Press, San Diego, in press (1994).
5. U. Marti, S.J. Burwen, and A.L. Jones, Biological effects of epidermal growth factor, with emphasis on the gastrointestinal tract and liver: an update, *Hepatology* 9: 126 (1989).
6. P. Kirkegaard, P.S. Olsen, E. Nexø, J.J. Holst, and S.S. Poulsen, Effect of vasoactive intestinal polypeptide and somatostatin on secretion of epidermal growth factor and bicarbonate from Brunner's glands, *Gut* 25: 1225 (1984).
7. C.L. Mynott, S.A. Pinches, A. Garner, and S.P. Shirazi-Beechey, Location and characteristics of epidermal growth factor binding to enterocyte plasma membranes, *Biochem. Soc. Trans.* 19: 307S (1991).
8. J.F. Thompson, Specific receptors for epidermal growth factor in rat intestinal microvillus membranes. *Am. J. Physiol.* 254: G429 (1988).
9. M-E. Forgue-Lafitte, M. Laburthe, M-C. Chamblier, A.J. Moody, and G. Rosselin, Demonstration of specific receptors for EGF-urogastrone in isolated rat intestinal epithelial cells, *FEBS Lett.* 114: 243 (1980).
10. N. Gallo-Payet and J.S. Hugon, Epidermal growth factor receptors in isolated adult mouse intestinal cells: Studies *in vivo* and in organ culture, *Endocrinology* 116: 194 (1985).
11. L.A. Jaeger and C.H. Lamar, Immunolocalization of epidermal growth factor (EGF) and EGF receptors in the porcine upper gastrointestinal tract, *Am. J. Vet. Res.* 53: 1685 (1992).
12. L.A. Scheving, R.A. Shiurba, T.D. Nguyen, and G.M. Gray, Epidermal growth factor receptor of the intestinal enterocyte - localization to laterobasal but not brush border membrane, *J. Biol. Chem.* 264: 1735 (1989).
13. J.E. Galán, J. Pace, and M.J. Hayman, Involvement of the epidermal growth factor receptor in the invasion of cultured mammalian cells by *Salmonella typhimurium*, *Nature* 357: 588 (1992).
14. C.H. Allan, D.L. Mendrick, and J.S.Trier, Rat intestinal M cells contain acidic endosomal-lysosomal compartments and express class II major histocompatibility complex determinants, *Gastroenterology* 104: 698 (1993).
15. H. Nagura, H. Ohtani, T. Masuda, M. Kimura, and S. Nakamura, HLA-DR expression on M cells overlying Peyer's patches is a common feature of human small intestine, *Acta Pathol. Jpn.* 41: 818 (1991).
16. A. Gebert and G. Hach, Differential binding of lectins to M-cells and enterocytes in the rabbit caecum, *Gastroenterology* 105, in press (1993).
17. T. Kato, A study of secretory immunoglobulin A on membranous epithelial cells (M cells) and adjacent absorptive cells of rabbit Peyer's patches, *Gastroenterol. Jpn.* 25: 15 (1990).
18. J. Pappo and R.L. Owen, Absence of secretory component expression by epithelial cells overlying rabbit gut-associated lymphoid tissue, *Gastroenterology* 95: 1173 (1988).

19. R.L. Owen and D.K. Bhalla, Cytochemical analysis of alkaline phosphatase and esterase activities and of lectin-binding and anionic sites in rat and mouse Peyer's patch M cells, *Am. J. Anat.* 168: 199 (1983).
20. P.A. Gonnella, K. Siminoski, R.A. Murphy, and M.R. Neutra, Transepithelial transport of epidermal growth factor by absorptive cells of suckling rat ileum, *J. Clin. Invest.* 80: 22 (1987).
21. W. Thornburg, L. Matrisian, B. Magun, and O. Koldovsky, Gastrointestinal absorption of epidermal growth factor in suckling rats, *Am. J. Physiol.* 246: G80 (1984).
22. M.H. Ulshen, L.E. Lyn-Cook, and R.H. Raasch, Effects of intraluminal epidermal growth factor on mucosal proliferation in the small intestine of adult rats, *Gastroenterology* 91: 1134 (1986).
23. M.D. Basson, I.M. Modlin, and J.A. Madri, Human enterocyte (Caco-2) migration is modulated *in vitro* by extracellular matrix composition and epidermal growth factor, *J. Clin. Invest.* 90: 15 (1992).
24. B. Daniele and A. Quaroni, Effects of epidermal growth factor on diamine oxidase expression and cell growth in Caco-2 cells, *Am. J. Physiol.* 261: G669 (1991).
25. J.G. Naglich, J.E. Metherall, D.W. Russell, and L. Eidels, Expression cloning of a diphtheria toxin receptor: identity with a heparin-binding EGF-like growth factor precursor, *Cell* 69: 1051 (1992).
26. N.A. Wright, R. Poulsom, G.W.H. Stamp, P.A. Hall, R.E. Jeffery, J.M. Longcroft, M-C. Rio, C. Tomasetto, and P. Chambon, Epidermal growth factor (EGF/URO) induces expression of regulatory peptides in damaged human gastrointestinal tissues, *J. Pathol.* 162: 279 (1990).

PLACE OF MALT IN THE IMMUNE DEFENCE SYSTEM

Ernst Heinen

Institute of Human Histology
University of Liege
Belgium

DEFINITION

Mucosa-associated lymphoid tissues (MALT) appear early in phylogenesis and ontogenesis. They give rise to primary lymph organs (fetal liver, thymus, bursa of Fabricius), to secondary lymph organs (tonsils, Peyer's patches, appendix), and to the diffuse immune system along the mucosae. However, MALT usually designates the areas where immunopoiesis and immune reactions occur, and thus the secondary lymph organs and the diffuse effector cells located along the mucosae. A mucosa is composed of an epithelial lining and a lamina propria rich in blood and lymph vessels; sometimes glands and smooth muscles are also found. Common features characterize mucosa-associated lymphoid tissues:
- heavy and continuous exposure to external antigens
- existence of antigen transfer mechanisms
- mainly Ig A production
- peculiar cell populations: B_1 cells, $\gamma \delta$ T cells, mast cells, M cells, etc.
- strong external influences: LPS, superantigens, lectins, etc.
- typical diseases: Crohn's disease, coeliac disease, lymphomas, etc.

COMPONENTS

The MALT system can be divided into different specialized parts:
- the upper respiratory tract with the attached tonsils (adenoids, tubar tonsils)
- bronchus-associated lymphoid tissue (BALT)
- glands (lacrimal, salivary, mammary)
- gut-associated lymphoid tissue (GALT), itself subdivided into:
  * the oral cavity (gingiva; palatine and lingual tonsils...)
  * the small intestine

* Peyer's patches
* the appendix
* the colon
- the urogenital tract
This illustrates the heterogeneity of MALT.

All along the mucosae, specialized areas produce effector cells: tonsils, Peyer's patches, the appendix, and follicles which arise locally (disseminated lymph follicles associated with T-dependent zones). From these secondary lymph organs, effector cells (precursors of plasma cells, sensitized T cells) spread out and populate the mucosae.

THE SECONDARY LYMPH ORGANS OF THE MALT

Tonsils, Peyer's patches, and the appendix form the major secondary lymph organs of the MALT system; their basic structure is the same, including:
- areas of antigen entry and presentation
- lymph follicles
- T-dependent zones
- areas for effector cell function
- blood and lymph vessels for cell migration and recirculation.

Secondary lymph organs develop where antigens can have selective access to the defence system. Entry, transport, and retention of antigen do not occur in a stochastic way but are controlled. For example, M cells are found only in the follicle-associated epithelium; they do not express MHC Cl II molecules but ensure transport of particulate antigens to lymphoid and accessory cells (Owen and Nemanic, 1978). Even tonsils possess M cells (Howie, 1980). Adherence of microorganisms to M cells can be mediated by lectin-sugar bonds (see Gebert and Hach, this volume). Antigen presentation probably occurs beneath the epithelium between dendritic cells and lymphoid cells; retention of antigen is insured in the form of immune complexes at the level of follicular dendritic cells in germinal centres. These complexes allow affinity selection and restimulation among B cells but apparently also selection of T cells inside the germinal centres and, indirectly, repeated activation of T cells in the T-dependent zones. Lymph follicles compose the main part of these lymph organs; their germinal centres usually develop in response to repetitive stimulation caused by the continuous arrival of antigens and bacterial, viral, and parasitic factors (LPS, superantigens, lectins). Tonsils mainly produce IgG-secreting B cells, the other organs deliver IgA B cells.

The T-dependent zones, frequently ignored, are essential lymphoid areas to which lymphoid and other leucocytes can home upon leaving high endothelial venules (HEV). They express selectins specific to the MALT system (Nakache et al. 1989). Inside these T-dependent zones, T and B cell activation occurs; the T cells can divide in situ whereas the B cells migrate to the germinal centres to become centroblasts, then centrocytes and memory B cells.

Effector cells leave the germinal centres and T-zones and migrate to areas where they differentiate (epithelium for T cells, subepithelial spaces for plasma cells). Most of these cells do not, however, remain in these organs, they pass into efferent lymphatics to recirculate or to home towards mucosae. Isolated follicles present the same features and are always associated with T-dependent zones (Heinen et al. 1990). These ever-associated lymphoid structures form a functional unit which is found multiplied in the larger secondary lymph organs of the MALT.

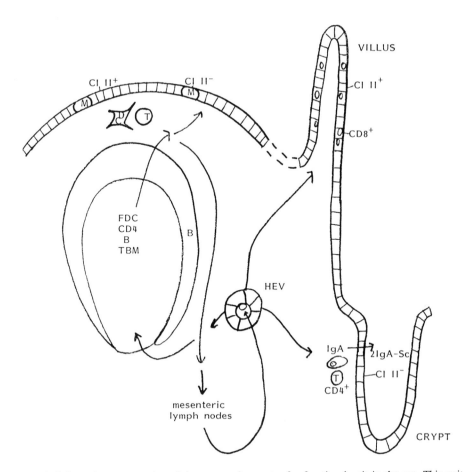

Figure 1. Schematic representation of the structural aspects of a functional unit in the gut. This unit comprises (1) a follicle, (2) an associated T-dependent zone, and (3) the follicle-associated epithelium. Follicular dendritic cells (FDC), CD4+ T cells, activated B cells, and tingible body macrophages (TBM) populate the germinal centre. High endothelial venules (HEV) allow the immigration of cells into the T-dependent zone. The follicle-associated epithelium covers the dome zone containing dendritic cells (DC), B, and T cells. This epithelium is composed of enterocytes expressing MHC Cl II molecules and of M cells capable of transferring particulate antigens. Lymphocytes having passed through the HEV can be activated by antigen that has penetrated the mucosa. T cells divide in the T-dependent zone after activation in contact with antigen-presenting cells. B cells move to the germinal centres where they divide and become B memory cells. The lymphoid cells emigrate via lymphatics towards draining lymph nodes or enter the epithelial or subepithelial areas to become effector cells. Lymphoid cells, after their passage through the draining lymph nodes where they can divide and/or further mature, recirculate and usually enter the mucosa (at the level of the crypts); B cells transform, in contact with CD4+ T cells and other cells, into plasma cells; CD8+ T cells settle in the villus epithelium and move, pushed by enterocytes, to the tip. Villus enterocytes are MHC Cl II+, crypt enterocytes are MHC Cl II- but express the receptor for dimeric IgA.

LOCATION OF EFFECTOR CELLS

Lymphoid effector cells do not migrate at random: where they go depends on the expression of selectins, of receptors for matrix molecules, and on their responsiveness to chemotactic and differentiating factors. IgG-forming B cells settle beneath the crypt epithelium of tonsils, the follicle-associated epithelium of Peyer's patches, or home to the bone marrow. Most IgA-secreting cells terminally differentiate along crypts or glandular ducts. They appear to be attracted by epithelia expressing the receptor for dimeric IgA, yielding, after transfer to the lumen, the secretory component. Interestingly IgA, which neutralize antigens outside tissues, are produced along the mucosae whereas IgG, capable of activating the complement cascade and thus of inducing inflammation, are found at the sites where the secondary lymph organs develop. The amount of secretory IgA delivered to the human adult gut lumen every day (40 mg/kg b.w.) exceeds the total daily delivery (30mg/kg b.w.) of IgG to the blood (Conley and Delacroix, 1987). IgA appear to perform different tasks: they form an immune barrier in preventing the adherence and absorption of antigens. Apparently, two additional functions for mucosal IgA are to neutralize intracellular microbial pathogens such as viruses directly within the epithelial cells and to bind antigens to the mucosal lamina propria for excretion into the lumen, thus discarding locally formed immune complexes (Mazanec et al., 1993).

Sensitized T cells home to epithelia, for example CD8[+] cells to the villi of the gut. These cells remain intimately attached to the epithelial cells and are thus carried along as the cells move towards the tips of the villi. Lymphokines produced by T cells act on epithelial cells (Beagley and Elson, 1992) but the latter, conversely, produce cytokines (IL1, IL6, TGF, etc.) which in turn act on the lymphoid cells (Bland et Kambarage, 1991). Villus enterocytes, but normally not crypt enterocytes, express MHC Cl II molecules at the brush border. The meaning of this is not clear. γδ T cells are present among these intraepithelial lymphocytes. In the lamina propria and the dome zone above follicles, more CD4 T cells than CD8 T cells are found, notably in contact with plasma cells. In the tonsils, along the subepithelial area (lamina propria beneath the crypts) many IL4- and IL6-producing cells have been detected by in situ hybridization (Bosseloir et al., 1990). These cytokines, notably produced by TH2 cells, induce the terminal differentiation of B cells to plasma cells, which are indeed numerous along the lympho-epithelial tissue of the crypts. Few NK or effector cells for ADCC populate the mucosa (Brandtzaeg et al., 1991).

PLACE OF THE MALT

Mucosa-associated lymphoid tissues form a defence system presenting peculiar features and are comparable to the systemic immune system. They produce more immunoglobulins than the latter and their lymphoid cell content is higher (Per Brantzaeg, 1989). They comprise specialized areas where immunopoiesis occurs (secondary lymph organs). Their effector cells (plasma cells, T cells) are dispersed all along the mucosa.

The MALT system produces its own defence cells which recirculate locally. Being connected to draining lymph nodes (cervical, pulmonary, and mesenteric), however, it participates in the general defence of the body and in the regulatory mechanisms which maintain a high degree of homeostasis. The MALT defence system is both effective and economical since, at strategic points, secondary lymph organs produce effector cells which seed all levels of the mucosa. These strategic points are located at sites where antigens are selectively transferred through the epithelium.

REFERENCES

1. K.V. Beagley and C.O. Elson, Cells and cytokines in mucosal immunity and inflammation, *Gastroent. Clin. N^{th} Amer*. 21: 347-366 (1992).
2. P.W. Bland and D.M. Kambarage, Antigen handling by the epithelium and lamina propria macrophages, *Gastroent. Clin. N^{th} Amer*. 20: 577-596 (1991).
3. A.L. Bosseloir E. Hooghe-Peters, E. Heinen, N. Cormann, C. Marcoty, C. Kinet-Denoël and L.J. Simar, IL6 and IL4: localization and production in human tonsils *in*: "Lymphatic tissues and in vivo immune responses", Ed. Imhof, Berrih-Aknin, Ezine, pp. 315-319, (1991).
4. P. Brandtzaeg, Overview of the mucosal immune system, *Curr. Top. Microbiol. Immunol*. 146: 13 (1989).
5. P. Brantzaeg, D.E. Nilssen, T.O. Rognum and P.S. Thrane, Ontogeny of the mucosal immune system and IgA deficiency, *Gastroent. Clin. N^{th} Amer*, 20: 397-439 (1991).
6. M.E. Conley and D.L. Delacroix, Intravascular and mucosal IgA: two separate but related systems of immune defense, *Ann. Intern. Med*. 106: 892-899 (1987).
7. E. Heinen, C. Kinet-Denoël, A. Bosseloir, N. Cormann and L.J. Simar, B cell microenvironments during antigen stimulation, *in*: "Molecular Biology of B cell developments", Ed. C. Sorg, Karger, Basel, pp. 24-60 (1990).
8. A.J. Howie, Scanning and transmission electron microscopy on the epithelium of human palatine tonsils, *J. Pathol*. 130: 91-98 (1980).
9. M.B. Mazanec, J.G. Nedrud, C.S. Kretzel and M.E. Lamm, A three-tiered view of the role of IgA in mucosal defense, *Immunol. Today*, 14: 430-435 (1993).
10. M. Nakache, E.L. Berg, P.R. Strecter and E.C. Butcher, The mucosal vascular addressin is a tissue-specific endothelial cell adhesion molecule for circulating lymphocytes, *Nature* 337: 179-181 (1989).
11. R.L. Owen and P. Nemanic, Antigen processing structures of the mammalian intestinal tract, *Scan. Electron Microsc*. 2: 367-378 (1978).

INDEX

Selfpeptides
  thymus, 21
  non follicular compartments,
          75
Spleen, transplantation, 57
Survival, centroblasts,
          centrocytes, 213

T cells
  MALT, 261
T-cell
  cytokine production, 219
  factors, 1
  memory phenotype, 179
  priming, 82
  selection, 21
Thymic
  lymphomas, 195
  nurse cells, cytokines, 4
Thymocytes
  alteration, 107
  apoptosis, 113
  newborns, 89
  proto-oncogene, 9
Thymus-dependent antibody
          responses, 75
Thymus
  differentiation, 30
  epithelium, 4
  fetal, 27
  gap-junctions, 155
  medullary cell activation,
          87
  neuroendocrine self, 21
  nurse cells, 1
  organ culture, 27
  perivascular structures, 143
TNF-α, 195
TNP
  immunization, 277
  specific memory, 39, 220,
          239
Tolerance, transfer, 46
Tonsils, 303
Transplantation, 58, 126
Tumor necrosis factor, 195